Tissue Engineering and Regenerative Medicine

The book emphasizes the technological advancements in tissue engineering related to biomaterials and biomanufacturing techniques. It further discusses important topics such as 3D bioprinting, process parameter optimization, Convolutional Neural Network (CNN) for stem cell imaging, diabetes risk prediction and Parkinson's disease detection using machine learning, telehealth systems, acute pancreatitis, and data-driven monitoring of chronic diseases.

This book:

- Explores the role of artificial intelligence in designing biomaterials, optimizing fabrication processes, and predicting tissue formation
- Focuses on technological advancements in tissue engineering related to biomanufacturing techniques and biomaterials
- Discusses the denture base acrylic resins, brain tumor detection, CNN for stem cell imaging and machine learning for diabetes risk prediction and Parkinson's disease detection
- Covers acute myocardial infarction, post-operative urinary retention, telehealth systems, graph convolutional network, and acute pancreatitis
- Explains the role of serum magnesium levels in febrile convulsions and Apache-II score and Ranson criteria with modified CT severity index

It is primarily written for senior undergraduates, graduate students, and academic researchers in the fields of manufacturing engineering, biomedical engineering, materials science, biomaterials, mechanical engineering, and production engineering.

Advances in Manufacturing, Design and Computational Intelligence Techniques

Series Editor: Ashwani Kumar

Senior Lecturer, Mechanical Engineering, at Technical Education Department, Uttar Pradesh, Kanpur, India

The book series editor is inviting edited, reference, and text book proposal submission to the book series. The main objective of this book series is to provide researchers a platform to present state-of-the-art innovations, research related to advanced materials applications, cutting edge manufacturing techniques, innovative design, and computational intelligence methods used for solving non-linear problems of engineering. The series includes a comprehensive range of topics and its application in engineering areas such as additive manufacturing, nanomanufacturing, micromachining, biodegradable composites, material synthesis and processing, energy materials, polymers and soft matter, non-linear dynamics, dynamics of complex systems, MEMS, green and sustainable technologies, vibration control, AI in power station, analog-digital hybrid modulation, advancement in inverter technology, adaptive piezoelectric energy harvesting circuit, contactless energy transfer system, energy efficient motors, bioinformatics, computer-aided inspection planning, hybrid electrical vehicle, autonomous vehicle, object identification, machine intelligence, deep learning, control-robotics-automation, knowledge-based simulation, biomedical imaging, image processing, and visualization. This book series compiled all aspects of manufacturing, design, and computational intelligence techniques from fundamental principles to current advanced concepts.

Thermal Energy Systems: Design, Computational Techniques, and Applications
Edited by Ashwani Kumar, Varun Pratap Singh, Chandan Swaroop Meena, and Nitesh Dutt

Tissue Engineering and Regenerative Medicine: Advances and Applications
Edited by Shailesh D. Kamble, Subhash Singh, Ashwani Kumar, and Gaurav Dwivedi

https://www.routledge.com/Advances-in-Manufacturing-Design-and-Computational-Intelligence-Techniques/book-series/CRCAIMDCIT?publishedFilter=alltitles&pd=published,forthcoming&pg=1&pp=12&so=pub&view=list?publishedFilter=alltitles&pd=published,forthcoming&pg=1&pp=12&so=pub&view=list

Tissue Engineering and Regenerative Medicine

Advances and Applications

Edited by
Shailesh D. Kamble
Subhash Singh
Ashwani Kumar
Gaurav Dwivedi

CRC Press
Taylor & Francis Group
Boca Raton New York London

CRC Press is an imprint of the
Taylor & Francis Group, an informa business

First edition published 2025
by CRC Press
2385 NW Executive Center Drive, Suite 320, Boca Raton FL 33431

and by CRC Press
4 Park Square, Milton Park, Abingdon, Oxon, OX14 4RN

CRC Press is an imprint of Taylor & Francis Group, LLC

ISBN: 978-1-032-88143-0 (hbk)
ISBN: 978-1-032-88144-7 (pbk)
ISBN: 978-1-003-53635-2 (ebk)

DOI: 10.1201/9781003536352

Typeset in Sabon
by SPi Technologies India Pvt Ltd (Straive)

Contents

Aim and scope

Tissue engineering and regenerative medicine constitute an interdisciplinary field dedicated to developing biological substitutes that can restore, maintain, or enhance tissue function. Evolving from biomaterials development, tissue engineering involves the synergistic combination of scaffolds, cells, and biologically active molecules to create functional tissues. The ultimate goal of tissue engineering is to fabricate constructs that can effectively replace, repair, or improve damaged tissues or organs. Examples of engineered tissues include artificial skin and cartilage. Regenerative medicine, a broader field, encompasses research on self-healing processes where the body utilizes its own systems, often with the aid of exogenous biological materials, to regenerate cells, tissues, and organs. This field is continually evolving and expanding beyond medical applications to include non-therapeutic uses such as biosensors for detecting biological or chemical threats and tissue chips for evaluating the toxicity of experimental medications.

The book *Tissue Engineering and Regenerative Medicine: Advances and Applications* aims to provide a comprehensive overview of the latest developments and applications in the field of tissue engineering and regenerative medicine. The book is designed to serve as a valuable resource for researchers, clinicians, students, and healthcare professionals interested in understanding the principles, techniques, and clinical implications of this rapidly evolving field. The book covers a wide range of topics, from fundamental concepts of tissue engineering to the most recent advancements in biomaterials, cell biology, and clinical applications. It explores the use of various bioprinting techniques, stem cell therapies, and decellularized matrices for tissue regeneration. Additionally, the book delves into ethical considerations and regulatory challenges associated with tissue engineering and regenerative medicine.

Recent advancements have empowered researchers to precisely manipulate cells and cellular constructs, facilitating the fabrication of biomimetic tissues and organs. While current tissue-engineered products may still lack certain critical functionalities, including vascular networks, innervation, and lymphatic systems, innovative strategies are being explored to address these limitations. Overall, this book aims to provide a comprehensive and up-to-date overview of the field of tissue engineering and regenerative medicine. By covering a wide range of topics and presenting the latest research findings, the book will be a valuable resource for medical and engineering professionals interested in this exciting and rapidly growing field.

Editors
Dr. Shailesh D. Kamble
Dr. Subhash Singh
Dr. Ashwani Kumar
Dr. Gaurav Dwivedi

Preface

The book *Tissue Engineering and Regenerative Medicine: Advances and Applications* undoubtedly provides valuable insights into the field, and it could benefit from a more in-depth exploration of the ethical implications surrounding stem cell research and tissue engineering. A more detailed discussion of the challenges and limitations associated with large-scale tissue and organ manufacturing, including scalability, cost-effectiveness, and long-term viability, would provide readers with a more nuanced understanding of the current state of the field. The book consists of 24 chapters. **Chapter 1** deals with the role of tissue engineering in real medical field. Tissue engineering plays an important role in patient treatment. Supplemental bladders, small arteries, skin grafts, cartilage, and even a full trachea have been implanted in patients, but the procedures are still experimental and very costly. While more complex organ tissues like heart, lung, and liver tissue have been successfully recreated in the lab, they are a long way from being fully reproducible and ready to implant into a patient. Tissue engineering and regenerative medicine are rapidly growing fields that aim to develop methods for replicating human tissues and organs. **Chapter 2** deals with the transformative potential of machine learning, AI, and computer vision in revolutionizing tissue engineering, paving the way for more efficient and personalized approaches to tissue regeneration. **Chapter 3** deals with various 3D bioprinting techniques employed in tissue engineering, highlighting their unique advantages and limitations for different tissue types. **Chapter 4** deals with the extraction and processing of natural biomaterials, such as collagen, chitosan, and silk fibroin, for their use in tissue engineering scaffolds and regenerative medicine applications. **Chapter 5** deals with the promising applications of advanced synthetic biomaterials in tissue engineering and regenerative medicine, highlighting their potential to revolutionize healthcare.

Chapter 6 presents a comparative study of three polishing techniques on two commonly used denture base acrylic resins. The findings provide valuable insights into the efficacy of each technique in achieving optimal surface finish and gloss. **Chapter 7** presents a comprehensive overview of the latest advancements in detecting cancer stem cells in brain tumors, highlighting the critical role they play in tumor initiation, progression, and recurrence. In continuation **Chapter 8** highlights into the innovative field of user-enabled brain tumor detection, exploring how advanced technologies are empowering individuals to play an active role in monitoring their own brain health. **Chapter 9** deals with the current limitations of CNNs in stem cell imaging and discusses potential future directions for AI research in this field, aiming to overcome these challenges and improve the accuracy and efficiency of stem cell analysis. **Chapter 10** deals with the evaluation of focal solid hepatic lesions using shear wave elastography, a non-invasive imaging technique that assesses tissue stiffness. This chapter explores the role of shear wave elastography in differentiating benign from malignant hepatic lesions, providing valuable insights for clinical decision-making.

Chapter 11 deals with predicting the risk of diabetes using machine learning techniques. **Chapter 12** evaluates the risk factors associated with coronary artery disease among patients with and without non-alcoholic fatty liver disease. **Chapter 13** investigates the association between blood sugar levels and patient outcomes in acute myocardial infarction (STEMI and NSTEMI) among non-diabetic individuals. The study aims to identify potential glycemic thresholds that may influence clinical outcomes. **Chapter 14** explores the application of machine learning algorithms in early detection of Parkinson's disease. By analyzing various clinical and physiological data, the study aims to develop accurate and efficient predictive models. **Chapter 15** focuses on strategies to prevent post-operative urinary retention in elderly male patients undergoing elective surgery. The study examines factors contributing to this condition and evaluates the effectiveness of different prevention methods.

Chapter 16 Explores the application of the Random Forest algorithm in predicting the outcomes of various diseases and demonstrates the effectiveness of this algorithm in providing accurate prognoses. **Chapter 17** investigates the attitudes and intentions of individuals in Uttar Pradesh regarding the adoption of telehealth services and provides valuable insights into the factors influencing the acceptance of telehealth in the region.

Chapter 18 Explores computational methods to identify potential drug candidates targeting the SARS-CoV-2 virus and discusses the advantages and limitations of in silico drug discovery for accelerating the development of COVID-19 treatments. In continuation **Chapter 19** presents a novel approach using graph convolutional networks to analyze X-ray images for early and accurate diagnosis of COVID-19 and evaluates the performance of the proposed method compared to traditional image analysis techniques.

Chapter 20 investigated the association between serum magnesium levels and febrile convulsions and found a significant correlation between low serum magnesium levels and an increased risk of febrile convulsions. **Chapter 21** compared the Apache-II score, Ranson criteria, and modified CT severity index in predicting the severity of acute pancreatitis and determined that the modified CT severity index was the most accurate predictor of disease severity.

Chapter 22 deals with comparing the accuracy of spot urine protein-to-creatinine ratio and 24-hour urine protein in diagnosing nephropathy in type 2 diabetic patients. **Chapter 23** explores the effectiveness of electrocardiogram in identifying the specific coronary artery responsible for occlusion in patients experiencing ST-segment elevation myocardial infarction. **Chapter 24** investigates the relationship between changes in optical coherence tomography (OCT) measurements after cataract surgery and the occurrence of intraoperative surgical complications.

Editors
Dr. Shailesh D. Kamble
Dr. Subhash Singh
Dr. Ashwani Kumar
Dr. Gaurav Dwivedi

Acknowledgments

The journey that led to the fruition of this book, *Tissue Engineering and Regenerative Medicine: Advances and Applications*, has been paved with invaluable contributions of numerous individuals and entities. We are immensely grateful to CRC Press for providing us with a platform to share our knowledge on clean energy. Their unwavering support and insightful guidance throughout the entire publishing process were instrumental in shaping this book into a valuable resource. Their commitment to excellence, from initial concept to final publication, significantly enhanced the overall quality of the work. Our sincere appreciation goes to the numerous contributors and reviewers who generously shared their expertise. Their diverse perspectives enriched every chapter, undeniably contributing to the depth and breadth of the content. Their illuminating feedback ensured the accuracy and comprehensiveness of this book, making it a vital reference for the scholarly community.

We dedicate this book to passionate and dedicated individuals whose tireless efforts are driving advancements in clean energy. Their relentless pursuit of innovation inspires us all. It is our hope that this work serves as a source of inspiration and a valuable reference for the scholarly community, furthering the collective effort toward a sustainable future. Finally, we recognize and honor the collaborative spirit that unites us all in the pursuit of excellence and progress within the dynamic intersection of engineering and technology. This book stands as a testament to the power of collaboration, and we are grateful to have been a part of this collective endeavor.

Editors
Dr. Shailesh D. Kamble
Dr. Subhash Singh
Dr. Ashwani Kumar
Dr. Gaurav Dwivedi

About the editors

Shailesh D. Kamble is working as Associate Professor in the Department of Artificial Intelligence and Data Science in Indira Gandhi Delhi Technical University for Women, Delhi, India. He received his Bachelor of Engineering degree in Computer Technology from Yeshwantrao Chavan College of Engineering, Nagpur, India under the Rashtrasant Tukadoji Maharaj Nagpur University, Nagpur, India. He received his Master of Engineering degree from Prof Ram Meghe Institute of Technology and Research, formerly known as College of Engineering, Badnera under Sant Gadge Baba Amravati University, Amravati, India. He received his doctoral degree in Computer Science Engineering from the Department of Computer Science Engineering, R.T.M. Nagpur University, Nagpur, India on 13 November 2018. He was working as Associate Professor in the Department of Computer Science and Engineering at Yeshwantrao Chavan College of Engineering, Nagpur, India. He has over 20 years of teaching and research experience. His current research interests include image processing, video processing, and language processing. He is the author or co-author of more than 70 scientific publications in International Journal, International Conferences, and National Conferences. He is a life member of ISTE, India and Fellow IE(I), India.

Subhash Singh is currently working as Associate Professor in the Department of Mechanical and Automation Engineering, Indira Gandhi Delhi Technical University for Women, New Delhi. He earned his B. Tech from KNIT, Sultanpur, 2003, and M. Tech from NIT Kurukshetra, 2007. He completed his Ph.D. from IIT Roorkee in 2017. Dr. Singh specializes in areas such as modification of nanomaterials, thin coating, fabrication of MMCs, synthesis of 2D Materials, FSP, and machining of biodegradable materials. He has published more than 40 research papers in various prestigious journals. He has also authored three books and 20 book chapters. He has completed three research projects.

Ashwani Kumar holds a Ph.D. in Mechanical Engineering, specializing in Mechanical Vibration and Design with a diverse and impressive career spanning over 14 years. He currently holds the position of Professor and Head of Department Mechanical Engineering (Gazetted Officer Group A) at the Technical Education Department Uttar Pradesh (under Government of Uttar Pradesh) in Kanpur, India. Prior to his current role, Dr. Kumar served as an Assistant Professor in the Department of Mechanical Engineering at Graphic Era University, Dehradun (ranked 52nd by NIRF India) from July 2010 to November 2013. Beyond his academic contributions, Dr. Kumar possesses extensive leadership and administrative experience. He has held numerous key positions within the education sector, including Coordinator for AICTE-Extension of Approval, Nodal Officer for PMKVY-TI Scheme (Government of India), Internal Coordinator – CDTP Scheme (Government of Uttar Pradesh), Industry Academia Relation Officer, Assistant Center Superintendent (ACS) – Institute Examination Cell, Zonal Officer for Joint Entrance Examination (JEE-Diploma), and Sector Magistrate for State Assembly and General Elections. Dr. Kumar is a passionate researcher and a prominent figure in the field of academic publishing. His dedication to knowledge dissemination is evident in his role as Series Editor for eight distinguished book series published by international publisher of repute. These series encompass a wide range of topics, titled as: Advances in Manufacturing, Design and Computational Intelligence Techniques/Renewable and Sustainable Energy Developments/Smart Innovations and Technological Advancements in Mechanical and Materials Engineering/Solar Thermal Energy Systems: Advancements in Engineering, Ergonomics, and Sustainable Development/Artificial Intelligence and Machine Learning for Intelligent Engineering Systems/Computational Intelligence and Biomedical Engineering/Renewable Green Technologies for Sustainable Energy Solutions. Dr. Kumar's editorial expertise extends beyond book series. He serves as Editor-in-Chief for the International Journal of Materials, Manufacturing and Sustainable Technologies (IJMMST, *ISSN: 2583-6625*), and Editor of the International Journal of Energy Resources Applications (IJERA, *ISSN: 2583-6617*). He has also been a guest editor for a special issue of Buildings titled as Sustainable Buildings, Resilient Cities and Infrastructure Systems (*ISSN: 2075-5309*, I.F. 3.1) and holds editorial board positions on eight international journals and acts as review board member of 20 prestigious (Indexed in SCI/SCIE/Scopus) international journals with high impact factor. Dr. Kumar's dedication to scholarship is further demonstrated by his prolific authorship of over 165+ articles in prestigious journals, book chapters, and conference proceedings. Additionally, he has co-authored or edited over 40+ books in Mechanical Engineering, Materials Science, and Renewable Energy Engineering. Dr. Kumar's achievements have been recognized with prestigious awards, including a Best Teacher award for excellence in academics and research.

He has also successfully guided 15 students through their B.Tech., MTech, and Ph.D. theses and currently serves as an external doctoral committee member at S.R.M. University, New Delhi. Dr. Kumar is actively involved in cutting-edge research, focusing on areas such as Artificial Intelligence and Machine Learning in Mechanical Engineering, Smart Materials and Manufacturing Techniques, Thermal Energy Storage, Building Efficiency, Renewable Energy Harvesting, Sustainable Transportation, and Heavy Vehicle Dynamics. He holds four patents and frequently participates in international conferences as an invited speaker, session chair, and member of advisory boards, review boards, and program committees. Dr. Kumar's ORCID ID is 0000-0003-4099-935X.

Gaurav Dwivedi has completed his B. Tech in Mechanical Engineering from IKGPTU Jalandhar, M. Tech in Energy Systems from IIT Roorkee and Ph.D. in the field of Renewable Energy (Biofuel) from IIT Roorkee, India. He has 12 years of teaching experience in the field of Mechanical & Energy Engineering and taught various subjects like IC Engine, Thermodynamics, Fluid Machinery, Bioenergy, and others at various Institute like VIT University Vellore and Amity University Noida. Currently, he is working as Assistant Professor in the Energy Centre at Maulana Azad National Institute of Technology, Bhopal India. His areas of interest are biodiesel production methodology, enhancement in fuel properties, and application of biofuel and hydrogen on engine operation. He has published more than 150 papers in various International Journals and conferences, along with more than 80 papers in SCI and Scopus Indexed Journal. He has published four books with International Publishers along with that he has contributed 12 book chapters. He recieved the Young Scientist award at NIT Trichy for his contribution in the field of renewable energy. He is an active member of Institution of Engineers, India and Solar Energy Society of India and IEEE. He also served as Guest Editor for International Journals like *Sustainable Energy Technology and Assessment* (SETA), *Materials Today* proceedings, and *Journal of Traffic and Transportation.* He has currently three running projects and more than 45 lakhs sponsored by DST and MPCST. He also featured in "Top 2% scientist of the world from India (all fields)" (2020,2021,2022,2023) by a survey conducted by Stanford University.

Contributors

Aditya Raj
United Institute of Technology
Prayagraj, India
New Horizon College of Engineering
Karnataka, India

Aiman Zakir
Indira Gandhi Delhi Technical University for Women
New Delhi, India

Akash Kumar Barik
United Institute of Technology
Prayagraj, India
New Horizon College of Engineering
Karnataka, India

Alok Srivastava
Indian Institute of Technology Delhi
New Delhi, India

Dr. Amol D. Langade
Department of Surgery
Krishna Institute of Medical Sciences
Krishna Vishwa Vidyapeeth (Deemed to be University)
Satara, Maharashtra, India

Amit Kumar Tiwari
Department of Computer Science and Engineering
United Institute of Technology
Prayagraj, India

Amar
Amity Business School
Amity University
Lucknow, Uttar Pradesh, India

Amit Kumar Tiwari
Computer Science and Engineering
United Institute of Technology
Prayagraj, Uttar Pradesh, India

Amol Bohite
Department of Radio-diagnosis
Krishna Institute of Medical Sciences
Krishna Vishwa Vidyapeeth (formerly known as KIMSDU)
Karad, India

Anil Singh
United Institute of Technology
Prayagraj, India

Arshad Khan
Department of Biological Science and Engineering
Maulana Azad National Institute of Technology
Bhopal, India

Ashish Mishra
Department of Computer Science and Engineering
United Institute of Technology
Prayagraj, India

Asif Tamboli
Department of Radio-diagnosis
Krishna Institute of Medical Sciences
Krishna Vishwa Vidyapeeth (formerly known as KIMSDU)
Karad, India

Ashwani Kumar
Technical Education Department Uttar Pradesh
Kanpur, India

Avni Dwivedi
Department of Computer Science and Engineering
United Institute of Technology
Prayagraj, India

Ayush Maurya
United Institute of Technology
Prayagraj, India

B. Meenkashi Sundaram
Department of Computer Science and Engineering
New Horizon College of Engineering
Bengaluru, India

C. Manjunatha Swamy
Department of Computer Science and Engineering
New Horizon College of Engineering
Bengaluru, India

Dr. D. B. Potdar
Department of Paediatrics
Krishna Institute of Medical Sciences
Krishna Vishwa Vidyapeeth (Deemed to be University)
Satara, Maharashtra, India

Dany P. John
Department of Medicine
Krishna Institute of Medical Sciences
Krishna Vishwa Vidyapeeth
Karad, India
Department of Cardiology
Krishna Institute of Medical Sciences
Krishna Vishwa Vidyapeeth (Deemed to be University)
Satara, Maharashtra, India

Deepika Khanna
School of Dental Sciences
Krishna Vishwa Vidyapeeth (formerly known as KIMSDU)
Karad, India

Desai Jabbar
Department of Pathology
Krishna Institute of Medical Sciences
Krishna Vishwa Vidyapeeth
Karad, India

Dr. Divya R. Brahmbhatt
Department of Pathology
Krishna Institute of Medical Sciences
Krishna Vishwa Vidyapeeth
Karad, India

Dr. G. G. Joag
Department of Paediatrics
Krishna Institute of Medical Sciences
Krishna Vishwa Vidyapeeth (Deemed to be University)
Satara, Maharashtra, India

Garima Shukla
Department of Computer Science and Engineering
United Institute of Technology
Prayagraj, India

Gaurav Dwivedi
Energy Centre
Maulana Azad National Institute of Technology
Bhopal, India

Gaurav Narain Singh
Department of Computer Science and Engineering
United Institute of Technology
Prayagraj, India

Dr Girish Gadre
Department of Ophthalmology
Krishna Institute of Medical Sciences
Krishan Vishwa Vidyapeeth (Deemed to be University)
Satara, Maharashtra, India

Harshit Bhatia
Department of Computer Science and Engineering
United Institute of Technology
Prayagraj, India

Hritik Dubey
Computer Science and Engineering
United Institute of Technology
Prayagraj, Uttar Pradesh, India

Ishita
United Institute of Technology
Prayagraj, India

Keerthana Balakrishnan
United Institute of Technology
Prayagraj, India
New Horizon College of Engineering
Karnataka, India

Khushhali M. Pandey
Department of Biological Science and Engineering
Maulana Azad National Institute of Technology
Bhopal, India

Dr. Komal Malik
Amity Business School
Amity University
Lucknow, Uttar Pradesh, India

Kriti Dwivedi
Department of Computer Science and Engineering
United Institute of Technology
Prayagraj, India

Lubna Zeenat
Department of Biological Science and Engineering
Maulana Azad National Institute of Technology
Bhopal, India

M. Sharanya
Department of Computer Science and Engineering
New Horizon College of Engineering
Bengaluru, India

Mohd Hasan Syed
Department of Computer Science and Engineering
United Institute of Technology
Prayagraj, India

Mohit Narayan Gupta
Computer Science and Engineering
United Institute of Technology
Prayagraj, Uttar Pradesh, India

Dr. Namita Srivastava
St. John's College
Agra, Uttar Pradesh, India

Dr. Mrs. Nanda J. Pati
Department of Pathology
Krishna Institute of Medical Sciences
Krishna Vishwa Vidyapeeth
Karad, India

Dr. Nitin Jadhav
Department of Medicine
Krishna Institute of Medical Sciences
Krishan Vishwa Vidyapeeth (Deemed to be University)
Satara, Maharashtra, India
Department of Medicine
Krishna Institute of Medical Sciences
Vishwa Vidyapeeth (formerly known as KIMSDU)
Karad, India

Pankaj Chauhan
Homi Bhabha Cancer Hospital and Research Centre
New Delhi, India

Pawan Kumar Tiwari
Computer Science and Engineering
United Institute of Technology
Prayagraj, Uttar Pradesh, India

Piyush Mishra
Department of Computer Science and Engineering
United Institute of Technology
Prayagraj, India

Pooja Bhati
Indira Gandhi Delhi Technical University for Women
New Delhi, India

Pradeep Yadav
United Institute of Technology
Prayagraj, India

Prafull Pandey
Computer Science and Engineering
United Institute of Technology
Prayagraj, Uttar Pradesh, India

Pratyush Puri
Computer Science and Engineering
United Institute of Technology
Prayagraj, Uttar Pradesh, India

Pronob Sanyal
School of Dental Sciences
Krishna Vishwa Vidyapeeth (formerly known as KIMSDU)
Karad, India

R. Suganya
United Institute of Technology
Prayagraj, India
New Horizon College of Engineering
Bangalore, Karnataka, India

Dr. Sujata R. Kanetkar
Department of Pathology
Krishna Institute of Medical Sciences
Krishna Vishwa Vidyapeeth
Karad, India

Dr. Ravendra Yadav
Department of Surgery
Krishna Institute of Medical Sciences
Krishna Vishwa Vidyapeeth (Deemed to be University)
Satara, Maharashtra, India

Dr. Ravindra Adikrao More
Department of Medicine
Krishna Institute of Medical Sciences
Vishwa Vidyapeeth (formerly known as KIMSDU)
Karad, India

Rohit Mishra
Department of Computer Science and Engineering
United Institute of Technology
Prayagraj, India

S. M. Soundarya
Department of Computer Science and Engineering
New Horizon College of Engineering
Bengaluru, India

Sanskriti Srivastava
United Institute of Technology
Prayagraj, India

Satyam Sangeet
Department of Chemistry
Indian Institute of Science Education and Research (IISER)
Kolkata, West Bengal, India

Shaik Arshid Banu
Department of Mechanical & Automation Engineering
Indira Gandhi Delhi Technical University for Women
New Delhi, India

Shalini Prajapati
Department of Biological Science and Engineering
Maulana Azad National Institute of Technology
Bhopal, India

Shreya Tiwari
Department of Radio-diagnosis
Krishna Institute of Medical Sciences
Krishna Vishwa Vidyapeeth (formerly known as KIMSDU)
Karad, India

Qazi Faiz
Department of Computer Science and Engineering
United Institute of Technology
Prayagraj, India

Shailesh D. Kamble
Department of Artificial Intelligence and Data Science
Indira Gandhi Delhi Technical University for Women
New Delhi, India

Sonvi Jain
Department of Mechanical and Automation
Indira Gandhi Delhi Technical University for Women
New Delhi, India

Stuti Narain
Department of Mechanical and Automation
Indira Gandhi Delhi Technical University for Women
New Delhi, India

Subhash Singh
Department of Mechanical and Automation
Indira Gandhi Delhi Technical University for Women
New Delhi, India

Sujey Rajesh Naik
Department of Computer Science and Engineering
New Horizon College of Engineering
Bengaluru, India

Tvisha Chawla
Department of Mechanical & Automation Engineering
Indira Gandhi Delhi Technical University for Women
New Delhi, India

V. E. Redkar
Department of Medicine
Krishna Institute of Medical Sciences
Krishan Vishwa Vidyapeeth (Deemed to be University)
Satara, Maharashtra, India

Vaishnavi Rukhaiyar
Department of Mechanical & Automation Engineering
Indira Gandhi Delhi Technical University for Women
New Delhi, India

Virendra C. Patil
Department of Medicine
Krishna Institute of Medical Sciences
Krishna Vishwa Vidyapeeth
Karad, India

Yatika Gori
Department of Mechanical Engineering, Graphic Era deemed to be University Dehradun, India

Chapter 1

Recent technological developments in tissue engineering

Stuti Narain, Sonvi Jain, Shailesh D. Kamble, Subhash Singh, Yatika Gori, and Ashwani Kumar

1.1 NEED FOR TISSUE ENGINEERING

Tissue engineering, a field with immense potential in 21st-century medicine, has evolved from creating bioengineered skin substitutes to a broad spectrum of tissue and organ applications [1]. Tissue Engineering and Regenerative Medicine (TERM) are often used together, reflecting their goal of repairing and replacing damaged tissues and organs using various cells, engineering, and materials science. This emerging field is focused on inventing alternative medicines or substitutes for tissue and organ restoration, addressing the challenges of an ageing society with prevalent chronic illnesses [2]. By integrating engineering and biological principles, TERM is paving the way for creating new tissues and organs and restoring injured or diseased tissues and organs.

Regenerative medicine's success hinges on its materials, primarily combinations of scaffolds, growth factors, and a select group of cells. These cells, including stem cells, fibroblasts, chondrocytes, and keratinocytes, play a crucial role in replacing damaged tissues and, importantly, accelerating the body's natural healing process. This practical application of regenerative medicine is shaping a promising future for healthcare, with its ability to enhance the body's natural healing process, ushering in a new era of medical treatment [3].

Although tissue engineering is considered a relatively new field in science and technology, its conception dates to the early 2500 BC, when the ancient Egyptians used prostheses. The first known depiction of tissue engineering occurred in 1933 when surgery was conducted on a pig to implant tumour cells wrapped in a polymer membrane. The idea of replacing tissues and improving the functionality of organs has been embedded in the human world since history [4, 5]. The history of tissue engineering is depicted in Figure 1.1.

The human body, with its lower regenerative possibility, continues to lose tissue and organs over age due to inherited deficiencies, trauma, and illnesses. The traditional approach of organ transplantation has also lost its appeal as it poses an immense public health challenge, with only a tiny

DOI: 10.1201/9781003536352-1

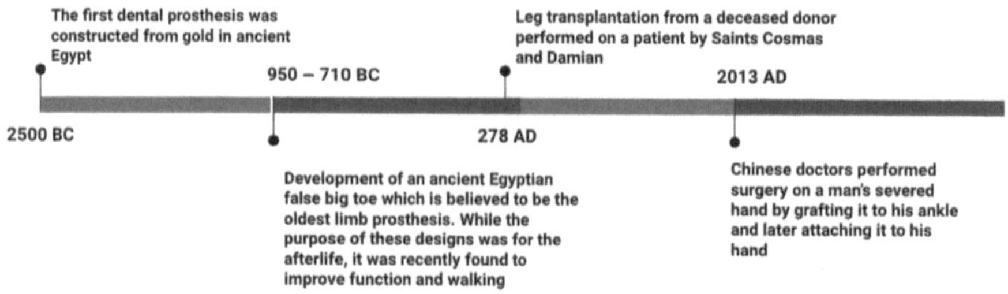

Figure 1.1 History of tissue engineering.

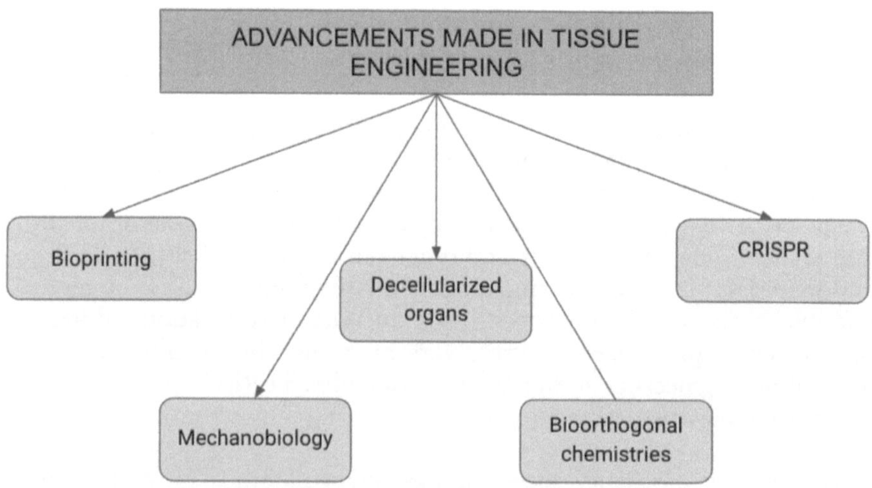

Figure 1.2 Advancements made in tissue engineering.

percentage of deserving patients receiving the help that they desperately need. A major challenge in traditional organ transplantation is the problem of immunological rejection of the donated body parts by the patient. Prompted by the scarcity of donor tissues and the limited regenerative capacity of specific tissues, such as the heart and domains of the nervous system, to heal themselves, tissue engineering techniques were developed as a promising solution to address organ shortages in transplantation. This interdisciplinary approach, which brings together the principles of engineering and biology, has been widely adopted since its inception, reflecting the collaborative spirit that underpins the field [3]. We can see in Figure 1.2 the various advancements of tissue engineering over the years.

1.1.1 Organ failure and tissue loss

Loss of tissues and organ failure can be attributed to injury, trauma, and the natural ageing process of the human body [6]. Cardiovascular diseases

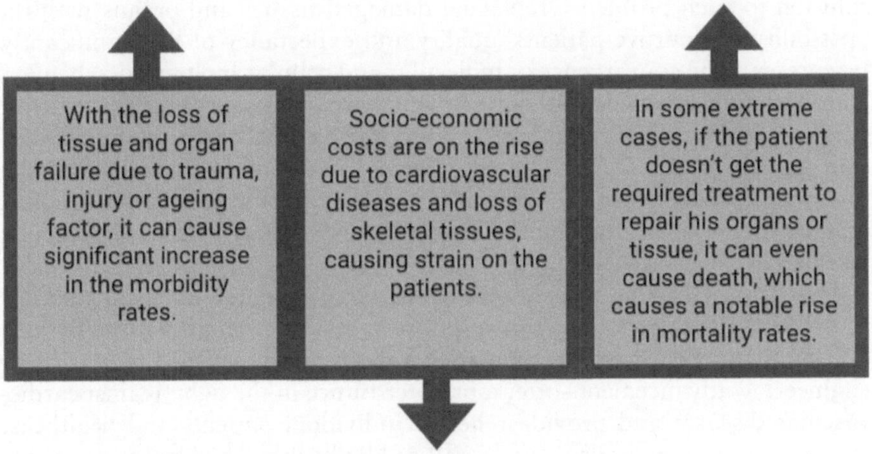

Figure 1.3 Problems faced due to organ failure and tissue loss.

continue to raise the mortality rates worldwide. In developed countries, myocardial infarction, stroke, and vascular diseases contribute to significant morbidity and mortality, resulting in thousands of deaths each year. According to a report from the American Heart Association in 2008, every 39 seconds, an average of one death emerged, leading to approximately 2,200 daily demises in the United States due to cardiovascular diseases, with black Americans being more susceptible than white Americans [7].

As we can see in Figure 1.3, there are various problems faced due to tissue loss and organ failure. Trauma, injury, disease, and ageing can lead to a substantial increase in skeletal tissue loss, morbidity, and an increase in patient complications. These evolving patient demographics and more complex clinical scenarios emphasize the need for new and improved skeletal regeneration methods. The current approaches, while valiant, face significant limitations and disadvantages, including but not limited to organ transplants to replace damaged tissues and restore lost skeletal tissue [8]. Transplantation faces the obstacle of immunological considerations, like the shortage of donor tissues and the possibility of the human body rejecting someone's organs. These limitations underscore the urgent need for new, more effective solutions [6].

The mortality and morbidity rates remain at an all-time high. By administering drugs to combat such diseases and lower the risk of organ failure, the body experiences several chemical reactions which cause autoimmune difficulties. Rather than treating the immediate illness, it leads to lupus, rheumatoid arthritis, or multiple sclerosis. With rapid developments and promising advancements in regenerative medicines and tissue engineering, there is hope for patients suffering from cardiovascular diseases and other ailments requiring tissue repair. Tissue engineering offers an alternative solution to such problems, replacing damaged tissues and organs with the possibility to improve patients' quality and expectancy of life significantly. It represents the convergence of molecular and cellular biology and chemical and mechanical engineering to create innovative approaches that accelerate patients' recovery and significantly reduce the medical and economic obligation among patients. In tissue engineering, particularly in cardiovascular disease, applying these innovative approaches promises to offer relief to many patients by addressing the challenges associated with cardiovascular diseases [6, 7].

This field of TERM takes benefit of the body's innate biological response to tissue damage, leveraging this response to restore organ functions by integrating living elements into the patients' body. These cardiovascular tissue engineering advancements offer a brighter future in the fight against cardiovascular diseases and provide relief to individual patients and healthcare systems, potentially improving overall public health. The impact of cardiovascular tissue engineering extends beyond individual patients. By addressing the challenges associated with cardiovascular diseases and offering new avenues for treatment, these advancements improve public health on a larger scale. Furthermore, by using the principles of tissue engineering in cardiovascular health, researchers and medical professionals can work towards developing more effective and personalized treatment options, ultimately improving outcomes for patients and the broader population [7].

1.1.2 Limitations of traditional transplant

Since organ transplantation has been incepted, it is considered a life-saving process for people who are suffering from the end stages of organ failure [9]. The journey of this medical practice has been marked by significant progress, offering hope and optimism for the future. Doctors treat tissue loss and organ failure by transplanting organs from the donor to the patient and performing surgery. The usage of mechanical devices like kidney dialyzers is also taken into practice. With continuous improvements seen in immunosuppressive drugs, there has been a tremendous increase in graft and short-term patient survival rates. Although the number of clinical tests in organ transplantation is growing annually, and these treatments have improved countless lives, this medical field faces several limitations [10–12].

Organ transplantation has many problems, and one of the most pressing issues is the severe lack of donor organs. With less than 3,000 donors for 30,000 patients annually, the organ demand far exceeds the supply. This imbalance poses a significant health challenge, with only a tiny percentage of patients receiving the transplantation. Many patients can spend years on the waiting list and, in extreme cases, may even lose their lives [3, 11]. The waiting time for transplants can even surpass five years, but the condition can be kept in check by dialysis [10]. Another common challenge is the patient's body's rejection of the donated organ due to

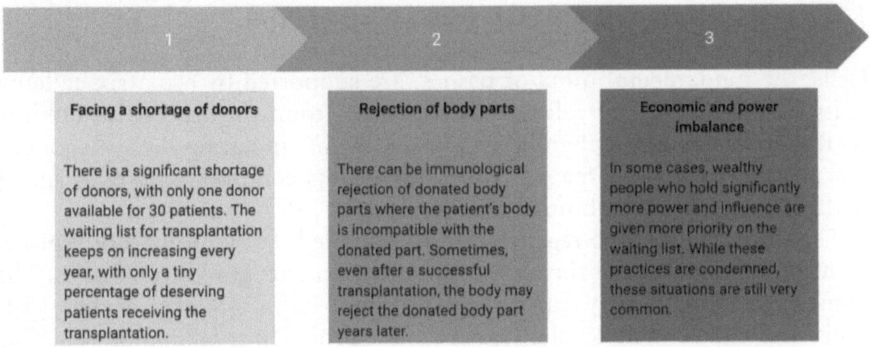

Figure 1.4 Disadvantages of traditional transplant.

immunological differences. Sometimes, the body may reject the donated organ after successful surgery, leading to more demand for new donors. This perpetuates a vicious cycle of more demand and low supply, underscoring the urgent need for a more equitable and ethical approach to organ transplantation [3, 9]. Figure 1.4 gives an overview of the disadvantages of traditional transplant.

Organ transplantation is not without its ethical issues. In developing nations, 'transplant tourism' cases occur, where tourists with more power and wealth are prioritized over the general public. This practice, while widely condemned, still takes place, leading to the exploitation of defenceless people [3]. The field also grapples with inferior long-term graft survival rates, a constant requirement for immunosuppressive medicine, and complications of immunological therapy, which can increase the risks of cardiovascular diseases and malignancy [10]. These complications can lead to an overall increase in the risk of infections. Surgical reconstruction can also result in life-long problems, with people who undergo treatment for incontinence often develop colon cancer [11].

Tissues and organs are immediately required for transplantation in accidents, natural disasters, and wars. However, the shortage of donors and differences in national economic powers and health infrastructures hamper patient treatment and stall research in this field [3]. Traditional transplantation is the prey of its own conquest. With increased outcomes, the demand has been surging, leading to a gap between the supply and consumption demand. Some approaches have been adopted to face this problem, like using organs from marginalized donors, which refers to older donors or those whose hearts do not beat. More recent immunosuppressive agents have been produced, and advances in surgical approaches have been made. However, despite all of these, the long-term results of transplantation methods continue to be poor, and patients have to go back to the waiting list for transplantation [10]. Considering these points, tissue engineering is the superior field for combating such problems.

1.2 PRINCIPLES OF TISSUE REGENERATION

Cells, the fundamental units of tissues, are supported by a matrix called a scaffold. All relaying of cell signals to the environment occurs through the scaffold, which starts a chain of responses. By manipulating these responses, it is possible to mend damaged tissues. Tissue regeneration requires an intact scaffold and cells of high proliferative capacity [3].

The principle of tissue regeneration is grounded on the process of replacement of damaged tissue through cell replication and growth of tissues. The tissue engineering triad as can be seen in Figure 1.5, is made up of cells, scaffolds, and signalling molecules that are implemented in combination [13]. The success of regenerative medicine hinges on the correct combination of scaffolds for cell proliferation and differentiation, signalling molecules and cells that replace or regenerate damaged tissue to its original state [3]. For tissue regeneration to occur, it is necessary to increase the population of cells and also reconstruct the extracellular matrix (ECM). The ECM plays a critical part in cell proliferation and cell differentiation for regeneration induction [14].

Cell sources, particularly stem cells, are the source of tissue generation. Stem cells are undifferentiated and can differentiate into specialized cells for organ regeneration. Stem cells are commonly sourced from the bone marrow (hematopoietic or mesenchymal). Stem cell fate is contingent on the carefully engineered microenvironment of the scaffold and the signalling molecules [13].

One of the critical principles of tissue regeneration is the indispensable role of blood supply. It is not only essential for providing oxygen and nutrients but also for delivering macrophages and phagocytic cells to the tissue, thereby creating a conducive local environment for cell proliferation. The growth factors are secreted, and the local ECM works as a scaffold through which tissue regeneration occurs [15].

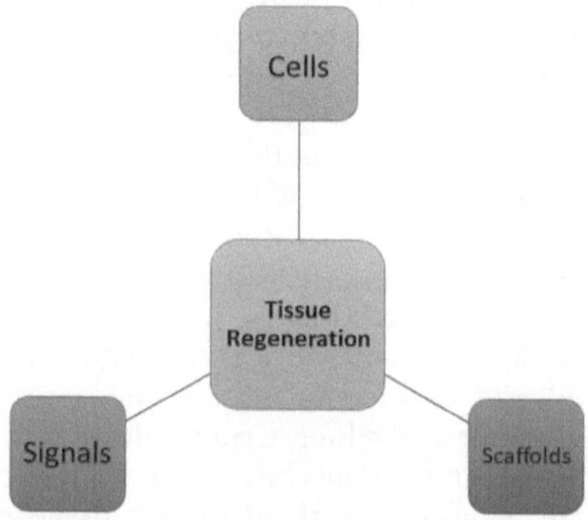

Figure 1.5 Triad of tissue regeneration: Cells, signals and scaffolds.

Tissue regeneration can be carried out in vitro or in vivo, although the final stage of implantation of synthesized tissue is in vivo [16].

1.2.1 Immune system

The immune system plays a critical role in the success of regenerative medicine implementations, as immune cells interact with donor cells and biomaterials. The immune response occurs through overlapping stages. Firstly, leukocytes are recruited to the site of tissue implantation and interact with the scaffold. This is followed by phagocyte recruitment. After phagocyte recruitment, lymphocytes accumulate at the site, which is known as the chronic inflammation phase [17]. The immune response can affect tissue regeneration positively and negatively, depending on the case [18]. Figure 1.6 gives a brief overview of the role of immune cells in tissue regeneration.

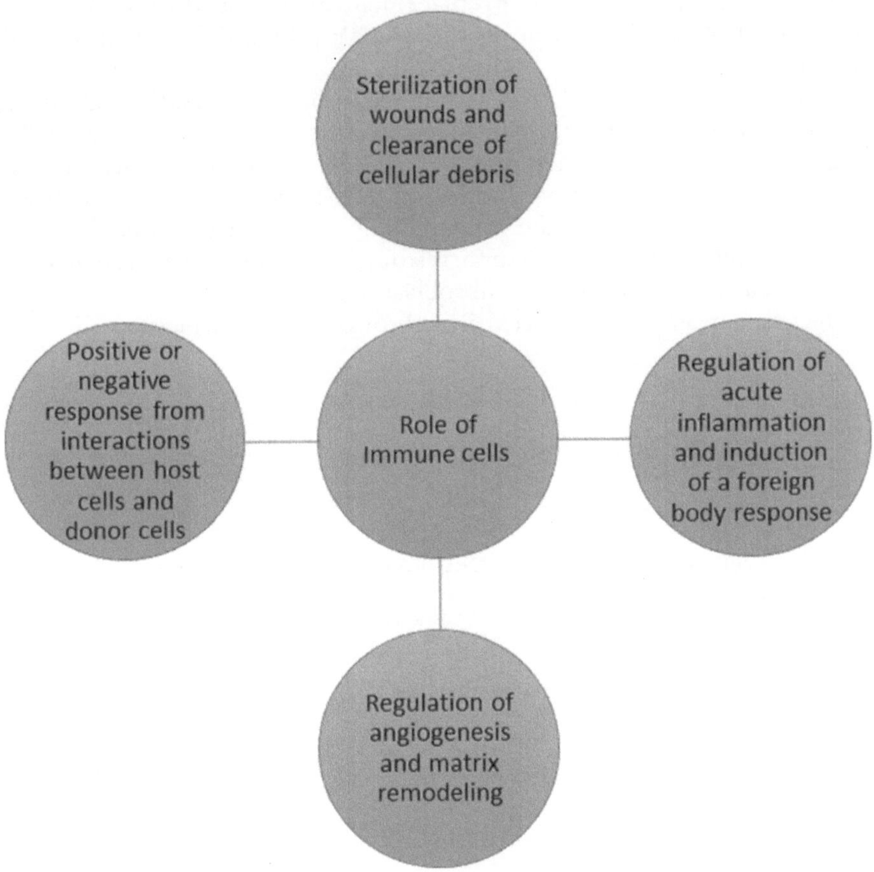

Figure 1.6 Role of immune cells in tissue regeneration.

1.2.2 Regeneration in the human body

The human body has a lower regenerative capacity limited to tissue repair than amphibians and reptiles that can regenerate complete body parts and organs. Tissue engineering employs engineering principles and biology of tissue regeneration in humans to damaged and diseased tissues and organs. The cornea and cartilage exhibit little to no regenerative capacity in humans, whereas the liver, bone marrow and lungs have high regenerative capacity [19]. The varying regenerative capacity of Labile, Quiescent and Permanent cells is mentioned in Figure 1.7.

1.2.3 Tissue regeneration vs. repair

When injured, tissue naturally responds with fibroblast deposition, which contributes to a combination of regeneration and scarring. Scaffolds act as a bridge for regeneration [17]. Tissue regeneration is characterized by the complete replacement of damaged tissue by new, undamaged cells, thus restoring the tissue's previous architecture and function.

Tissue repair is a natural process that occurs in two ways: through tissue regeneration or by healing, which results in scar formation. Generally, repair refers to collagen deposition at the damaged site to form a scar. Tissue regeneration and repair both lead to the restoration of interrupted continuity sustained by acute injury. While tissue regeneration leads to complete functional and structural restoration of lost tissue, repair only leads to scar formation through fibroblast deposition [16].

The tissue regeneration process goes through the following steps:

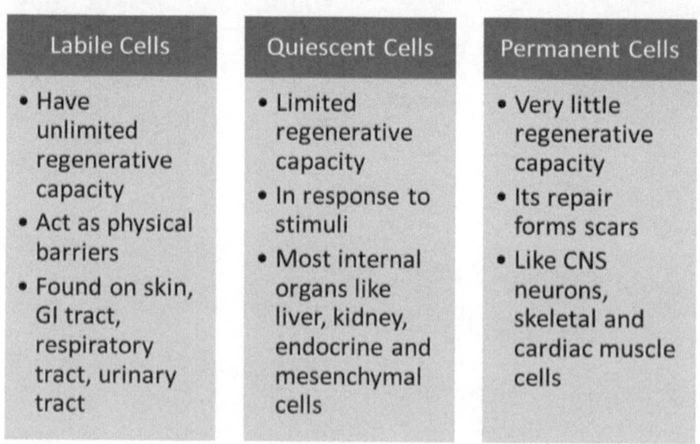

Figure 1.7 Different cell types have different capacity for regeneration [19].

i. In the first crucial step, the epidermal cells migrate to the injury site, forming the apical epidermal cap, which is a thick covering of the injury site [16].
ii. The undifferentiated fibroblast cells then cluster under the apical epidermal cap, forming a blastema. The blastema is a cluster of stem cells that are able to differentiate into any tissue or organ [16].
iii. The blastema receives oxygen and nutrients from the new blood capillary network, and the stem cells undergo mitosis [16].

Tissue repair occurs through a process called healing, which is comprised of four overlapping stages:

A. *Homeostasis*: The first phase of the response concerns maintaining homeostasis. A fibrin clot controls active bleeding. Vasoconstriction isolates the wound site, followed by vasodilation to initiate the inflammatory response [17].
B. *Inflammatory response*: The second phase prevents infection as immune cells course through the bloodstream to reach the damaged site. Bacteria and debris removal occurs through phagocyte recruitment [17].
C. *Proliferation*: This phase is concerned with reconstituting the wound site. It consists of four phases: revascularization or angiogenesis, collagen deposition, granulation, tissue formation, cell growth and contraction, where the wound becomes smaller through myofibroblasts [17].
D. *Remodelling*: In this phase, the tissue function and strength are restored through collagen remodelling [17].

Tissue regeneration constitutes proliferation, macrophage activation matrix remodelling and recruitment of cells to reduce inflammation. Aberrant tissue repair results from the continued actions of inflammatory cells and impaired regeneration. The determining factor for scar deposition or resolution is the interaction between macrophages and myofibroblasts [20].

1.2.4 The hallmark events of tissue regeneration

The human body's regenerative capacity varies greatly. The central nervous system and the heart exhibit little to no regeneration. The liver and lungs demonstrate slow cell turnover, whereas the skin and blood exhibit active renewal [18].

Tissue regeneration occurs through a series of events that will be further explained. These include inflammation, tissue formation and maturation.

1.2.4.1 Inflammation

This is the first phase of tissue regeneration. Wound healing occurs, and blood rushes to the injury site. Immune cells are recruited, affecting the repair process. The immune system strongly affects the repair process in mammals.

Immune cells:

a) restore homeostasis by clearing cellular debris,
b) remodel the ECM,
c) produce cytokines and growth factors [18].

The scaffold provides an environment for seeding stem cells and an early orientation for tissue [15]. The transition to regeneration must be rapid for good regeneration outcomes, to prevent complex diseases, and to ensure repair [20].

1.2.4.2 Tissue formation

Stem cells, activated by injury, differentiate into two daughter cells. One stem cell undergoes self-renewal, and the other differentiates. The differentiated stem cell regenerates the lost cells as proliferation generates new cells. In general, dedifferentiation occurs in the same lineage [21].

The regeneration process occurs through the following steps:

- Homeostatic regeneration: Each lineage replenishes its population through its stem cells in homeostatic conditions.
- Quiescent stem cells undergo self-renewal and generate progenitors that multiply and differentiate into required cells [21].

These sequential regeneration events lead to tissue formation. A key prerequisite for this is extracellular matrix remodelling. This involves the rate-limiting activity of metalloproteinases (MMPs) and tissue inhibitors of metalloproteinases (TIMPs) for ECM degradation and preservation [17].

1.2.4.3 Maturation

The maturation step involves an interplay of mesenchymal cells with tissue-resident and immune cells. The regenerated tissue finally matures to a functional state [20].

It is necessary to note that the local environment plays a crucial role in tissue regeneration. Low oxygen and inadequate circulation can hinder the recruitment of progenitor cells. The formation of scar tissue also inhibits mammalian tissue regenerative processes [15].

1.3 COMPONENTS OF TISSUE ENGINEERING: CELLS, SCAFFOLDS, AND SIGNALLING MOLECULES

The tissue regeneration triad of cells, scaffolds and signalling molecules constitute an interplay of factors that influence tissue regeneration outcomes.

1.3.1 Cells

Almost every tissue in the body, including the brain, liver, circulating blood, heart, skin, fat, kidney, and muscle, has various types of progenitor cells [22]. Stem cells can differentiate into other cells of various types in response to injury and grow into over 200 types of cells [23]. Stem cells undergo asymmetric replication and replace the lost cells through maturation. When stem cells undergo mitosis, one daughter cell continues to remain a stem cell, and the other differentiates and becomes a mature cell to fulfil the needs of the tissue it is in. Stem cells may be unipotent, multipotent or totipotent, depending on the types of cells they can differentiate into. Stem cells are usually present in small, discrete populations. A high stem cell population is necessary for tissue regeneration [21].

Stem cells reside in a microenvironment known as the niche and are activated on the instance of changes in the niche. This can include injury or trauma. Various types of stem cell niches can be found in different body parts, as explained later in Section 1.3.1. Scaffolds can be functionally, biologically and chemically engineered to emulate the niche. Stem cell populations are sustained by a suitable scaffold that provides oxygen and nutrient access and neovascularization. Endogenous stem cells have a lower risk of rejection, infection and tumour formation as compared to exogenous stem cells [18].

1.3.2 Scaffold

Scaffolds provide structural support and act as delivery vehicles for cells and drugs [24]. They also physically separate the stem cell population from host cells and the intercellular matrix [18].

An ideal scaffold is one that can closely mimic the properties of the extracellular matrix. For a scaffold to be ideal, it must be biologically compatible and non-toxic, and its matrix must be easily degradable by host cells. The scaffold's composition, porosity and stiffness significantly affect cell activity [18]. The scaffold's porosity should support cell growth, water absorption and oxygen transfer. This ensures that tissue regeneration is promoted [24]. The artificial microenvironment of the scaffold must assist in neovascularization and the permeability of nutrients [22].

Most scaffolds are constructed from polymers, bio-ceramics or hybrid materials, depending on their biocompatibility [24]. Even though naturally occurring biomaterials like collagen are more closely compatible with the native cellular milieu, they restrict versatility in the design of scaffolds and showcase batch-to-batch variations upon isolation [25]. The various criteria for designing scaffolds are discussed in later sections. The characteristics of different biomaterials used for scaffold fabrication are also discussed.

Scaffolds may be implanted, like hydrogel, nanofibre, or macroporous scaffolds, or injected, like polymer nanoparticle colloidal gel, microparticle colloidal gel or hydrogel. While implantable scaffolds have better shape, tuneable biocompatibility and strength than injectable scaffolds, they are also more invasive [18].

1.3.3 Signalling molecules

Tissue regeneration is controlled by cell-to-cell communication. This is achieved through signalling molecules like growth factors, cytokines, chemokines, small modulus and genes, which play an essential role in controlling the microenvironment for regeneration. The delivery of these biomolecules results in the direction of cell migration and delivery [22].

Three methods that can be used to incorporate signalling molecules in the scaffold are bulk encapsulation, surface attachment and bio-membrane coating [18].

1.3.4 Cell sources for tissue engineering

In the tissue engineering triad of cells, scaffolds and signals, the cells are the first and foremost requirement as a source for new tissue regeneration. Cells may be sourced from tissue that may be xenogeneic (from a different species), allogeneic (from the same species but a different member), syngeneic (from another individual with the same genetics) or autologous (from the same individual). Most applications are syngeneic or autologous due to immune responses [25].

1.3.4.1 Sequence of differentiation

Stem cells are a type of undifferentiated, immature cells that are able to differentiate into specialized cell types [13]. The differentiation and dedifferentiation of stem cells occur in a sequence. A stem cell undergoes mitosis to produce two daughter cells. One is a daughter stem cell (self-renewal), which maintains the stem cell population. The other daughter cell is differentiated into specialized cells. Then, the dedifferentiation of this stem cell gives new desired cells that form new tissues [21].

A great deal of research has been done to understand the nature of stem cells and to preserve and expand them in vitro for implantation [15]. Endogenous stem cells are adult stem cells that can auto-renew and differentiate into multiple other cell types. The extracellular matrix must be modelled after the stem cell niche, which is an instructive microenvironment made using biomaterials. Biochemical and biophysical cues guide and instruct the stem cells for migration and proliferation [18].

1.3.4.2 Sources of stem cells

Stem cells can be derived from various sources within the human body. This includes

- the amniotic fluid,
- umbilical cord tissue,
- fat tissue,
- central nervous system,
- bone marrow,
- retina,
- and skin.

1.3.4.3 Types of stem cells

Generally, stem cells are of two types: pluripotent (embryonic stem cells) or multipotent and unipotent (adult stem cells). Other stem cell types include totipotent stem cells, HSCs, ESCs and MSCs [23].

1.3.4.3.1 Pluripotent stem cells

Pluripotent cells have the potential to develop into almost all cell types. These cells include ESCs, cells isolated from endoderm, mesoderm and ectoderm germ layers. Embryonic stem cells are also pluripotent; however, their applications are limited due to ethical reasons [23].

1.3.4.3.2 Multipotent stem cells

They have less proliferative potential than pluripotent and totipotent cells. However, they can still produce a variety of cells in a closely related family of cells. For example, mesenchymal stem cells (MSCs) and HSCs are multipotent [23].

1.3.4.3.3 Totipotent stem cells

Totipotent cells, with their remarkable potential to develop into any kind of cell in the organism, are a fascinating area of study. They can develop into primary germ cell layers of the embryo and the placenta [23].

1.3.4.3.4 Unipotent stem cells

Unipotent stem cells can create cells with only one lineage of differentiation. Muscle stem cells are an example of this. In adult stem cells, unipotent stem cells have the lowest proliferative potential [23].

1.3.4.3.5 The stem cell niche

The stem cell niche plays a crucial role in anchoring the cells inside the tissue, keeping them undifferentiated and quiescent. It generally consists of cells, the extracellular matrix and soluble factors.

The different types of stem cell niches and where they are located can be understood with the help of Table 1.1 [18].

1.3.4.4 Mesenchymal stem cells

Mesenchymal stem cells in adults can be found in bone marrow and used for organ regeneration [13].

Mesenchymal stem cells have the following characteristics:

- Derived from: MSCs are derived from skin, fat and bone marrow. Most generally, they are derived from bone marrow and gingiva.
- Differentiate into: MSCs differentiate into connective tissue cells for remodelling bone, fat and vascular tissue.
- Multipotency: MSCs exhibit self-renewal and differentiate into multiple cell types, such as osteoblasts, chondrocytes, monocytes and adipocytes [13].

Stem cells alone cannot undergo tissue regeneration. Controlling the local environment through regulators like growth factors is essential for good stem cell fate [13]. The regeneration process hinges upon good scaffolding techniques and controls through signalling molecules, discussed in the next two sections.

1.3.5 Biomaterials as scaffolds

As we have read in the earlier sections, scaffolds play a significant role in the domain of tissue engineering. They are highly porous materials that aim to regenerate damaged organs and tissues when combined with the body's cells. These scaffolds work as a template for the regeneration of tissues and help evolve new tissues. They are implanted with cells and crucial growth factors and exposed to biophysical stimuli that take the shape of a bioreactor. These can be either grown in vitro for synthesizing tissues embedded in

Table 1.1 Types of stem cell niches found in different locations in the human body

Location in the body	*Type of stem cell niche*
Bone marrow	HSC and MSC niches
Ovaries and testes	Germline stem cell (GSC) niches
Epithelia (hair follicles, skin, intestinal crypts and cornea)	Epithelial stem cell niches
Brain	Neural stem cell niches
Skeletal Muscle	Satellite stem cell niches
Teeth	Dental pulp stem cell niches
Tumours	Cancer stem cell niches

the wound site or implanted directly into the injured site, where the in vivo technique is used to regenerate tissues using the body's system.

There are several conditions which must be kept in mind while creating or specifying the usefulness of scaffolds for usage in tissue engineering, which are:

a) Biocompatibility
b) Biodegradability
c) Mechanical properties
d) Scaffold architecture
e) Manufacturing technology

While the five criteria discussed in detail in Figure 1.8 are crucial, the most significant factor for the success of research in this domain is the preference for the biomaterial with which the scaffold is to be fabricated. This choice is a critical determinant of the scaffold's performance and its ability to support tissue regeneration [26].

Over the previous 50 years, the domain of tissue engineering has witnessed remarkable evolution in the definition and use of biomaterials. Tissue engineering integrates engineering principles with biology, typically consisting of biomaterials, bioactive materials and cells. The definition of a biomaterial has evolved according to its needs and applications, marking significant progress in the field. Earlier, the main goal of a biomaterial was to check whether the mechanical and material properties were the same while being consistent with the functional outcome of the native issue without causing any damage to the tissue or evoking a detrimental host response. For example, the early biomaterials consisted of materials like bone cement, stainless steel, and Dacron, as they were inert and induced a predictable yet harmless body response [27]. With time, biomaterials are now planned to interact

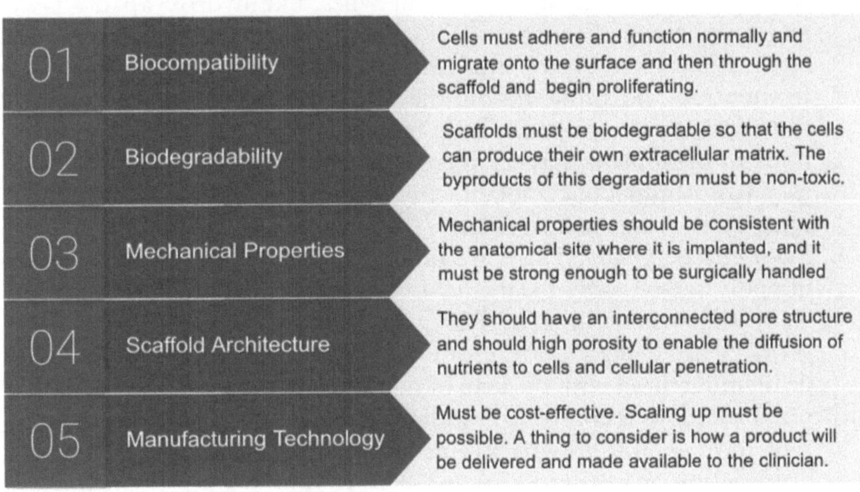

Figure 1.8 Criteria for designing scaffolds.

with biological strategies and assess and replace tissues and organs of the body [26].

Within the domain of tissue regeneration, biomaterials play a crucial role. They provide the necessary support along with scaffolding for the growth of cells, a key aspect of tissue engineering. The extracellular matrix, or the ECM, refers to the secretion of materials by the cells which support the tissues and organs. It acts as the template for biomaterials and provides physical support and spatial organization. ECM comprises structural proteins, for example, collagen, elastin, cell adhesion proteins like fibronectin and laminin, and glycans like proteoglycans [27]. Bio-based materials possess several favourable properties, like a unique chemical structure, non-toxicity, and recyclability, which give them an edge in today's materials sector [28].

Several methods are used to produce such interconnected porous scaffolds, including, but not limited to, fibre bonding and extrusion, 3-D printing, electrospinning and particle aggregation. These techniques enable the development of biodegradable scaffolds, which are classified into two practices: (i) solvent-based and (ii) melt-based. Methods which are solvent-based require very stringent and thorough verifications to ensure no remaining toxic residual solvents after processing scaffolds. On the other hand, melt-based processing does not involve solvents. However, mild temperatures are required to ensure that the biomaterials are not thermally degraded [1].

Generally, three types of biomaterials are commonly used to fabricate scaffolds: ceramics, synthetic polymers and natural polymers. The characteristics of these biomaterials are given in Figure 1.9. All these biomaterials have different properties, advantages and drawbacks, and because of this, composite scaffolds are becoming more common. Let us study them in more detail.

A. ***Ceramics***: Although not generally used for soft tissue regeneration, ceramic biomaterials are of several types, like hydroxyapatite (HA) and tri-calcium phosphate (TCP), which are being used widely for applications like bone renewal. Since ceramics enhance osteoblast differentiation and proliferation, they must react with osteogenic cells for bone regeneration. Ceramic biomaterials have multiple applications in orthopedic surgery to replenish bone defects. They are also used to cover metallic implant exteriors, which helps enhance implant integration with the host bone.
B. ***Synthetic Polymers***: There are numerous synthetic polymers, including polystyrene, poly-l-lactic acid, also known as PLLA, polyglycolic acid, which is written as PGA, and poly-dl-lactic-co-glycolic acid (PLGA), are being used to create scaffolds. All of these materials can be manufactured with the help of tailored architecture. Their degradation procedure is controlled by altering the polymer itself. These materials have several drawbacks, including the concern surrounding the degradation process of PLLA and PGA as they degrade by hydrolysis. During that process, they produce carbon dioxide as a byproduct.

Ceramics	Synthetic Polymer	Natural Polymer
• High Young's modulus • Low elasticity • Hard brittle surface • Good biocompatibility due to their chemical and structural similarity to the mineral phase of native bone. • Difficulty of shaping for implantation • Difficult to control degradation rate	• Can be fabricated with a tailored architecture • Degradation rate can be controlled • Risk of rejection due to reduced bioactivity • Degradation by hydrolysis produces carbon dioxide • Lowering of local pH results in cell and tissue necrosis.	• Biologically active • Promotes excellent cell adhesion and growth • Biodegradable • Host cells can produce their own extracellular matrix to replace the degraded scaffold • Poor mechanical properties

Figure 1.9 Characteristics of various biomaterials.

C. ***Natural Polymers*:** This is the third type of biomaterial in which biological materials like collagen, several proteoglycans and alginate-based substrates along with chitosan are used for the production of scaffolds. While these materials provide excellent cell growth and are biologically active, fabricating scaffolds from biological materials which have homogeneous structures poses various challenges. Because of their poor mechanical properties, natural polymers have limited use in load-bearing orthopaedic applications [26].

Over the years, research has been conducted on biomaterials, including polyhydroxyalkanoates (PHAs), alginite and chitin, to develop unexplored constructs for both bio and non-bio sectors. They comprise excellent properties like biocompatibility and non-toxicity and are non-immunogenic, which make them suitable for simulating the extracellular matrix, promoting cell adhesion and cell interaction and improving overall mechanical strength. They also generate different tissues like cartilage, bone and skin [28]. The most critical estimation of scaffold materials is the host response to the scaffold material and not their composition, shape or mechanical properties. Irrespective of how the material behaves during the implantation, it is more important how it feels and reacts 1, 5 or 10 years after the implantation [27].

1.3.6 Signalling molecules for cell guidance and differentiation

Tissue Engineering and Regenerative Medicine comprises numerous methodologies and approaches. One critical element is the usage of a cell population that will give rise to fresh tissue formation with the interaction of the resident cells of the tissue to be revived. The cell's essence and differentiation stage vary with different strategies and procedures used in TERM, along with the whole number of cells used for transplantation and the tissues that are required for processes like biopsy along with posterior cell isolation [1]. While the preparation and differentiation of the cell are multistep processes that consume much time, the output of the target cell type is usually lower. Due to this, the differentiation of stem cells utilizing biomaterials has evolved into an active research subject in recent years. This method of controlled differentiation using biomaterials has several advantages, like supplying a biomimetic environment, which helps improve the differentiation's effectiveness. It also helps reduce the processing stages for tissue fabrication by incorporating the process of cell differentiation and incorporation and enables the accompanying differentiation of numerous cell styles in a single platform for engineering complex tissues [2]. Some of the factors influencing stem cells can be seen in Figure 1.10.

For processes like cell differentiation and guidance to be carried out successfully, a deep understanding of the role of signalling molecules is imperative. These external signals in the stem cell environment play a key part in delivering cues and regulating the fate decision of these stem cells, which are adept at both repeated self-renewal and producing specialized, differentiated progeny. These signals control the stem cells' proliferation or differentiation into a desired phenotype. Incorporating these signals into tissue regeneration methods is crucial for the successful exposure of stem cells. The exact spatial and temporal representation of the elements directing stem cells is significant during embryogenesis, along with natural healing events. Distinct types of cell populations respond differently to individual signals, as can be seen in mesenchymal, neural and endothelial stem cell populations [29]. Table 1.2 gives an outline of the response of various stem cells to different signals.

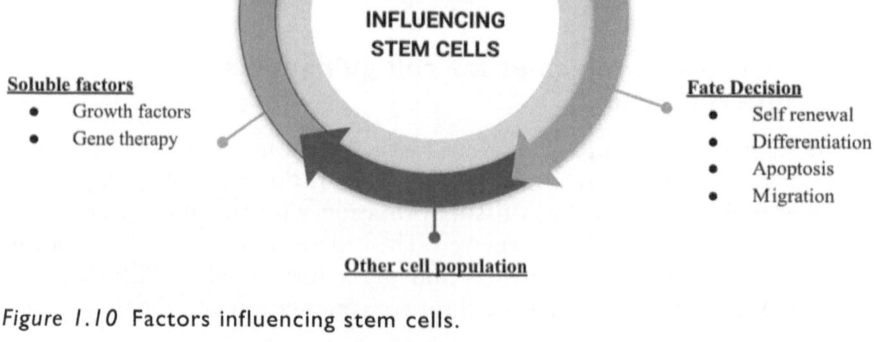

Figure 1.10 Factors influencing stem cells.

We have read in the earlier sections about extracellular matrix (ECM). The ECM is vital in organ morphogenesis and maintains the structure and function of both tissues and cells. It is a combination of structure and functional macromolecules. While it plays an essential role during the growth and evolution of organs and tissues, it transmits signals from different sources to migrating and differentiating cells. Tissue engineering cannot function without providing external signals to the cell populations to stimulate differentiation and proliferation of the cells. These external characteristics are generated from:

- growth factors
- cell–ECM interaction
- cell–cell interactions
- physical–chemical and mechanical stimuli [30]

Until now, we have understood that the intention of tissue engineering is to restore and resurrect impaired tissues and organs using three fundamental materials: scaffolds, cells, and growth factors, which may or may not be used together. However, the success of any approach of TE depends on the efficient integration of these three components. Scaffolds, along with having to provide the needed mechanical and structural support, also have to direct and maintain differentiation, migration, and proliferation. This can only be accomplished if the scaffolds provide biological signals that help guide and control the cell functions.

TE scaffold can be used as a control release platform by incorporating signalling molecules in 3-D scaffolds, which can be achieved through dispersal in the matrix. It can also take place through immobilization by electrostatic exchanges and covalent bonding to the scaffold. This can also be achieved through a gene-mediated approach by inducing nucleic acid encoding into target cells for a distinctive protein signal, yielding tissue regeneration. Here, each cell acts as a single reference point for releasing the signalling protein in this method. Below are some different types of signals commonly used within scaffolds.

1.3.6.1 Interspersed signals

As the name suggests, signalling molecules are incorporated within scaffolds by incorporating them into the scaffolds. While this method has various disadvantages, it is still being used everywhere. Many of these techniques use hydrogel-based scaffolds, simultaneously acting as a scaffold and also as a controlled delivery platform. Some examples of scaffolds include natural hydrogel-based scaffolds like collagen, fibrin, and chitosan and synthetic hydrogel-based scaffolds like poly(ethylene glycol) (PEG). Natural materials tend to experience a cell-related degradation shape, whereas synthetic materials tend to lack cellular recognition but can be easily controlled in macro and microscopic properties.

Table 1.2 Response of Stem Cells to Different Signals

Mesenchymal stem cell populations (MSC)	• **Soluble Factors**: MSCs can be differentiated down to multiple mesenchymal lineages when exposed to soluble factors • **Growth Factors**: Delivery of multiple growth factors has a synergistic effect on new tissue formation • **Gene Therapy**: These can be genetically modified to produce bioactive factors themselves • **Insoluble Factors**: Microarchitectural features of a biomaterial can also give signals to MSCs
Neural stem cell populations (NSC)	• **Soluble Factors**: These can expand when exposed to soluble factors like mitogen • **ECM**: NSC fate can be modulated by the presence of ECM molecules and cell surface receptors during morphogenesis • **Gene Therapy**: Overexposing genes that are used to encode these transcription factors can change the fate of these NSCs • **Other Cells**: Vascular cells can impact NSC fate, i.e. when cultured in the presence of endothelial cells, NSCs continue to proliferate without differentiating
Endothelial precursor cell populations (EPC)	• **Soluble Factors**: The number of cells per ml of peripheral blood increases when EPCs come in contact with soluble factors • **Gene Therapy**: Helps in reducing cell senescence • **Insoluble Factors**: ECM provides attachment signals along with homing cues for endothelial precursors

1.3.6.2 Immobilized signals

Polymer scaffolds are altered to interact with signalling molecules, which interferes with their diffusion out of the polymer medium and, therefore, prolongs their release. Immobilization of signals can be done through reversible connection with the binding, such as binding and de-binding kinetics, and irreversible binding with the polymer. On the other hand, cues can also be given upon degradation of a linking tether or the matrix, which in turn immobilizes the molecule within the scaffold. Some critical determinants of the amount of bound signal along with the release profile include how many binding sites there are, the degradation rate of the scaffold and the association of these signals for such sites.

1.3.6.3 Signal delivery from cells

A different and much more refined technique for controlling the process, overcoming the shortcomings of tissue regeneration, and evoking the preferred biological responses within the scaffold relies on the use of nucleic acid-releasing systems. These acids consist of sequences encoding distinctive proteins, which are generated in the target cells and, therefore, deliver the preferred proteins. Moreover, oligonucleotides can also be used instead of nucleic acid-releasing systems to give rise to anomalous gene expression in a particular form in antisense and interference therapies, which are based on silencing RNA [31].

It is now clear that different biological processes demand a steady flow of signals from the surrounding ECM environment to function correctly and satisfy precise genetic programmes. To achieve the purpose of tissue engineering, which is replacing the damaged tissues of living organisms with healthy ones, it is crucial to merge the use of cells with scaffolds (natural or synthetic) onto which the cells must grow and evolve as if they are in their native tissue. Thus, cells must receive signals from the environment to function smoothly and carry out processes like differentiation and proliferation [30].

1.4 CONCLUSION

Tissue engineering is a rapidly advancing field with numerous applications in medicine. This chapter introduces the vast domain of tissue engineering to new readers. The need for tissue engineering and regenerative medicine has evolved from the limitations of organ transplantation such as donor shortages, economic imbalance and rejection of donated parts. The principles of tissue regeneration are discussed along with the difference between regeneration and repair. The series of events consisting of tissue regeneration are inflammation, tissue formation and maturation. A combination of cells, scaffolds and signalling molecules determines the success or failure of tissue regeneration. Each of these components are introduced and then further discussed in detail. Advancements in tissue engineering have revolutionized healthcare and biotechnology.

REFERENCES

[1] Salgado, A. J., Oliveira, J. M., Martins, A., Teixeira, F. G., Silva, N. A., Neves, N. M., ... & Reis, R. L. (2013). Tissue engineering and regenerative medicine: past, present, and future. *International review of neurobiology*, *108*, 1–33.

[2] Zorlutuna, P., Vrana, N. E., & Khademhosseini, A. (2013). *The Expanding World of Tissue Engineering: The Building Blocks and New Applications of Tissue Engineered Constructs. IEEE Reviews in Biomedical Engineering*, 6, 47–62. doi:10.1109/rbme.2012.2233468

[3] Dzobo, K., Thomford, N. E., Senthebane, D. A., Shipanga, H., Rowe, A., Dandara, C., ... & Motaung, K. S. C. M. (2018). Advances in regenerative medicine and tissue engineering: innovation and transformation of medicine. *Stem cells international*, *2018*(1), 2495848.

[4] Hench, L., & Jones, J. (Eds.). (2005). *Biomaterials, artificial organs and tissue engineering*. Elsevier.
[5] Hasan, A. (Ed.). (2017). *Tissue engineering for artificial organs: regenerative medicine, smart diagnostics and personalized medicine*. John Wiley & Sons.
[6] Risbud, M. (2001). Tissue engineering: implications in the treatment of organ and tissue defects. *Biogerontology*, 2, 117–125.
[7] Nemeno-Guanzon, J. G., Lee, S., Berg, J. R., Jo, Y. H., Yeo, J. E., Nam, B. M., ... & Lee, J. I. (2012). Trends in tissue engineering for blood vessels. *BioMed Research International*, *2012*(1), 956345.
[8] Black, C. R., Goriainov, V., Gibbs, D., Kanczler, J., Tare, R. S., & Oreffo, R. O. (2015). Bone tissue engineering. *Current Molecular Biology Reports*, *1*, 132–140.
[9] Kuntz, K., Weinland, S. R., & Butt, Z. (2015). Psychosocial challenges in solid organ transplantation. *Journal of Clinical Psychology in Medical Settings*, *22*, 122–135.
[10] Lechler, R. I., Sykes, M., Thomson, A. W., & Turka, L. A. (2005). Organ transplantation—how much of the promise has been realized?. *Nature Medicine*, *11*(6), 605–613.
[11] Langer, R., & Vacanti, J. P. (1993). Tissue Engineering. *Science*, *260*(5110), 920–926. http://www.jstor.org/stable/2885618
[12] Knight, S. R., Morris, P. J., Schneeberger, S., & Pengel, L. H. (2016). Trial design and endpoints in clinical transplant research. *Transplant International*, *29*(8), 870–879.
[13] Yadav, S., Chamoli, S., Kumar, P., & Maurya, P. K. (2023). Structural and functional insights in polysaccharides coated cerium oxide nanoparticles and their potential biomedical applications: A review. *International Journal of Biological Macromolecules*, 125673, https://doi.org/10.1016/j.ijbiomac.2023.12567
[14] Tabata, Y. (2004). Tissue regeneration based on tissue engineering technology. *CongenitalAnomalies*,*44*(3),111–124.doi:10.1111/j.1741-4520.2004.00024.x
[15] Gupta, P., Gupta, H., Kairamkonda, M., Kumar, N., & Poluri, K. M. (2022). Elucidating the lactic acid tolerance mechanism in vaginal clinical isolates of Candida glabrata. *Medical Mycology*, *60*(6), myac042. https://doi.org/10.1093/mmy/myac042
[16] Yannas, I. V. (2001). *Tissue and organ regeneration in adults*. Springer.
[17] Atala, A., Irvine, D. J., Moses, M., & Shaunak, S. (2010). Wound healing versus regeneration: Role of the tissue environment in regenerative medicine. *MRS Bulletin*, *35*(8), 597–606.
[18] Xia, H., Li, X., Gao, W., Fu, X., Fang, R. H., Zhang, L., & Zhang, K. (2018). Tissue repair and regeneration with endogenous stem cells. *Nature Reviews. Materials*, *3*(7), 174–193. doi:10.1038/s41578-018-0027-6
[19] Coffman, J. A., Rieger, S., Rogers, A. N., Updike, D. L., & Yin, V. P. (2016). Comparative biology of tissue repair, regeneration and aging. *Npj Regenerative Medicine*, *1*(1). doi:10.1038/npjregenmed.2016.3
[20] Forbes, S. J., & Rosenthal, N. (2014). Preparing the ground for tissue regeneration: from mechanism to therapy. *Nature Medicine*, *20*(8), 857–869. doi:10.1038/nm.3653
[21] Rodriguez, A. M., & Kang, J. (2020). Regeneration enhancers: Starting a journey to unravel regulatory events in tissue regeneration. *Seminars in Cell & Developmental Biology*, *97*, 47–54. doi:10.1016/j.semcdb.2019.04.003

[22] Lee, S., Yoo, J., & Atala, A. (2016). *Fundamentals of in situ tissue regeneration*. Elsevier eBooks (pp. 3–17). doi:10.1016/b978-0-12-802225-2.00001-5

[23] Rajabzadeh, N., Fathi, E., & Farahzadi, R. (2019). Stem cell-based regenerative medicine. *Stem Cell Investigation*, 6, 19. doi: 10.21037/sci.2019.06.04

[24] Eltom, A., Zhong, G., & Muhammad, A. (2019). Scaffold techniques and designs in tissue engineering functions and purposes: A review. *Advances in Materials Science and Engineering*, *2019*, 1–13. doi:10.1155/2019/3429527

[25] Marler, J. J., Upton, J., Langer, R., & Vacanti, J. P. (1998). Transplantation of cells in matrices for tissue regeneration. *Advanced Drug Delivery Reviews*, *33*(1–2), 165–182. doi:10.1016/s0169-409x(98)00025-8

[26] O'Brien, F. J. (2011). Biomaterials & scaffolds for tissue engineering. *Materials Today*, *14*(3), 88–95.

[27] Keane, T. J., & Badylak, S. F. (2014, June). Biomaterials for tissue engineering applications. In *Seminars in pediatric surgery* (Vol. 23, No. 3, pp. 112–118). WB Saunders.

[28] Bedian, L., Villalba-Rodríguez, A. M., Hernández-Vargas, G., Parra-Saldivar, R., & Iqbal, H. M. (2017). Bio-based materials with novel characteristics for tissue engineering applications – A review. *International Journal of Biological Macromolecules*, *98*, 837–846.

[29] Alsberg, E., von Recum, H. A., & Mahoney, M. J. (2006). Environmental cues to guide stem cell fate decision for tissue engineering applications. *Expert Opinion on Biological Therapy*, *6*(9), 847–866.

[30] Rosso, F., Giordano, A., Barbarisi, M., & Barbarisi, A. (2004). From cell–ECM interactions to tissue engineering. *Journal of Cellular Physiology*, *199*(2), 174–180.

[31] Biondi, M., Ungaro, F., Quaglia, F., & Netti, P. A. (2008). Controlled drug delivery in tissue engineering. *Advanced Drug Delivery Reviews*, *60*(2), 229–242.

Chapter 2

The future of tissue engineering: Integrating ML, AI, and computer vision

Tvisha Chawla, Vaishnavi Rukhaiyar, Shaik Arshid Banu, and Subhash Singh

2.1 MACHINE LEARNING AND AI FOR BIOMATERIAL DESIGN: A SYSTEMATIC APPROACH

Tissue engineering is a multifaceted field, focused on creating new tissue using principles from cell biology, materials science, reactor engineering, and clinical research. Biomaterials, encompassing metals, ceramics, plastics or even living cells and tissues, are substances designed to interact with biological systems for diagnostic purposes. Modern data science, particularly artificial intelligence (AI) and machine learning (ML), is driving the discovery and testing of innovative biomaterials. While ML applications in biomaterials development are still emerging, existing models have optimized mechanical properties in biomedical implants, predicted fracture behavior in ceramics, and contributed to nanomaterial development [1, 2].

Recent advancements in tissue engineering have unveiled the potential for groundbreaking developments in the creation of biomaterials tailored for specific biomedical applications [3, 4]. The pursuit of optimal biomaterials, characterized by biocompatibility and mechanical robustness, has spurred extensive research and investigation. Traditional material design methods, while valuable, often necessitate prolonged trial-and-error cycles, hindering the rapid progression of tissue engineering. An AI-driven material design approach for tissue engineering, integrating generative adversarial networks (GANs) and high-throughput experimentation (HTE), has emerged [5]. This methodology combines synthetic data generation, dimensionality reduction through principal component analysis (PCA), and model evaluation using random forest classifiers, a widely employed supervised learning algorithm that will be explored in detail later in this chapter [6–8].

2.1.1 Generative design of biomaterials with machine learning

Material research, though capable of revolutionizing society, is hindered by extended research timelines. Machine learning has emerged as a promising solution to this challenge, demonstrating accuracies comparable to

DOI: 10.1201/9781003536352-2

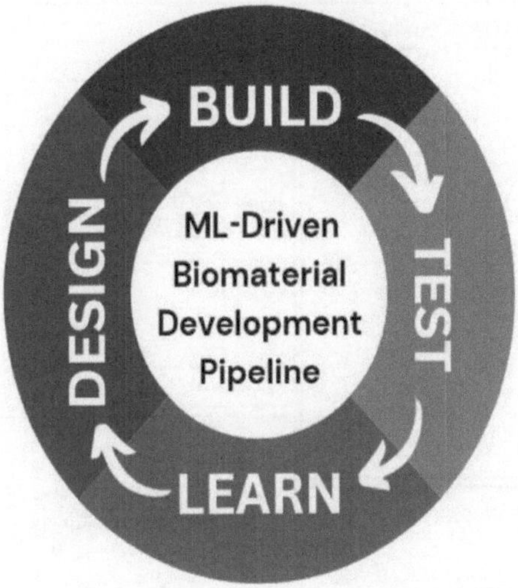

Figure 2.1 Materials are initially conceptualized with specific chemical and physical attributes derived from thorough design and comprehensive material analysis. Subsequent to construction, these materials undergo rigorous testing for desired properties via automated laboratory processes.(Data collected from these tests is correlated with the original design parameters and integrated into a machine learning framework.ML excels at analyzing voluminous and intricate datasets, enabling the identification of critical performance factors and forecasting the behavior of future iterations.These models serve as valuable tools in the creation of materials with predetermined functionalities.)

other computational methods. Generative models, in particular, are gaining attention due to their ability to approximate high-dimensional probability distributions, enabling the generation of novel data, such as biomaterial structures, through sampling from these approximated distributions. While materials science has primarily focused on conventional and deep learning algorithms and their applications, a comprehensive understanding of the underlying principles of three generative model classes: recurrent neural networks (RNNs), variational autoencoders (VAEs), and generative adversarial networks (GANs), is crucial for advancing materials discovery.

Since the true probability distribution (P(x, y)) is unknown, supervised learning models resort to an empirical estimation of integral states using a training dataset. This essentially involves building a model based on labeled data where inputs (x) and desired outputs (y) are known. Common supervised learning algorithms used in materials science include random forests, support vector machines, and neural networks. These algorithms learn patterns from the training data to make predictions on new, unseen data.

Neural networks, the foundation of many generative models, excel at handling highly non-linear and dynamic data, unlike random forests or

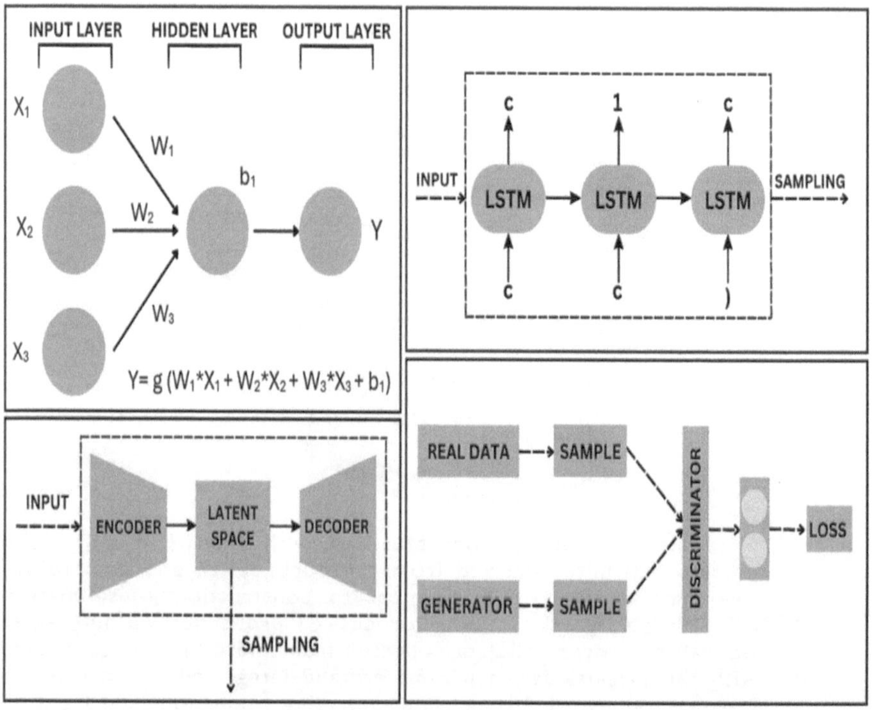

Figure 2.2 A machine learning approach can replace the time-consuming process of accumulating vast amounts of domain knowledge by shifting the focus to the relatively simpler task of collecting extensive datasets known as the "training set" for training machine learning algorithms. Machine learning models can be categorized into supervised, unsupervised, and reinforcement learning. Supervised learning involves algorithms that utilize externally provided data instances to derive hypotheses for predicting future outcomes on unseen data. In the materials domain, supervised learning techniques are primarily employed for predicting material properties and screening extensive databases.

support vector machines. Deep neural networks, with their numerous hidden layers, enhance predictive capabilities but at the cost of increased computation time [9–11].

Unlike supervised learning where models map inputs to desired outputs, generative models aim to learn an underlying representation of the data. This representation allows them to perform tasks like generating new data or making decisions. This is particularly valuable in unsupervised learning, where data lacks labels. The model's goal is to implicitly capture the data distribution, enabling the generation of novel materials or optimization of existing ones in the context of materials research. Recurrent neural networks (RNNs), variational autoencoders (VAEs), and generative adversarial networks (GANs) are the most prominent examples of generative models used in this field [12–14].

Recurrent Neural Networks: Recurrent neural networks, a specialized type of neural network, excel at identifying patterns within sequential data and are widely used for sequence modeling and generation. For example, daily COVID-19 cases over a three-month period can be considered sequential data with numerical patterns. RNNs operate in cycles, transmitting information back to themselves, which facilitates learning from sequential data. However, traditional RNN training methods face challenges with long sequences due to compounding errors. This issue is addressed by employing special units called long short-term memory (LSTM) units.

Variational Autoencoders: Variational autoencoders (VAEs) extract fundamental features from input data through compression and decompression. This feature extraction process can be likened to normal mode analysis, providing insights into underlying collective variables describing the low-dimensional hidden features captured by the VAEs encoding and decoding stages. Historically, this approach faced challenges, including model dependence on data structure, the need for complex approximations, and reliance on computationally demanding techniques. Newer generative model classes, like VAEs, address many of these limitations.

Generative Adversarial Networks: As the name implies, a generative adversarial network (GAN) is a generative model designed to compete against an adversarial model, often termed a discriminative model, and is essentially a classifier capable of distinguishing between real and generated data samples. Initially, the discriminator easily differentiates between real and fake data, but with each training cycle, the generator improves, producing more realistic content. Eventually, the generated data becomes so realistic that the discriminator's ability to differentiate becomes random, signaling the end of the training process. GANs have been successfully applied to various tasks, including generating high-quality human faces, converting aerial images to maps, and transforming black and white images into color images [9, 10].

2.1.2 Machine learning-driven material property prediction

Materials science traditionally relies on experiments and simulations to characterize materials, with properties like structure and behavior dictating potential applications. However, the ever-growing volume of data from these experiments and simulations is becoming increasingly difficult to manage and analyze. This has spurred the development of new data-driven methods to uncover patterns in structure–property relationships across various timescales. As an alternative to traditional trial-and-error or physical metallurgy approaches, machine learning (ML) methods are gaining traction for property prediction and material design, offering a more efficient way to generate material property information [15–17].

Big data and machine learning (ML) approaches are proving to be powerful tools in materials science. This field revolves around four key elements:

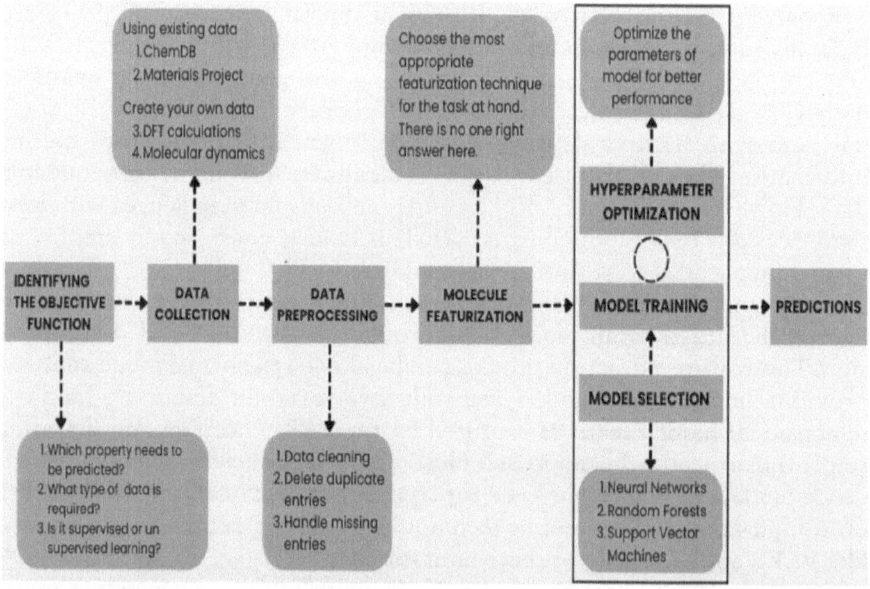

Figure 2.3 Workflow schematic for developing a ML model from a materials research perspective. Identifying the objective function, along with data handling and curation, as well as molecular featurization, has emerged as two of the most significant challenges to the success of these models. Each step is critical for smooth working and functioning of the model.

processing, structure, properties and performance. While the exact relationships between these elements remain under debate, ML can shed light on their intrinsic connections within the process-structure-property-performance chain. Additionally, these approaches aim to achieve high-throughput identification and quantification of essential material properties.

Mechanical properties, heavily influenced by processing parameters and resulting microstructures, are particularly crucial for precise prediction and control. In essence, ML methods for material property prediction involve analyzing and mapping the (often non-linear) relationships between material properties and their related characteristics. This knowledge extraction happens through existing experimental or simulation data. Since experimental testing helps in understanding materials better, the following sections will explore how ML can be utilized for metallic material characterization [18–21].

Corrosion: Recent ML advancements have shown promise in enhancing corrosion detection, aiding human inspectors and reducing inspection time and costs for civil structures. ANN-based image processing for corrosion detection is a popular approach. Fang et al. introduced a hybrid method combining genetic algorithms and support vector regression to forecast atmospheric corrosion depth of metallic materials. Inputs for the support vector regression include temperature, wetness duration, exposure time, sulfur dioxide concentration, and chloride concentration. The outputs are predicted corrosion depths for specific metallic materials.

Creep: Creep, a metal deformation occurring below yield strength at elevated temperatures, is a focus for ML modeling. Chatzidakis et al. compare general regression neural networks, ANNs, and Gaussian processes to predict creep rupture. Shin et al. employ five ML models: random forest, linear regression, k-nearest neighbor, kernel ridge and Bayesian ridge, to predict Larson-miller parameters representing creep behavior. Through optimization and feature selection, relevant factors are identified and models are evaluated.

2.1.3 AI-assisted biomaterial optimization for tissue specificity

While traditional experimental approaches offer valuable insights into tissue composition and organization, machine learning and AI are emerging

ALGORITHM	BRIEF INTODUCTION	ADVANTAGE	DISADVANTAGE	REPRESENTATIVE APPLICATIONS
Regression Analysis	It can find regression equations and predict dependent variables	Deeply developed and widely used in many occasions	Needs large amounts of data and may cause overfitting in practical applications	Machine learning with systematic density-functional theory calculations: application to melting temperatures of single and binary component solids
Naive Bayes classifier	It can classify data into several categories following the highest possibility	Only a small amount of data is needed to obtain essential parameters	The feature independence hypothesis is not always accurate	A naive-Bayes classifier for damage detection in engineering materials
Support Vector Machine	SVM can find a hyperplane to divide a group of points into two categories	It has great generalization ability and can property handle high-dimension datasets	SVM is not very appropriate for multiple classification problems	PVP-SVM: sequence-based prediction of phage virion proteins using a support vector machine
Decision Tree and Random Forest	By splitting source datasets into several subsets, all data will be judged and classified	The calculating processes are easy to comprehend. Also, it can handle large amounts of data	It is difficult to obtain a high performance decision tree or a random forest. Also, the overfitting problem may occur	High-throughput machine-learning-driven synthesis of full-Heusler compounds
Artificial Neural Networks	By imitating neuron activities, ANN can automatically find underlying patterns in inputs	ANN has great self-improving ability, great robustness and high fault tolerance	Its inner calculation progresses are very difficult to understand	Learning from the Harvard Clean Energy Project: the use of neural networks to accelerate materials discovery
Deep Learning	Originated from ANN. It aims to build a neural network to analyze data by imitating the human brain	It has the best self-adjusting and self-improving abilities compared with other ML methods	As a new trend in ML, deep learning has not yet been well studied. Many defects are still unclear	Artificial intelligence in neuropathology: deep learning-based assessment of tauopathy

Figure 2.4 Explaining the different types of machine learning algorithms briefly.

as powerful tools for analyzing and interpreting tissue-specific data. Deep learning methods can predict how individual mutations might affect gene expression, splicing, and disease phenotypes across different tissues. Network-based approaches can capture relationships between biomolecules and integrate large datasets to model molecular circuits and identify tissue-specific functionality and regulation. This integration of high-resolution, large-scale multiomics data with interpretable machine learning models holds great promise for unraveling the complexities of multicellular organisms.

The development of AI technology has revolutionized biomedicine. By simulating, extending, and expanding human intelligence, AI has led to new research theories, methods, and technologies. Advancements in machine learning, particularly deep learning based on neural networks, have paved the way for AI applications in biomaterial development and healthcare research. These applications range from biomaterial design, disease prediction, and intervention, optimization of biomaterials, processing, and validation of large clinical data, algorithms in matching patients for trials, with the ultimate goal of optimizing clinical trials and decision-making. Thereby, this emerging technology possesses the potential to improve eminently basic and translational research in biomaterials and biomedicine [22, 23].

This has driven the development of a related field termed "computational biomaterials," which focuses on the use of AI in biomaterial design and optimal biomaterials prediction. The most active interest of researchers refers to making use of AI with respect to the simulation and prediction of ideal biomaterial structures, physicochemical properties, bioactivity, and other key features. Design of Experiments (DoE) techniques are also known for optimization and statistical quality control but are increasingly applied in the systematic development of biomaterials.

More broadly within biomedicine, AI algorithms and machine learning models are enabling single-cell analysis, image detection, bioprocess design, biomarker discovery, and large-scale genomic data analysis. AI-powered diagnostics are streamlining disease screening, reducing test times and numbers, and aiding clinical decision-making, ultimately improving diagnostic precision and treatment efficiency. By integrating biochip technology with AI, healthcare professionals can efficiently gather, analyze, and interpret data, addressing the ever-growing complexity of clinical information. This data analysis, enabled by AI, can support evidence-based approaches to patient care and biomaterial optimization [11, 12].

2.2 COMPUTER VISION-ASSISTED BIOPRINTING – ENHANCING PRECISION AND CONTROL

Bioprinting, a promising additive manufacturing technique with significant potential in biomedicine, faces a key hurdle: inaccurate shae formation, especially for high-resolution applications. Fortunately, the manufacturing field's adoption of computer vision for process control offers a solution. By integrating computer vision, bioprinting can achieve the accuracy, resolution, and cell viability required for advanced biomedical research.

There are three main bioprinting methods: inkjet, laser extrusion, and stereolithography. Extrusion-based printing, popular for applications like bone scaffold printing, suffers from limitations in resolution. This factor significantly affects the performance of bone scaffolds, highlighting the need for advancements in high-resolution bioprinting techniques.

Computer vision offers a revolutionary approach to tackling the limitations of low accuracy and resolution in extrusion-based bioprinting. This technology has evolved significantly in recent years, transitioning from basic binary image processing to handling large, high-resolution datasets. This advancement is fueled by advancements in artificial intelligence, microelectronics, big data, and deep learning.

Beyond image processing, computer vision encompasses the collection and analysis of various data streams during the bioprinting process. High-speed cameras, thermocouples, pressure sensors, and microphones work together to capture a comprehensive picture of the printing process, including visuals, temperature, pressure, and sound. This data is then stored and

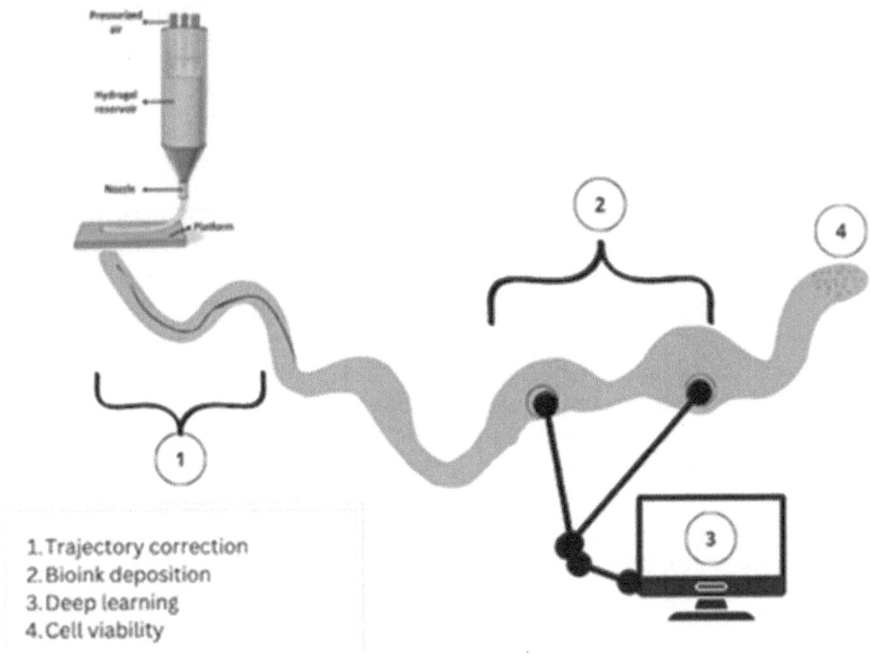

Figure 2.5 Typical cases of computer vision optimizing the bioprinting process to improve the final bone bioprinting quality.

analyzed by a computer to identify defects in real time. This valuable information can be fed back into the bioprinting algorithm, enabling closed-loop process control and ensuring optimal printing outcomes [24, 25].

Given the prevalence of printing defects in additive manufacturing, including extrusion-based bioprinting, implementing computer vision and process control to rectify errors is crucial across industries such as biomedicine and aerospace. For instance, bone scaffold failures often stem from localized stress concentrations during porous scaffold creation. By employing computer vision to gather stress data and optimize the stress distribution, scaffold quality can be significantly enhanced. Non-destructive evaluation through computer vision involves capturing numerous images of defects during the bioprinting process to identify and address issues proactively.

Sophisticated image analysis techniques, particularly those employing deep learning architectures, are revolutionizing how we examine visual data. Convolutional Neural Networks (CNNs), a prime example, excel at pinpointing specific image elements. These networks can be trained to decipher intricate patterns within medical scans, such as determining tissue age from standardized radiographs. This same approach is applicable to the realm of bioprinting. By exposing CNNs to a vast array of labeled bioprinted structures, they can learn to identify and classify structural anomalies, such as internal defects or porosity, which are critical factors in evaluating the overall efficacy of bioprinted constructs [13].

2.2.1 Real-time bioprinting monitoring with computer vision

The burgeoning field of bioprinting offers immense potential to create biomimetic structures and living tissues, thanks to the ever-expanding array of biomaterials and printing technologies. To elevate the capabilities of both bioprinting and its resulting constructs, computer vision is being harnessed to optimize relevant processes, materials, and mechanical and biological functionalities. Existing research suggests that both traditional machine learning and computer vision can be employed for this purpose. While machine learning leverages features extracted from image or numerical data to build predictive models, computer vision directly utilizes images to develop segmentation or classification models. These advancements pave the way for a new era of bioprinting characterized by stable and reliable printing processes, precise control over fiber deposition and layer stacking, and ultimately, bioprinted constructs with superior designs and improved cellular performance [26, 27].

The rapidly increasing repertoire of biomaterials and printing technologies exponentially increases the complexity for creating intricate biological constructs. Such a process indeed requires extreme attention to material composition, printing parameters, and interdependent effects on the final product. The traditional approaches, relying on mathematical modeling and experimentation of these, have proved highly inefficient for finding an optimum path through this complex landscape. The increasing research in addressing the challenge at hand is hence finding a synergistic approach in machine learning and computer vision, which presents a far more efficient and comprehensive strategy for unleashing the real potentials of bioprinting.

As illustrated in (b) deep learning, a powerful subset of computer vision is revolutionizing image analysis tasks. Unlike traditional machine learning methods, deep learning excels at automatically identifying key features within images, eliminating the need for manual feature extraction. This makes it particularly well-suited for complex tasks like classification, segmentation, and object detection in various image applications. CNNs are a prime example of deep learning models achieving remarkable success in these areas. However, deep learning often requires access to large-scale datasets for optimal performance [14, 15].

2.2.2 Closed loop control of bioprinting processes using machine vision

Extrusion-based bioprinting, a cornerstone of the field, has seen a surge in efforts to establish robust quality control protocols. This pursuit aims to streamline the intricate process of parameter optimization for diverse bioinks, ensuring consistent and reliable outcomes across different research environments. Ultimately, this will accelerate the clinical translation of bioprinted products.

Machine learning presents a promising avenue for achieving these goals. By training algorithms on extensive datasets, researchers can develop intelligent systems capable of real-time process monitoring and predictive optimization. These kinds of systems can find and correct the mistakes before reflecting on the final product, saving the precious resources and thus becoming economic. Integration of machine learning with bioprinting has. the potential to revolutionize the field.

New trends in AI bring new life to the extrusion-based bioprinting process—it is highly complex by nature in terms of control and automation. For example, Fu et al. studied the use of an SVM in refining the printing settings, where a 3D map could be obtained that indicates, for the most part, which combinations of the parameters would likely result in a high-quality print. In another example, Rubero et al. presented a way to iterative use of Bayesian optimization. The process entailed printing the lattice structures with the random parameters, then classifying them visually based on quality to use in building a probability model. Additionally, research has investigated the use of AI for anomaly detection and localization [1]. Studies printed infill patterns at different speeds while capturing images. Machine learning models, including SVMs and CNNs, were

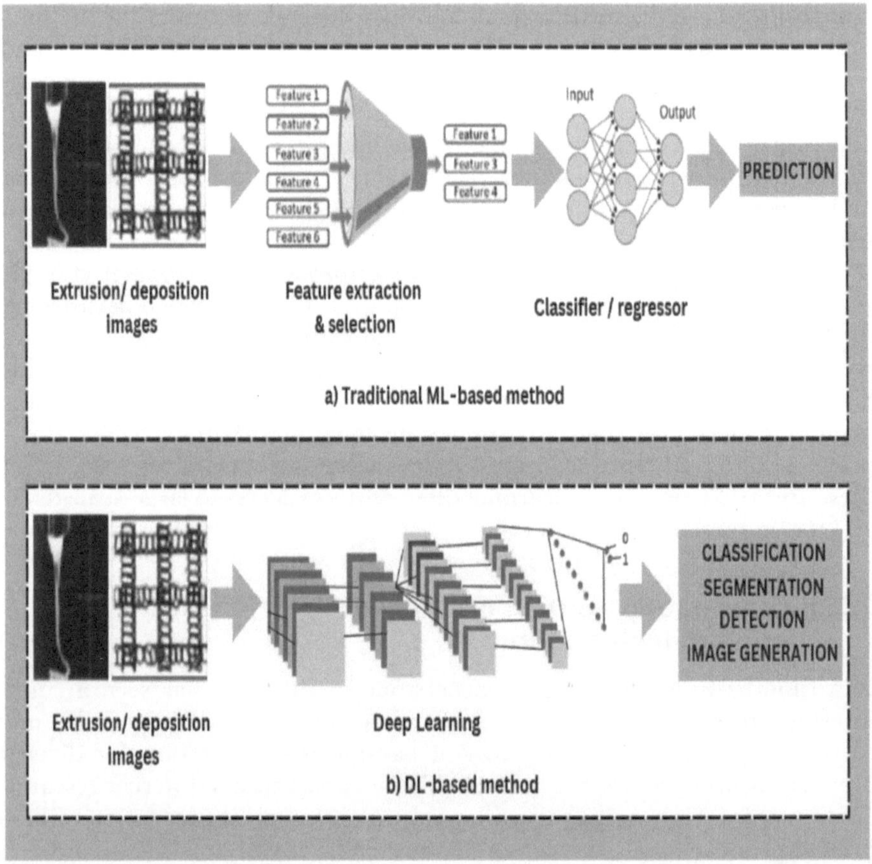

Figure 2.6 The traditional machine learning approaches shown in (a) depend on handcrafted features for image analysis. These features are extracted from image data based on expert knowledge and experience, such as identifying shapes, edges, colors, and textures. The choice of features plays a crucial role in achieving accurate predictions. Common traditional machine learning methods, such as Support Vector Machines (SVMs) and K-Nearest Neighbors, use these features to build classification or regression models for various prediction tasks.

then tested for automatic print classification. CNNs emerged as the most effective approach for anomaly detection in this specific dataset.

While initial studies show promise for AI-powered quality control in extrusion bioprinting, significant hurdles remain. A truly autonomous system requires the ability to analyze prints and adjust parameters in real time, eliminating manual intervention. Additionally, quality assessment must extend beyond the initial layers and encompass the entire 3D scaffold structure for accuracy. Finally, the ideal system should not only optimize parameters but also continuously monitor printing for on-the-fly adjustments and quality control [16].

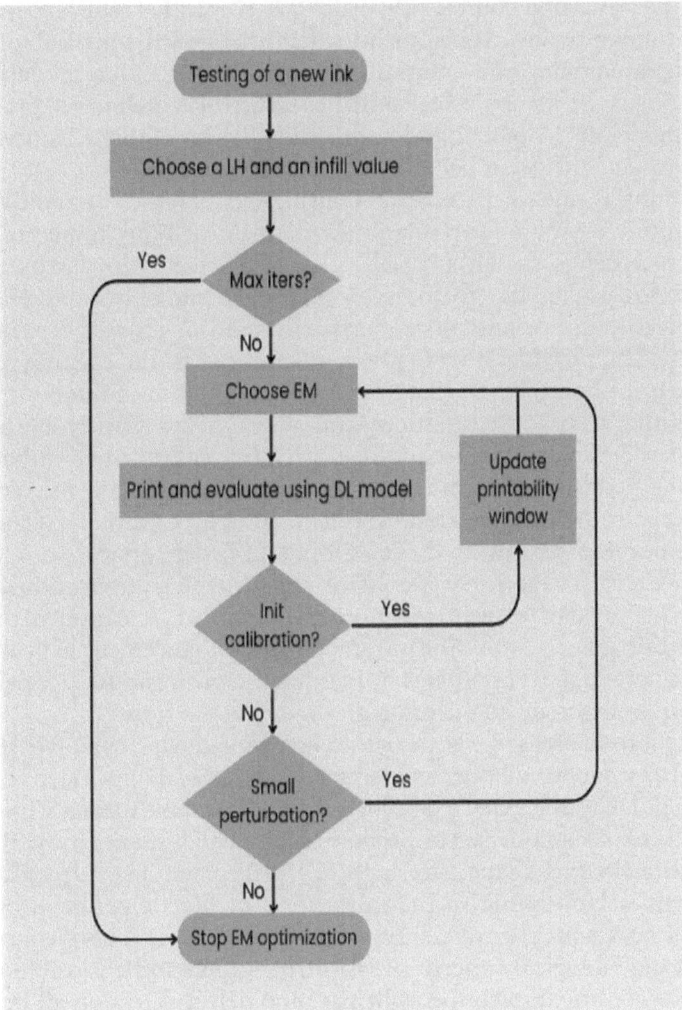

Figure 2.7 Schematic representation of the process of testing new ink, starting from parameter selection to an evaluation step with the deep learning model including key decisions of important options at the steps of iterations, calibration, and perturbations to ensure optimal performance of the printing process according to updates of the printability window with the results of the evaluation.

2.2.3 Computer vision-guided bioprinting for complex tissue architectures

Advances in in vitro tissue models have significantly enhanced our understanding of drug and chemical interactions. These models offer unparalleled control over cellular composition, extracellular matrix, environmental factors, and structural complexity, which are crucial for replicating the intricacies of human tissues. 3D bioprinting has emerged as a pivotal technology in this field, enabling the creation of sophisticated tissue models. Recent breakthroughs in machine learning have further accelerated progress by refining model development and application, with notable advancements in cancer, cardiac, muscular, hepatic, and bone tissue research.

Bioprinting is one of the most promising technologies in additive manufacturing and shows great potential in the field of bony implantation and repair. Nevertheless, the broad application of this technology in bone studies is currently restricted due to complex shapes. Fortunately, rapid progress in computer vision, a technology increasingly used in process control within manufacturing, provides a wide range of solutions to the existing problems. Trying to print bones with cell cultures by computer vision in bone research improves the accuracy, resolution, and cell viability greatly by orders of magnitude. The role of this technology in overcoming current limitations for bioprinting precision is cardinal for enabling further use in the technology of bone repair and regeneration. Recently, computer vision has gained considerable development in bone bioprinting. In order to tackle a wide range of challenges related to process control, deep learning applications, and cell viability assessment, current technology is applied. It captures the visual data of printing to optimize the parameters for enhancement in print quality and efficiency. Such technologies hold immense promises for acceleration in research in bone tissue engineering and redefine the future.

Applications in areas like bone tissue engineering, which involves the regeneration of any damaged bone, have seen an exponential increase in research in bioprinting due to the expected accuracy and affordable means. This additive manufacturing technique has advantages such as high specificity, with control over factors such as shape, size, and cell placement. The use of computer vision enables bioprinting in the fabrication of biocompatible scaffolds or grafts that bear a number of cell types and biomaterials. This technology is a replica of the biological concept of vision, hence making it possible to recognize objects, re-orient, pick the right size, and defect detection all in the concept of the printing process. These functionalities greatly enhance the attainment of precise control required for successful bone implantation.

Thus, bioprinting has great potential not only in in vitro research but also in in vivo clinical applications. With its applications in creating tissue models for drug testing and the study of disease being very promising, its final goal will be to develop functional tissues suitable for transplantation. Having said that, despite all the great advancements, bioprinting obviously still faces numerous obstacles, with a number of challenges to be worked out with innovative solutions. A prime example is bone bioprinting, where a focused effort has been given to enhancing the scaffold structural properties by developing and modifying bioinks. Despite significant advancements in bioprinting, achieving consistent and high-quality bone scaffolds remains a challenge. To address this, precise data collection and real-time process control are essential. Computer vision, a technology increasingly adopted in manufacturing, offers a promising solution. By integrating computer vision, researchers can optimize printing parameters and monitor the process, leading to substantial improvements in the final product's structural and biological properties [28, 29].

2.3 FROM DATA TO DESIGN: MACHINE LEARNING AND ARTIFICIAL INTELLIGENCE FOR BIOMANUFACTURING OPTIMIZATION

Biomanufacturing processes use AI and ML to optimize and streamline the large amount of data generated in study and research of tissue engineering. It involves integration of appropriate cell sources, growth factors to regenerate functional tissue, and supportive biomaterial scaffolds [1], but it is also challenging to find the most optimized combination to a particular application due to the large number of variables that are involved, from cell type

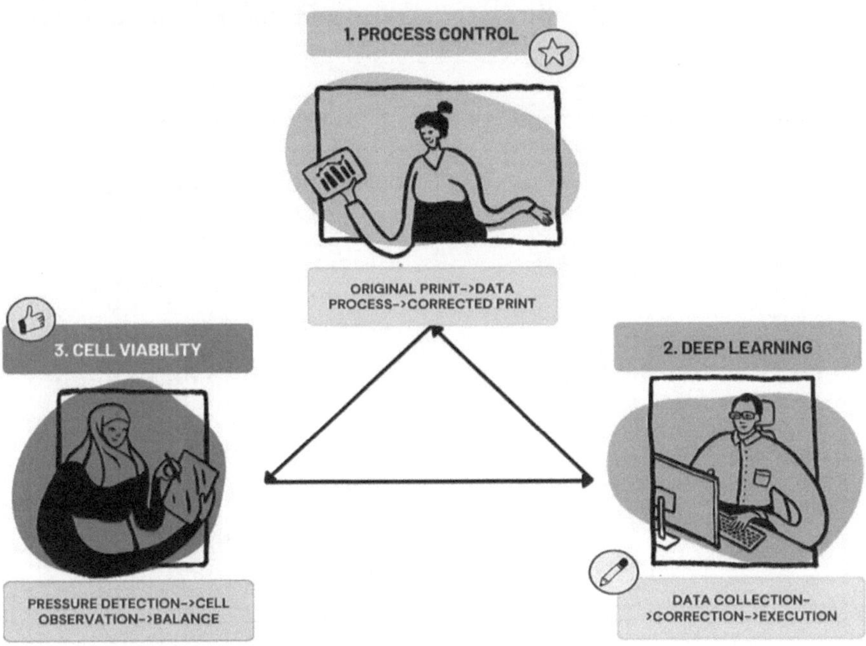

Figure 2.8 Recent advancements in computer vision are transforming bone bioprinting. This technology offers a multipronged approach to enhance the field. Firstly, it facilitates precise process control. This includes monitoring and correcting bone scaffold trajectory and width during printing, leading to higher resolution bioprinted structures. Secondly, deep learning algorithms, particularly CNNs, are emerging as powerful tools for image analysis in computer vision [17, 18].

and culture conditions to bioreactor parameters and scaffold design. Design of Experiments (DoE) methodologies are widely employed for optimization tasks, contributing significantly to statistical quality control and systematic randomization in experiment planning. However, their application is primarily focused on analyzing and optimizing quantitative data. DoE methods may not be as well suited for handling complex data types like images or high-dimensional datasets.

2.3.1 Machine learning for bioprinting process parameter optimization

Bioprinting involves the fabrication of complex and heterogeneous tissue constructs, which is an important technique in tissue engineering. Bioprinting process includes various parameters that have to be optimized to get desired cell properties, and viability and machine learning algorithms enable data-driven optimization of these process parameters.

The usage of ML is becoming a strong methodology in different stages of 3D bioprinting for the fabrication of more sophisticated tissue-engineered constructs. A recent study by Lee et al. explored the application of ML in

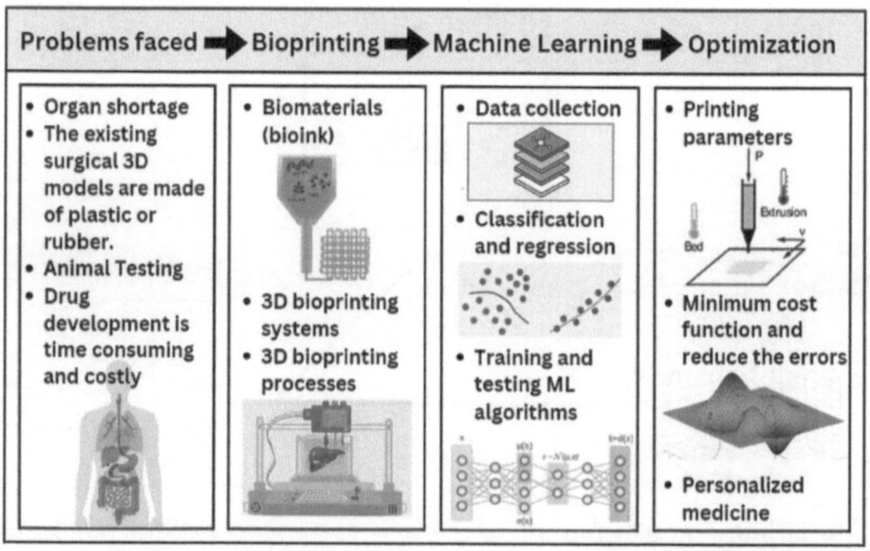

Figure 2.9 Machine learning and artificial intelligence offer considerable potential for data analysis, providing greater flexibility in terms of data that can be used for optimization and prediction in biomanufacturing. Recent advances have involved the application of ML for material optimization, classification, and image segmentation. In particular, there has been recent interest in bringing ML approaches to optimize and automate the fabrication processes and provide predictions relating to the material behavior under certain parameters [19].

designing 3D printable bioinks using natural biomaterials. Their research focused on analyzing the connections between the bioink's rheological properties (flow and deformation characteristics) and its printability using ML techniques. In this regard, the relative least general generalization (RLGG) algorithm—a unique ML algorithm for classification problems—was utilized. Finally, to cross-check the results obtained from the ML process and to attempt at predicting of printability from this bioink's composition, further analysis using multiple regression was carried out. This study revealed a universal relationship between the bioink's mechanical properties and its printability. Notably, the findings suggest that a high elastic modulus (resistance to deformation) improves the bioink's ability to maintain its shape after printing, while printing successfully occurs below a critical yield stress (the point where the bioink transitions from elastic to plastic behavior).

Bioprinting involves the precise arrangement of cells, biomaterial and other biological elements to create functional tissue structures. The success of bioprinting relies heavily on optimizing various parameters which include bioink composition, printing parameters, and post-processing conditions.

1. Bioink composition: Bioink composition refers to the makeup of bioink used for printing and includes factors like crosslinking density and polymer concentration. This composition has a crucial role in determining final properties of tissue construct. [2, 3].
2. Printing parameters: These parameters include nozzle diameter, extrusion pressure, printing speed, etc. The diameter of the nozzle influences resolution and precision of the printed features while the

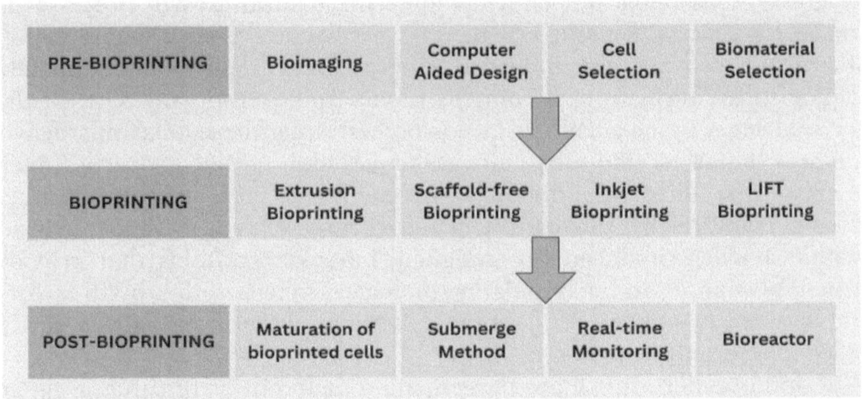

Figure 2.10 Three stages: pre-bioprinting, bioprinting, and post-bioprinting and considerations in fabricating the tissue/organ constructs. Pre-bioprinting relates to the properties of the bioprinting structure. Determining the appropriate bioink for bioprinting relates to the printability and biocompatibility. Post-printing helps in determining the quality of printed outcomes.

printing speed affects the shear stresses and structural integrity of the whole construct. The applied extrusion pressure during bioprinting is the determining factor for flow rate and deposition of material [2, 3].

3. Post-processing conditions: After initial printing, post-processing conditions are needed for complete maturation and stabilization of the construct. Crosslinking, where additional ionic/covalent bonds are formed between polymer chains, enhances the mechanical stability and shape fidelity of printed tissue. Further, incubation and culture of the bioprinted construct in a bioreactor promotes cellular proliferation, differentiation and the development of functional tissue properties [3, 4].

Inadequate or suboptimal parameter settings result in defects such as unstable structures, low cell viability, and lack of tissue functionality. Thus, efficient optimization of these parameters is crucial for creation of reliable and reproducible engineered tissues [4, 5].

In order to optimize the processes for tissue engineering, it is essential to have models that can establish connections between the parameters to be optimized and forecast the structural and performance results based on physical and chemical processes. Design of Experiments (DoE) techniques are widely utilized for optimization, as well as serving a crucial function in statistical quality control and systematic randomization for planning experiments.

2.3.2 AI-powered bioreactor design and control

Engineering tissues involve using cells and biomaterials to create functional structures. Observing and understanding the natural growth processes is crucial for successful tissue design. This necessitates precise manipulation of critical parameters that influence cell growth and remodeling, ultimately leading to the formation of complex tissues and even organs. One of the key challenges tissue engineers face is orchestrating the cellular microenvironment signals to efficiently cultivate tissues with specific properties, such as anisotropy (directional organization) and hierarchical structure (distinct layers). Traditionally, this can be achieved through two methods. In vivo (within a living organism) by designing bioactive scaffolds that provide structural support and manipulating biological signals with growth factors and in vitro (in a controlled laboratory setting) within a specialized device called a bioreactor.

AI and optimal control are burgeoning to help power research in tissue regeneration while fast-tracking our learning processes for such complex undertakings. With these technologies, it is now possible for researchers to peep further into the dynamics of tissue growth and develop ways to design bioreactors more effectively, with easier management [30–32].

Micro and small bioreactors are instrumental in both bioprocess development and tissue engineering. In bioprocess development, they optimize pre-production manufacturing through ultra-scale down and microfluidic techniques. Tissue engineering benefits from bioreactors by enabling the recreation of in vivo conditions for studying cell physiology, expanding cells for clinical applications, modeling disease states, and developing new treatments more effectively than traditional in vitro culture. This technology also holds promise for reducing animal testing in pharmacological research. Bioreactor design plays a critical role in determining tissue function. The structure and organization of cells within the bioreactor must closely mimic their natural environment in the body (in vivo) to ensure optimal cell survival and ultimately the desired functionality. This "one size fits all" approach cannot be applied, as different tissues have unique requirements.

To effectively model these complexities in a bioreactor, it's essential to consider not only the correct cell types but also the mechanical structures that replicate the desired function. Current bioreactors often contain either dingle-cell type constructs which consist of cells with a uniform identity or co-cultures which combine cells of different types, such as epithelial and endothelial cells. Dynamic bioreactors using simple convection techniques enhance mass transfer within the system. This fluid flow ensures efficient movement of essential nutrients and waste products throughout the cell cultures.

Standard industry practices outline a three-phase lifecycle for validating biopharmaceutical manufacturing processes: initial process design, comprehensive qualification, and ongoing verification. The efficacy and reliability of analytical methods used in the continuous verification phase necessitate a deep understanding of the manufacturing process.

To address these complexities, we employed supervised and unsupervised machine learning models using data from diverse fed-batch bioprocesses under varying oxygen conditions (normoxic and hypoxic) [20–22].Our approach involved a two-step process:

1. Anomaly detection: Utilizing an isolation forest model to identify unusual patterns during the batch phase of the bioprocess.
2. Predictive modeling: Employing a random forest model to forecast necessary operator interventions during the semi-automated fed-batch phase under oxygen-limited conditions.

2.3.3 Data-driven monitoring of chronic diseases

Chronic illnesses, including diabetes, asthma, heart conditions, and cancer, are the leading causes of death globally, accounting for a substantial 70% of fatalities annually. The financial burden of managing these conditions is immense, with healthcare expenditures dedicated to chronic disease treatment consuming a disproportionate 86% of total healthcare costs, as reported by the Centers for Disease Control and Prevention. In the United States, the prevalence of chronic diseases is alarming, affecting over 140

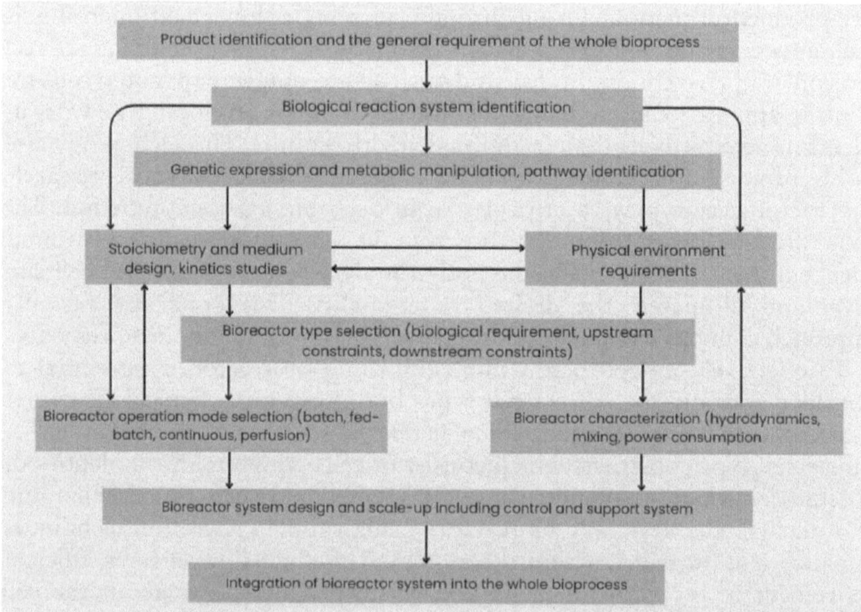

Figure 2.11 Schematic representation of the process and the scope of bioreactor engineering.

million individuals and projected to an increase by at least 10 million cases per decade. This increasing patient population has directly increased health expenses as well, such that more than 75% of the total expense related to national health is for chronic care (CDC, 2014). All these pose a big problem for the healthcare system, and without solutions, it would only mean that costs and delivery are not optimized. Information systems and data analytics will change healthcare. These will be able to provide valuable insights into developing appropriate strategies.

The convergence of these advanced technologies with the Internet of Things (IoT), sensors, wearable devices, social media platforms, mobile applications, and genomics, further accelerated by the aggregate changes taking place in the electronic health records space, is quickly changing the landscape of data about the patient and wellness, changing its nature, volume, and velocity in a uniquely deep way. At the same time, artificial intelligence and analytical breakthroughs have brought a new paradigm to the potential of this data-rich milieu.

The Internet of Things has brought human health data generation to an all-time high. This network of devices spans from hospital equipment and patient monitors to wearable technology, in-home sensors, and even ingestible sensors. Such devices create copious amounts of granular real-time data on just about every conceivable measure and, if combined, the added value far exceeds the sum of their stand-alone utility. It certainly adds up quickly, and much of this could be analyzed quickly enough to offer immediate alerts and interventions. Sensor technologies have undergone a dramatic metamorphosis—from fixed-location sensors to wearable sensors, and now even swallowable ones. Such sensors feature expanded capabilities for basic measurements and recording with seamless web integration, data sharing, and even AI-driven analysis [23, 24].

Chronic disease management is an integrated approach comprising of screenings, check-up and follow-ups, treatment monitoring, patient education, and care collaboration. Recent technological advances in tools and techniques may provide some promising solutions to these hurdles. New business models can be envisioned that would be built around tracking, monitoring, and analyzing the data from sensors that would be pertinent to preventing and managing chronic illnesses. Additionally, leveraging data analytics holds immense potential for:

1. Cost-effective treatment: Through the analysis of the treatment data, the analysts will be able to establish which care alternatives manage chronic diseases cost-effectively.
2. Preventive care and lifestyle modification: Through the profile analysis of a patient, one can establish that which ones need preventive measures or lifestyle modification.
3. Fraud detection: Analytics will facilitate the identification of fraudulence and abuse in treating chronic diseases.
4. Value-based care: Collection and dissemination of data regarding medical procedures will help both patients and providers in selecting protocols that not only are cost-effective but also return the best outcomes.
5. Profile diseases: Advanced analytics projects and avoids adverse events for chronic diseases.
6. Treatment adherence: Payers are enabled to assess adherence of patients to prescribed medication courses and treatment programs.
7. Population Health Trends: Determination of trends related to better population health and well-being.

Furthermore, advancements in computational methods offer the potential to develop novel algorithms for aggregating diverse health datasets across various scales. This can significantly contribute to a more holistic understanding of chronic disease progression and treatment effectiveness.

Comprehensive profiling of the patient, including clinical data, biological information, contextual knowledge, and environmental factors, forms the basis for informed decisions. Advanced decision support can be based on this. With these elements now in consideration, information system enables in developing extensive knowledge frameworks for reasoning in insights derivation from individual and population data for optimal delivery of patient-centered care in line with evidence-based practices. Information systems are further capable of enabling the development of extensive knowledge frameworks in reasoning for insights derivation from both individual and population data in the health sector, which pushes the potential of innovative technologies even further toward assisted and automated healthcare discovery through secondary health data.

The last ten years have seen an exponential increase in digital health information. This is data locked up in electronic health records and, recently, a mountain of "real-world" data contributed through mobile devices and different kinds of sensors. Similarly, the field of AI has undergone some notable changes, especially regarding AI development and deployment. Lately, deep learning approaches have been developed as effective tools for

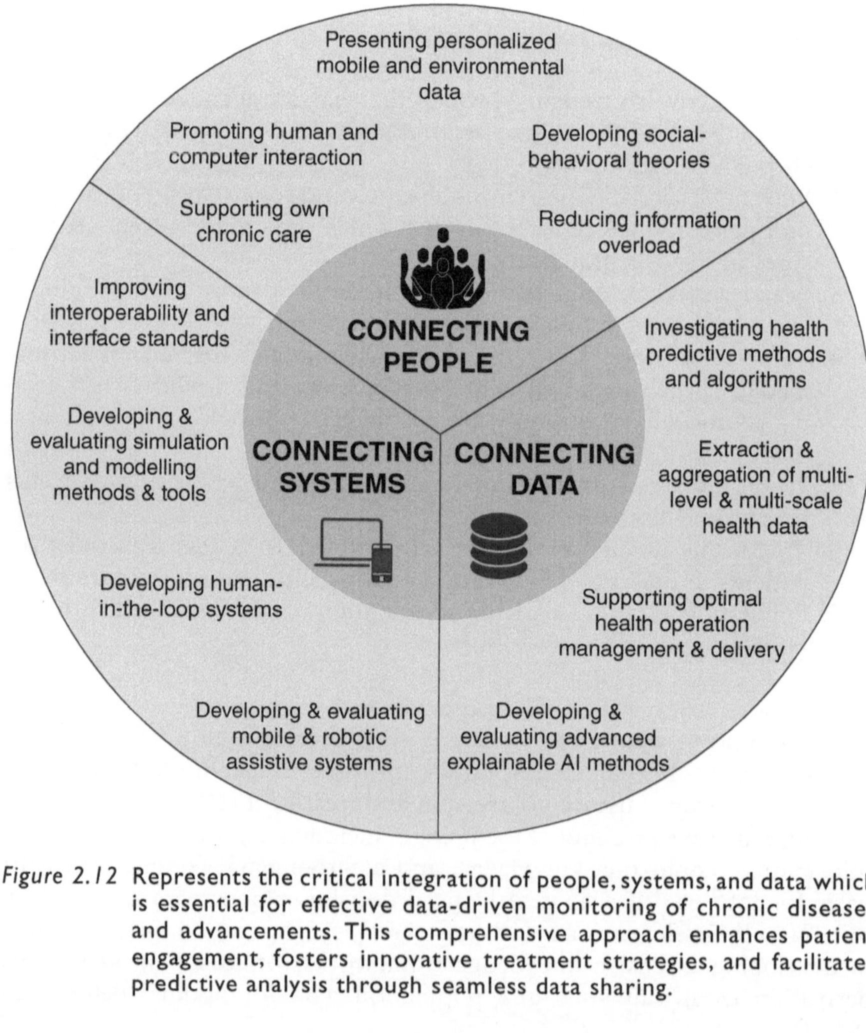

Figure 2.12 Represents the critical integration of people, systems, and data which is essential for effective data-driven monitoring of chronic diseases and advancements. This comprehensive approach enhances patient engagement, fosters innovative treatment strategies, and facilitates predictive analysis through seamless data sharing.

a wide variety of successes shown in the most diverse application areas. The effectiveness of these methods is based on their capability to build very complex structures with many hierarchies and to effectively capture long-range dependencies in the data [33–35].

2.4 CONCLUSION

As such, bioprinting holds enormous health innovation potential and allows for the production of complex tissues and organs for transplantation, drug discovery, and disease modeling. Challenges in the field still persist on issues regarding process optimization, quality consistency, and a solution to developing the complexity of natural tissues, among others. ML is becoming a powerful tool to overcome these limitations and reach the full potential of bioprinting.

One of the exciting uses of ML in bioprinting is in process optimization. Traditional techniques bring in a trial-and-error method to identify a set of printing parameters that make up the optimal strategy for printing a particular bioink. Machine learning algorithms, such as Support Vector Machines and deep learning models, now have the potential to sort through these large datasets of printing results to identify the optimal parameters with a lot more accuracy and in less time. This saves time and resources but at the same time brings in more consistency and quality of prints.

Another very promising application area has to do with the use of ML approaches for quality control in bioprinting. Deep neural networks also belong to a specific class of ML models that boast unlimited potential in real-time anomaly detection during the printing process. This enables early intervention, correction, and hence minimizes the chances of printing failures and material waste. Other than that, generative models such as Variational Autoencoders (VAEs) and Generative Adversarial Networks (GANs) allow the design of novel bioinks with targeted properties.

In conclusion, by putting ML and bioprinting together, brighter perspectives are foreseen on overcoming the current challenges and accelerating progress in this field. From optimization of printing parameters and quality control to designing new biomaterials, ML offers a versatile toolbox for both researchers and engineers. As the field further evolves, we should expect even more innovations using ML as our guide for such eventual wide application of bioprinting in personalized medicine and tissue regeneration.

REFERENCES

[1] Bakhshandeh, B., Zarrintaj, P., Oftadeh, M. O., Keramati, F., Fouladiha, H., Sohrabi-Jahromi, S., & Ziraksaz, Z. (2017). Tissue engineering; strategies, tissues, and biomaterials. *Biotechnology and Genetic Engineering Reviews*, *33*(2), 144–172. https://doi.org/10.1080/02648725.2018.1430464

[2] Shin, Jaemyung & Lee, Yoonjung & Li, Zhangkang & Hu, Jinguang & Park, Simon & Kim, Keekyoung. (2022). Optimized 3D bioprinting technology based on machine learning: A review of recent trends and advances. *Micromachines*, *13*. https://doi.org/10.3390/mi13030363

[3] Ouyang, Liliang & Yao, Rui & Zhao, Yu & Sun, Wei. (2016). Effect of bioink properties on printability and cell viability for 3D bioplotting of embryonic stem cells. *Biofabrication*, *8*. 10.1088/1758-5090/8/3/035020

[4] Krishna, Devara Venkata & Sankar, Mamilla Ravi. (December 2023). Persuasive factors on the bioink printability and cell viability in the extrusion-based 3D bioprinting for tissue regeneration applications. *Engineered Regeneration*, *4*(4), 396–410.

[5] Zeqing, Jin, Zhizhou, Zhang, Xianlin, Shao & Gu, Grace X. (2023). Monitoring anomalies in 3D bioprinting with deep neural networks. *ACS Biomaterials Science & Engineering*, *9* (7), 3945–3952. https://doi.org10.1021/acsbiomaterials.0c01761

[6] Travis A. Meyer, Cesar Ramirez, Matthew J. Tamasi, and Adam J. Gormley. A user's guide to machine learning for polymeric biomaterials, *ACS Polymers Au* 2023 *3* (2), 141–157, https://doi.org/10.1021/acspolymersau.2c00037

[7] McDonald, S.M., Augustine, E.K., Lanners, Q. et al. (2023). Applied machine learning as a driver for polymeric biomaterials design. *Nature Communications*, *14*, 4838. https://doi.org/10.1038/s41467-023-40459-8

[8] Stewart, C.E., Kan, C.F.K., Stewart, B.R. et al. (2020). Machine intelligence for nerve conduit design and production. *Journal of Biological Engineering* 14, 25. https://doi.org/10.1186/s13036-020-00245-2

[9] Menon, Dhruv and Ranganathan, Raghavan. (2022). A generative approach to materials discovery, design, and optimization. *ACS Omega*, *7* (30), 25958–25973. https://doi.org/10.1021/acsomega.2c03264

[10] Kim, Seonghwan, Schroeder, Charles M., and Jackson, Nicholas E. (2023). Open macromolecular genome: Generative design of synthetically accessible polymers. *ACS Polymers Au*, *3* (4), 318–330. https://doi.org10.1021/acspolymersau.3c00003

[11] Shuyan Han, and Jun Wu. (June 2024). Artificial intelligence (AI) meets biomaterials and biomedicine. *Smart Materials in Medicine*, *5*(2), 251–255.

[12] Krishna, Devara Venkata, Mamilla Ravi Sankar. (November 2023). Machine learning-assisted extrusion-based 3D bioprinting for tissue regeneration applications, *Annals of 3D Printed Medicine*, *12*, 100132.

[13] Liu, C., Wang, L., Lu, W. et al. (2022). Computer vision-aided bioprinting for bone research. *Bone Research*, *10*, 21. https://doi.org/10.1038/s41413-022-00192-2

[14] Sun, Wenhuan, and Webster-Wood, Victoria. (2022). An integrated computer vision system for real-time monitoring and control of long-fiber embedded hydrogel 3D printing. *70*, 376–381.

[15] Sun, J., Yao, K., An, J., Jing, L., Huang, K., and Huang, D. (2023). Machine learning and 3D bioprinting. *International Journal of Bioprinting*, *9*(4), 717. https://doi.org/10.18063/ijb.717

[16] Bonatti, A.F., Vozzi, G., Chua, C.K., and Maria, C. (2022). A deep learning quality control loop of the extrusion-based bioprinting process. *International Journal of Bioprinting*, *8*(4), 620. https://doi.org/10.18063/ijb.v8i4.620

[17] Liu, C., Wang, L., Lu, W. et al. (2022). Computer vision-aided bioprinting for bone research. *Bone Research*, *10*, 21. https://doi.org/10.1038/s41413-022-00192-2
[18] Xiang, Y., Miller, K., Guan, J. et al. (2022). 3D bioprinting of complex tissues in vitro: State-of-the-art and future perspectives. *Archives of Toxicology*, *96*, 691–710. https://doi.org/10.1007/s00204-021-03212-y
[19] Al-Kharusi, G., Dunne, N.J., Little, S., and Levingstone, T.J. (2022). The role of machine learning and design of experiments in the advancement of biomaterial and tissue engineering research. *Bioengineering*, *9*(10), 561. https://doi.org/10.3390/bioengineering9100561
[20] Mitra, S., and Murthy, G.S. (2022). Bioreactor control systems in the biopharmaceutical industry: a critical perspective. *Syst Microbiol and Biomanuf*, *2*, 91–112. https://doi.org/10.1007/s43393-021-00048-6
[21] Ondracka, Andrej, Gasset, Arnau, García-Ortega, Xavier, Hubmayr, David, van Wijngaarden, Joeri, Montesinos-Seguí, José Luis, Valero, Francisco, Manzano, Toni. (2023). CPV of the future: AI-powered continued process verification for bioreactor processes. *PDA Journal of Pharmaceutical Science and Technology*, 77(3), 146–165. https://doi.org/10.5731/pdajpst.2021.012665
[22] Selden, C., and Fuller, B. (2018). Role of bioreactor technology in tissue engineering for clinical use and therapeutic target design. *Bioengineering*, *5*(2), 32. https://doi.org/10.3390/bioengineering5020032
[23] Bardhan, I., Chen, H., and Karahanna, Elena. (2020). Connecting systems, data, and people: A multidisciplinary research roadmap for chronic disease management. *MIS Quarterly: Management Information Systems*, 44, 185–200. https://doi.org/10.25300/MISQ/2020/14644
[24] Goh, G.D., Sing, S.L. & Yeong, W.Y. (2021). A review on machine learning in 3D printing: Applications, potential, and challenges. *Artificial Intelligence Review*, *54*, 63–94. https://doi.org/10.1007/s10462-020-09876-9
[25] Shin, J., Lee, Y., Li, Z., Hu, J., Park, S.S., Kim, K. (2022). Optimized 3D bioprinting technology based on machine learning: A review of recent trends and advances. *Micromachines*, *13*, 363. https://doi.org/10.3390/mi13030363
[26] Shankar, A. (2023). Efficient data interpretation and artificial intelligence enabled IoT based smart sensing system. *Artificial Intelligence Review*, 56(12), 15053–15077. https://doi.org/10.1007/s10462-023-10519-y
[27] Devi, S., Garg, H., & Garg, D. (2023). A review of redundancy allocation problem for two decades: Bibliometrics and future directions. *Artificial Intelligence Review*, 56(8), 7457–7548, https://doi.org/10.1007/s10462-022-10363-6
[28] Barnawi, A., Gaba, S., Alphy, A., Jabbari, A., Budhiraja, I., Kumar, V., & Kumar, N. (2023). A systematic analysis of deep learning methods and potential attacks in internet-of-things surfaces. *Neural Computing and Applications*, 35(25), 18293–18308, https://doi.org/10.1007/s00521-023-08634-6
[29] Swain, S., Bhushan, B., Dhiman, G., & Viriyasitavat, W. (2022). Appositeness of optimized and reliable machine learning for healthcare: a survey. *Archives of Computational Methods in Engineering*, 29(6), 3981–4003. https://doi.org/10.1007/s11831-022-09733-8
[30] Singh, J., Wazid, M., Das, A. K., Chamola, V., & Guizani, M. (2022). Machine learning security attacks and defense approaches for emerging cyber physical applications: A comprehensive survey. *Computer Communications*, 192, 316–331, https://doi.org/10.1016/j.comcom.2022.06.012

[31] Alrashed, F. A., Alsubiheen, A. M., Alshammari, H., Mazi, S. I., Al-Saud, S. A., Alayoubi, S., ... & Dhiman, G. (2022). Stress, anxiety, and depression in pre-clinical medical students: Prevalence and association with sleep disorders. *Sustainability*, *14*(18), 11320. https://doi.org/10.3390/su141811320

[32] Wazid, M., Singh, J., Das, A. K., Shetty, S., Khan, M. K., & Rodrigues, J. J. (2022). ASCP-IoMT: AI-enabled lightweight secure communication protocol for internet of medical things. *IEEE Access*, *10*, 57990–58004, https://doi.org/10.1109/ACCESS.2022.3179418

[33] Diwakar, M., Singh, P., Ravi, V., & Maurya, A. (2023). A non-conventional review on Multi-modality-based Medical Image Fusion. *Diagnostics*, *13*(5), 820. https://doi.org/10.3390/s23063287

[34] Yadav, S., Chamoli, S., Kumar, P., & Maurya, P. K. (2023). Structural and functional insights in polysaccharides coated cerium oxide nanoparticles and their potential biomedical applications: A review. *International Journal of Biological Macromolecules*, 125673, https://doi.org/10.1016/j.ijbiomac.2023.12567

[35] Ahmad, W., & Kumar, S. (2024). T axus wallichiana leaf extract-mediated microwave-assisted one-pot biosynthesis of MgO NPs for biomedical and photocatalytic applications. *Emergent Materials*, 7(3), 1081–1090. https://doi.org/10.1007/s42247-023-00612-x

Chapter 3

3D bioprinting techniques for tissue engineering applications

Ashwani Kumar, Yatika Gori, Subhash Singh, and Gaurav Dwivedi

3.1 INTRODUCTION

Tissue engineering represents a revolutionary approach to address the growing demand for organ and tissue transplants. By combining biocompatible materials, cells, and supporting structures, researchers aim to fabricate functional tissues that can repair or replace damaged ones in the human body. In this endeavor, 3D printing, also known as additive manufacturing, has emerged as a powerful tool with immense potential. This technology allows for the precise creation of complex 3D structures, offering significant advantages for tissue engineering applications [1, 2]. One of the primary roles of 3D printing in tissue engineering lies in the fabrication of scaffolds. Scaffolds are porous structures that mimic the natural extracellular matrix (ECM) – the complex network that provides structural support and biochemical cues for cell growth and differentiation. Traditional scaffold fabrication techniques often lack the ability to create intricate architectures with controlled porosity and internal channels. 3D printing overcomes these limitations by enabling the design and production of scaffolds with high precision and tailored properties [3].

Researchers can utilize 3D printing to create scaffolds with interconnected pores that facilitate cell migration, vascularization (blood vessel formation), and nutrient transport within the engineered tissue [3]. This level of control over scaffold design allows for the creation of microenvironments that closely resemble native tissues, promoting optimal cell function and tissue regeneration. 3D printing technology has evolved beyond simply fabricating scaffolds. Bioprinting, a specialized form of 3D printing, allows for the precise deposition of living cells alongside biocompatible materials, potentially leading to the creation of functional tissues. This technique offers several advantages over traditional cell seeding methods [4]. Bioprinting enables the creation of complex cell patterns within the scaffold, mimicking the natural cellular organization of tissues. Additionally, bioprinting can potentially improve cell viability by minimizing the shear stress experienced by cells during the deposition process [4].

DOI: 10.1201/9781003536352-3

Table 3.1 shows the recent advancements in bioprinting materials, often referred to as bioinks, hold significant promise for tissue engineering

Table 3.1 Recent technological developments in tissue engineering [1–16]

Authors	*Area of focus*	*Key results*
Chimene et al. [1]	Bioinks for Neural Tissue	Development of bioinks for 3D printing of neural tissue models.
Jakus et al. [2]	3D Printing of Organs	Potential of 3D printing for creating human tissues and organs for transplantation.
Li et al. [3]	Cell-laden Bioinks	Engineering and applications of cell-laden bioinks for 3D bioprinting.
Murphy et al. [4]	3D Printing Applications	Overview of 3D printing applications in tissue engineering, medical devices, and drug delivery.
Xu et al. [5]	Bioinks for Functional Tissues	Recent progress in bioinks for 3D bioprinting of functional tissues.
Boneschansky et al. [6]	Personalized Bone Tissue Grafts	3D printing for creating personalized bone tissue grafts for craniofacial reconstruction.
Gao et al. [7]	3D Bioprinting in Precision Medicine	The role of 3D bioprinting in precision medicine.
Murphy et al. [8]	3D Bioprinting of Tissues and Organs	Overview of 3D bioprinting for tissue and organ creation.
Hosseini et al. [9]	3D Bioprinting for Vascularization	Utilizing 3D bioprinting for vascularization of tissue engineering constructs.
Khalil et al. [10]	Bioprinting of Complex Organs	Challenges and opportunities in bioprinting complex organs.
Liu et al. [11]	3D and 4D Printing for Tissue Engineering	Applications of 3D and 4D printing of polymers for tissue engineering.
Ozbolat et al. [12]	3D Printing in Medicine	Current applications and future perspectives of 3D printing in medicine.
Wang et al. [13]	4D Bioprinting for Regenerative Medicine	Potential of 4D bioprinting for regenerative medicine.
Mandrycky et al. [14]	3D Bioprinting for Complex Tissues	3D bioprinting for engineering complex tissues.
Xu et al. [15]	Inkjet Printing for Tissue Constructs	Inkjet printing for fabrication of functional tissue constructs using mesenchymal stem cells and biomaterials.
Benninghoff et al. [16]	Biomimetic Scaffolds for Tissue Engineering	3D printing techniques for creating biomimetic scaffolds in regenerative medicine.

applications. Bioinks are biocompatible materials designed to encapsulate and deliver cells while maintaining their viability and functionality. Researchers are actively developing bioinks that mimic the properties of the ECM, providing essential biological cues for cell growth and differentiation. A major challenge in tissue engineering is the need for personalized constructs that match the specific needs of each patient. 3D printing offers a unique solution by enabling the creation of patient-specific scaffolds and tissues. Medical imaging techniques, such as CT scans, can be used to generate digital models of a patient's anatomy. These models can then be employed to 3D print customized scaffolds that perfectly fit the size and shape of the defect site [5–7]. The potential integration of a patient's own cells into the bioprinting process holds promise for personalized tissue engineering. By utilizing a patient's cells, the risk of immune rejection after implantation can be significantly reduced. This approach could pave the way for the creation of fully functional, patient-specific tissues for transplantation.

Despite the remarkable progress, 3D printing for tissue engineering applications still faces certain challenges. One major hurdle lies in the development of bioinks that can fully replicate the complex composition and functionality of the natural ECM. Additionally, efficient vascularization of engineered tissues remains a challenge, as large and complex tissues require a network of blood vessels to deliver nutrients and oxygen throughout the construct [9, 10]. Researchers are actively exploring new biomaterials and bioprinting techniques to address these limitations. The field of 4D printing, which incorporates the time dimension into the printing process, is also gaining traction. 4D-printed scaffolds can transform over time, potentially leading to the creation of engineered tissues that can mature and adapt within the body [11, 12].

3D printing has revolutionized the field of tissue engineering, offering unprecedented control over scaffold design, cell placement, and ultimately, tissue functionality. The ability to create patient-specific constructs with biocompatible materials and living cells holds immense promise for regenerative medicine. As research continues to advance, 3D printing has the potential to transform the way we treat organ failure and tissue defects, offering new hope for patients in need [13–16].

3.2 3D PRINTING TECHNOLOGIES FOR TISSUE ENGINEERING

3.2.1 Extrusion-based bioprinting

Extrusion-based bioprinting is a prominent technique within the field of 3D bioprinting. Figure 3.1 shows that it functions by pushing bioink, a mixture of cells and biocompatible materials, through a nozzle layer by layer to create 3D structures. This approach offers several advantages for tissue

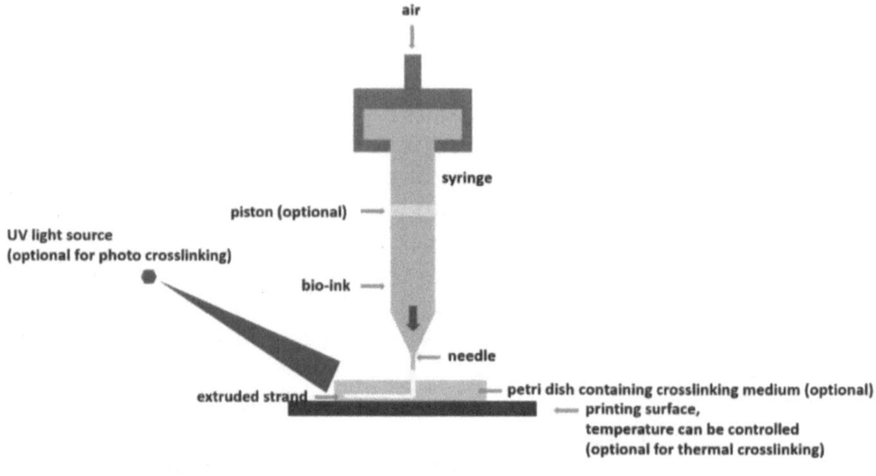

Figure 3.1 Schematic of extrusion-based bioprinting [17] (Open Access, Compound, MDPI).

engineering applications [4]. Compared to other bioprinting techniques, extrusion-based printing utilizes simpler setups, translating to lower costs. This makes it a more accessible option for research and development. The extrusion process generally exerts minimal stress on the cells within the bio-ink, leading to a high rate of cell survival during printing. This is crucial for maintaining the functionality of the engineered tissue. Ozbolat et al. [12] discuss the use of 3D printing techniques in medicine, including extrusion-based bioprinting, and mention their scalability for creating larger tissue constructs. Extrusion-based printing can handle a wide range of biomaterials with varying viscosities. This allows for the creation of scaffolds with diverse properties, mimicking the complexity of natural tissues. It can be readily scaled up to create larger constructs, making it suitable for engineering tissues of various sizes [16].

Compared to other techniques like inkjet printing [5], extrusion-based printing [4] offers lower resolution. This can limit the ability to create highly intricate structures needed for some tissues. Despite its advantages in cell viability, the extrusion process can still exert some shear stress on the cells. This can potentially affect cell function and differentiation. Printing large and complex tissues often necessitates the creation of internal channels for blood vessel formation (vascularization). However, extrusion-based printing may face challenges in achieving this effectively. Mandrycky et al. [14] discuss the use of 3D bioprinting for engineering complex tissues, acknowledging the limitations of extrusion-based printing in terms of resolution but emphasizing its potential for various tissue types. Research on extrusion-based bioprinting has yielded promising results. Scientists have successfully printed various tissues, including skin, bone, and cartilage. Additionally, advancements are being made in bioink development to better mimic the natural extracellular matrix, further enhancing the potential of this technology for tissue engineering.

3.2.2 Inkjet-based bioprinting

Inkjet-based bioprinting is a revolutionary technique that utilizes inkjet technology to deposit biological materials, such as cells and bioinks, onto a substrate in a highly controlled and precise manner. This approach has immense potential for tissue engineering, regenerative medicine, and drug discovery. The process begins with the preparation of a specialized "ink," which typically consists of a suspension of cells, biomaterials, and often growth factors or signaling molecules [18]. The ink is formulated to be compatible with the inkjet nozzle and to maintain cell viability and functionality. The prepared ink is then loaded into a cartridge and ejected from the nozzle in a controlled manner. This ejection process is governed by piezoelectric technology, which applies a voltage to a piezoelectric crystal to generate vibrations that force the ink out. By precisely controlling the droplet size, placement, and deposition rate, it's possible to create complex three-dimensional (3D) structures. The bioprinted layers are often allowed to solidify or crosslink before additional layers are deposited [19].

Inkjet bioprinting has numerous applications in the biomedical field. In tissue engineering, it can be used to create functional tissues and organs, such as skin, cartilage, and bone, for transplantation. Additionally, it can be employed to develop 3D tissue models for drug testing and toxicity screening, enabling more accurate and efficient drug development. Furthermore, inkjet bioprinting offers the potential for personalized medicine by tailoring treatments based on individual patient characteristics and disease states [20]. By creating miniature organ models, known as "organs-on-a-chip," researchers can study disease mechanisms and drug responses in a more physiologically relevant environment. Inkjet-based bioprinting represents a significant advancement in tissue engineering and regenerative medicine. Its ability to create complex, functional structures with high precision and cell viability makes it a valuable tool for a wide range of biomedical applications [21].

3.2.3 Laser-assisted bioprinting

Laser-assisted bioprinting is a revolutionary technique that utilizes laser technology to deposit biological materials, such as cells and bioinks, onto a substrate. This method offers precise control over the deposition process, enabling the creation of complex 3D tissue structures with high resolution and cell viability. The process begins with the preparation of a bioink, which is typically a suspension of cells, biomaterials, and growth factors. This bioink is similar to the one used in inkjet bioprinting [22–24]. A laser beam is then directed onto a thin layer of the bioink. The interaction between the laser and the bioink causes localized heating or phase changes, leading to the ejection of a droplet. By precisely controlling laser parameters like intensity, wavelength, and pulse duration, researchers can manipulate the droplet size and placement, ensuring accurate deposition of the biological material. Laser-assisted bioprinting has numerous applications in the biomedical field. In tissue engineering, it can be used to create functional tissues and organs, such as skin, cartilage, and bone, for transplantation. Additionally, it can be employed to develop 3D tissue models for drug testing and toxicity screening, enabling more efficient drug development [25–27].

Furthermore, laser-assisted bioprinting offers the potential for personalized medicine by tailoring treatments based on individual patient characteristics and disease states (Table 3.2). By creating miniature organ models, known as "organs-on-a-chip," researchers can study disease mechanisms and drug responses in a more physiologically relevant environment. Laser-assisted bioprinting represents a significant advancement in tissue engineering and regenerative medicine. Its ability to create complex, functional structures with high precision and cell viability makes it a valuable tool for a wide range of biomedical applications [30–32].

3.3 APPLICATIONS OF 3D PRINTING IN TISSUE ENGINEERING SCAFFOLDS

3D printing has revolutionized the field of tissue engineering by enabling the fabrication of highly customizable and complex scaffolds for tissue regeneration. These scaffolds serve as a structural support for cells, providing a suitable environment for them to proliferate, differentiate, and produce extracellular matrix.

3.3.1 Bone and cartilage regeneration

3D printing has revolutionized the field of tissue engineering, particularly in the realm of bone and cartilage regeneration. By enabling the fabrication of highly customizable and complex scaffolds, 3D printing offers a promising solution for addressing bone and cartilage defects. One of the key advantages of 3D-printed scaffolds is their ability to mimic the intricate geometries and varying pore sizes found in natural bone and cartilage. This customization enhances cell infiltration and tissue formation, as cells can interact with a more biologically relevant environment. Moreover, the porous structure of 3D-printed scaffolds facilitates the diffusion of essential nutrients and oxygen, promoting cell survival and growth. These scaffolds can be designed to incorporate bioactive materials, such as growth factors and osteoconductive substances, which can stimulate bone and cartilage regeneration. By combining these features, 3D-printed scaffolds provide a

Table 3.2 Comparative study of 3D printing technologies

Technique	*Main highlights*	*Advantages*	*Disadvantages*	*Applications*
Extrusion-based Bioprinting [4, 5, 12, 14, 16]	Deposits biomaterial through a nozzle using mechanical pressure.	Can handle a wide range of biomaterials. High throughput.	Lower resolution compared to other techniques. Potential for cell damage during extrusion.	Tissue engineering, organ-on-a-chip models, drug delivery systems.
Inkjet-based Bioprinting [18–21]	Ejects droplets of biomaterial using piezoelectric or thermal technology.	High resolution, precise control over droplet placement. Minimal cell damage.	Limited to biomaterials with suitable viscosity. Lower throughput compared to extrusion-based bioprinting.	Tissue engineering, drug screening, organ-on-a-chip models.
Laser-assisted Bioprinting [26, 27]	Uses laser energy to induce localized heating or phase changes in the biomaterial, leading to droplet ejection.	High resolution, precise control over droplet placement. Minimal cell damage.	Can be challenging to control the laser parameters. Limited to biomaterials that can be processed with laser energy.	Tissue engineering, drug screening, organ-on-a-chip models.
Stereolithography (SLA) [28]	Cures liquid photopolymer resin layer-by-layer using a UV laser.	High resolution, complex geometries possible.	Requires specialized photopolymer resins. Can be time-consuming for large structures.	Tissue engineering, dental prosthetics, prototyping.
Digital Light Processing (DLP) [29]	Projects a digital pattern onto a photopolymer resin bath, curing the exposed areas.	High resolution, faster curing times compared to SLA.	Requires specialized photopolymer resins. Can be limited in build volume.	Tissue engineering, dental prosthetics, prototyping.

supportive framework for tissue regeneration, offering a potential solution for various bone and cartilage disorders [33–36].

3.3.2 Skin and wound healing applications

3D printing offers unparalleled flexibility in designing scaffolds that precisely match the contours of irregular wound surfaces. This customization enhances wound healing by providing a supportive structure that promotes cell migration, proliferation, and differentiation. Layered scaffolds, fabricated through 3D printing, can be designed to deliver different types of cells or biomaterials sequentially. This approach mimics the natural structure and function of skin, providing a more biologically relevant environment for tissue regeneration. For instance, a layered scaffold might incorporate a dermal layer containing fibroblasts and an epidermal layer containing keratinocytes. By incorporating antimicrobial agents into the scaffold material, 3D printing can help prevent infections, a common complication in wound healing. These antimicrobial agents can be embedded within the scaffold structure or released in a controlled manner to maintain a sterile environment. Overall, 3D printing enables the creation of skin and wound healing scaffolds that are highly customizable, biocompatible, and effective in promoting tissue regeneration [37–40].

3.3.3 Printing of organs and complex tissues

3D printing has revolutionized the field of tissue engineering by enabling the creation of miniature organ models, known as "organs-on-a-chip." These models mimic the physiological functions and microenvironments of real organs, providing a valuable platform for studying disease mechanisms, drug interactions, and toxicity testing. By integrating multiple cell types and extracellular matrix components into a 3D-printed scaffold, researchers can create highly complex and functional organ models. For example, a liver-on-a-chip model can be used to study drug metabolism and toxicity, while a heart-on-a-chip model can be used to investigate cardiac function and disease progression [28, 29, 41, 42].

The ability to fabricate complex 3D structures with precise control over pore size, cell distribution, and material properties makes 3D printing an ideal tool for creating tissues like liver, heart, and kidney. These tissues often exhibit intricate architectures and require specific microenvironments to function properly. 3D printing allows for the customization of scaffolds to match the desired tissue structure, promoting cell differentiation, proliferation, and extracellular matrix production. The integration of vascular networks into tissue scaffolds is crucial for providing essential nutrients, oxygen, and waste removal to the cells. 3D printing enables the fabrication of vascular channels within the scaffold, mimicking the natural blood supply to organs. These channels can be designed to have varying diameters, branching patterns, and flow rates, allowing for the simulation of different physiological conditions. By incorporating vascular networks into tissue scaffolds, researchers can create more physiologically relevant and functional organ models [43–46].

3.3.4 Drug delivery and biosensing applications

3D-printed scaffolds can be designed to incorporate drug-loaded microparticles or channels that allow for the controlled release of therapeutic agents. This controlled release can improve drug efficacy by ensuring that the drug is delivered to the target tissue at the appropriate rate, reducing the risk of under- or overdosing. Additionally, controlled release can minimize systemic side effects by limiting the exposure of the drug to healthy tissues. By integrating biosensors into the scaffold material, 3D printing can create platforms for real-time monitoring of tissue function and detection of disease biomarkers. These biosensors can be designed to measure parameters such as pH, temperature, oxygen levels, and the presence of specific molecules. This information can be used to assess tissue health, track disease progression, and evaluate the effectiveness of therapeutic interventions [47, 48].

3D-printed scaffolds can be tailored to individual patients' needs, providing personalized drug delivery and tissue regeneration solutions. For example, scaffolds can be designed to match the specific anatomy and physiology of a patient's wound or defect. Additionally, scaffolds can be loaded with drugs that are specifically chosen to address the patient's unique medical condition. This personalized approach can improve treatment outcomes and reduce the risk of complications [49–51].

3.4 DISCUSSION AND CONCLUSION

3D printing has revolutionized the field of tissue engineering by offering unprecedented control over scaffold design and fabrication. This technology enables the creation of customized scaffolds with intricate geometries, tailored pore structures, and the incorporation of bioactive materials. These advancements have significantly improved the potential for tissue regeneration and have addressed many of the limitations associated with traditional tissue engineering methods. One of the key advantages of 3D printing is its ability to produce scaffolds with complex and patient-specific designs. This customization is essential for replicating the natural architecture and function of various tissues and organs [52–54]. Additionally, 3D printing allows for the precise control of scaffold properties, such as porosity, mechanical strength, and biodegradability, which are crucial for promoting cell growth, differentiation, and extracellular matrix production. By addressing the challenges of traditional tissue engineering methods, such as limited control over scaffold structure and difficulty in incorporating bioactive materials,

3D printing has opened up new possibilities for tissue regeneration [55, 56]. This technology has the potential to accelerate the development of innovative treatments for a wide range of diseases and injuries, including bone fractures, cartilage defects, skin wounds, and organ failure. As 3D printing technology continues to advance, we can expect to see even more sophisticated and functional scaffolds being developed. The integration of bioprinting with other emerging technologies, such as stem cell engineering and nanotechnology, will further enhance the capabilities of this powerful tool. In conclusion, 3D printing is poised to play a pivotal role in shaping the future of tissue engineering and regenerative medicine [57–59].

REFERENCES

1. Chimene, D., Gentile, P., Vernoni-Scagliotti, M., Vitale, F., & Druschler, S. (2020). Bioinks for 3D printing of neural tissue models. *Biomaterials Science*, 8(8), 2150–2163.
2. Jakus, A. E., Rizzino, A. R., Kang, H., Malone, M. E., Rohde, R. A., & Wolf, M. T. (2020). 3D printing of human tissues and organs for transplantation. *Nature Biotechnology*, 38(6), 602–612.
3. Li, J., Wu, C., Xiong, Z., Mao, Y., Qian, Z., & Yin, J. (2020). Engineering and applications of cell-laden bioinks for 3D bioprinting. *Science China Technological Sciences*, 63(12), 2674–2685.
4. Murphy, S. V., & Skoog, S. A. (2022). 3D printing: Applications in tissue engineering, medical devices, and drug delivery. *AAPS PharmSciTech*, 23(2), 2249–2261. DOI: 10.1208/s12249-022-02249-2
5. Xu, T., Luo, Y., Wang, X., Liu, J., & Cheng, H. (2021). Recent progress in bioinks for 3D bioprinting of functional tissues. *Journal of Materials Science & Technology*, 76(2), 247–266.
6. Boneschansky, P. C., Jansen, J. A., & Richards, R. G. (2020). 3D printing of personalized bone tissue grafts for craniofacial reconstruction. *Trends in Biotechnology*, 38(7), 787–796.
7. Gao, T., Liu, H., & Yan, X. (2019). 3D bioprinting in precision medicine. *Engineering in Medicine and Biology Magazine, IEEE*, 38(3), 74–80.
8. Murphy, S. V., & Atala, A. (2014). 3D bioprinting of tissues and organs. *Nature Biotechnology*, 32(8), 773–785.
9. Hosseini, V., Parkhurst, A. M., & Sultan, A. S. (2020). 3D bioprinting for vascularization of tissue engineering constructs. *Trends in Biotechnology*, 38(5), 507–522.
10. Khalil, S., Sun, W., & Mao, Y. (2020). Bioprinting of complex organs: Challenges and opportunities. *Science Bulletin*, 65(20), 1305–1314.
11. Liu, X., Zhang, G., Yan, X., & Zhu, J. (2019). 3D and 4D printing of polymers for tissue engineering applications. *Frontiers in Bioengineering and Biotechnology*, 7, 142, DOI: 10.3389/fbioe.2019.00142
12. Ozbolat, I. T., & Goepfert, J. (2020). 3D printing in medicine: Current applications and future perspectives. *Current Opinion in Biotechnology*, 63, 88–95.
13. Wang, W., Lin, S., Li, J., Liu, X., & Sun, W. (2018). 4D bioprinting for regenerative medicine. *Regenerative Biomaterials*, 7(1), 1–15.

14. Mandrycky, C., Wang, Z., Kim, K., & Shakesheff, K. (2016). 3D bioprinting for engineering complex tissues. *Biotechnology Advances*, 34(4), 422–434, DOI: 10.1016/j.biotechadv.2016.02.002
15. Xu, T., Wu, W., Ruan, Y., Song, W., Kong, C., Mao, Y., ... Li, D. (2020). Inkjet printing of mesenchymal stem cells and biomaterials for fabrication of functional tissue constructs. *Journal of Materials Science & Technology*, 36(7), 1640–1648, DOI: 10.1016/j.jmst.2019.12.022
16. Benninghoff, A. D., Rath, S. N., & Rajan, S. D. (2020). Toward biomimetic scaffolds for tissue engineering: 3D printing techniques in regenerative medicine. *Frontiers in Bioengineering and Biotechnology*, 8, 588, DOI: 10.3389/fbioe.2020.588832
17. Mahmood, M.A. (2021). 3D printing in drug delivery and biomedical applications: A state-of-the-art review. *Compounds*, 1, 94–115. DOI: 10.3390/compounds1030009
18. Ng, W. L., Huang, X., Shkolnikov, V., Suntornnond, R., & Yeong, W. Y. (2023). Polyvinylpyrrolidone-based bioink: influence of bioink properties on printing performance and cell proliferation during inkjet-based bioprinting. *Bio-Design and Manufacturing*, 6(6), 676–690.
19. Huang, X., Ng, W. L., & Yeong, W. Y. (2024). Predicting the number of printed cells during inkjet-based bioprinting process based on droplet velocity profile using machine learning approaches. *Journal of Intelligent Manufacturing*, 35(5), 2349–2364.
20. Li, Xinda, Boxun Liu, Ben Pei, Jianwei Chen, Dezhi Zhou, Jiayi Peng, Xinzhi Zhang, Wang Jia, and Tao Xu. (2020). Inkjet bioprinting of biomaterials. *Chemical Reviews*, 120(19), 10793–10833.
21. Xu, H., Martinez Salazar, D. M., Shahriar, M., & Xu, C. (2022). Investigation and characterization of cell aggregation during and after inkjet-based bioprinting of cell-laden bioink. *Journal of Manufacturing Science and Engineering*, 144(10), 104501.
22. Wazid, M., Singh, J., Das, A. K., Shetty, S., Khan, M. K., & Rodrigues, J. J. (2022). ASCP-IoMT: AI-enabled lightweight secure communication protocol for internet of medical things. *IEEE Access*, *10*, 57990–58004, 10.1109/ACCESS.2022.3179418
23. Prasad, Arbind, Kumar, Kishor, Ashwani, & Gajrani, Kumar (2022). *Biodegradable composites for packaging application*. Taylor & Francis (CRC Press). DOI: 10.1201/9781003227908
24. Kumar, Ashwani, Gori, Yatika, Kumar, Avinash, Meena, Chandan Swaroop, & Dutt, Nitesh (2022). *Advanced materials for biomedical applications*. Taylor & Francis (CRC Press). DOI: 10.1201/9781003344810
25. Arbind Prasad, Ashwani Kumar, Gupta, Manoj (2023). *Advanced materials and manufacturing techniques in biomedical applications*. Wiley Scrivener. DOI: 10.1002/9781394166985
26. Ventura, R. D. (2021). An overview of laser-assisted bioprinting (LAB) in tissue engineering applications. *Medical Lasers; Engineering, Basic Research, and Clinical Application*, 10(2), 76–81.
27. Guillotin, Bertrand, Souquet, Agnès, Catros, Sylvain, Duocastella, Martí, Pippenger, Benjamin, Bellance, Séverine, Bareille, Reine et al. (2010). Laser assisted bioprinting of engineered tissue with high cell density and microscale organization. *Biomaterials*, 31(28), 7250–7256.

28. Huang, J., Qin, Q., & Wang, J. (2020). A review of stereolithography: Processes and systems. *Processes*, 8(9), 1138.
29. Kadry, H., Wadnap, S., Xu, C., & Ahsan, F. (2019). Digital light processing (DLP) 3D-printing technology and photoreactive polymers in fabrication of modified-release tablets. *European Journal of Pharmaceutical Sciences*, 135, 60–67.
30. Kumar, Abhishek, Kumar, Avinash, & Kumar, Ashwani (2024). *Applications of biotribology in biomedical systems*. Springer Nature. DOI: 10.1007/978-3-031-58327-8, ISBN 978-3-031-58326-1.
31. Bhoi, Sandeep, Prasad, Arbind, Kumar, Ashwani, Sarkar, Rudra Bubai, Mahto, Bidyanand, Meena, Chandan Swaroop, & Pandey, Chandan (2022). Experimental study to evaluate the wear performance of UHMWPE and XLPE material for orthopedics application. *Bioengineering*, 9, 676. DOI: 10.3390/bioengineering9110676
32. Gangwar, Arun Kumar Singh, Sudhakar Rao, P., & Kumar, Ashwani (2021). Biomechanical design and analysis of femur bone. *Materials Today: Proceedings*, 44(Part 1), 2179–2187, ISSN 2214-7853. DOI: 10.1016/j.matpr.2020.12.282
33. Gangwar, Arun Kumar Singh, Sudhakar Rao, P., Kumar, Ashwani, & Patil, Pravin P., 2019, Design and analysis of femur bone: BioMechanical aspects. *Journal of Critical Reviews*, 6(4), 133–139, ISSN-2394-5125.
34. Gruene, Martin, Unger, Claudia, Koch, Lothar, Deiwick, Andrea, & Chichkov, Boris (2011). Dispensing pico to nanolitre of a natural hydrogel by laser-assisted bioprinting. *Biomedical Engineering*, 10, 1–11.
35. Kumar, A., Kumar, A., Kumar, A., Choudhari, A., Gupta, A. K., & Faisal, S. (2024). Chapter 01: Introduction to biotribology: A science of surface interaction. In A. Kumar, A. Kumar, A. Kumar (Eds.), *Applications of biotribology in biomedical systems* (pp. 01–26). Springer Nature Switzerland. DOI: 10.1007/978-3-031-58327-8_1
36. Chowdhury, N., Faisal, S., Kumar, A., Choudhari, A., Gupta, A. K., Kumar, A., & Kumar, A. (2024). Chapter 02: Characterization of hydrogel properties in the advancement of bio-tribology. In A. Kumar, A. Kumar, & A. Kumar (Eds.), *Applications of biotribology in biomedical systems* (pp. 27–78). Springer Nature Switzerland. DOI: 10.1007/978-3-031-58327-8_2
37. Pal, A., Gour, R., Kumar, A., Kumar, A., Kumar, A., & Chowdhury, N. (2024). Chapter 05: Tribological measurement of human skin. In A. Kumar, A. Kumar, A. Kumar (Eds.), *Applications of biotribology in biomedical systems* (pp. 149–165). Springer Nature Switzerland. DOI: 10.1007/978-3-031-58327-8_5
38. Kumar, A., Gajjar, P., Gudadur, K. S., Kumar, A., Gupta, A. K., Choudhari, A., Chowdhury, N., & Kumar, A. (2024). Chapter 06: Tribological hurdles in biomedical manufacturing: A comprehensive examination. In A. Kumar, A. Kumar, A. Kumar (Eds.), *Applications of biotribology in biomedical systems* (pp. 167–198). Springer Nature Switzerland. DOI: 10.1007/978-3-031-58327-8_6
39. Tortorella, Silvia, Greco, Pierpaolo, Valle, Francesco, Barbalinardo, Marianna, Foschi, Giulia, Lugli, Francesca, Dallavalle, Marco, Zerbetto, Francesco, Bortolotti, Carlo Augusto, & Biscarini, Fabio (2022). Laser assisted bioprinting of laminin on biodegradable PLGA substrates: Effect on neural stem cell adhesion and differentiation. *Bioprinting*, 26, e00194.

40. Guillotin, B., Catros, S., & Guillemot, F. (2014). Laser assisted bio-printing (LAB) of cells and bio-materials based on laser induced forward transfer (LIFT). In *Laser technology in biomimetics: Basics and applications* (pp. 193–209). Springer Berlin Heidelberg.
41. Heidari, M., Thangavel, S., Rahmanivahid, P., Khashehchi, M., Kumar, A., Kumar, A., & Kumar, A. (2024). Chapter 07: Navigating the landscape: Cutting-edge biomedical manufacturing techniques. In A. Kumar, A. Kumar, A. Kumar (Eds.), *Applications of biotribology in biomedical systems* (pp. 199–216). Springer Nature Switzerland. DOI: 10.1007/978-3-031-58327-8_7
42. Gour, R., Baliyan, N., Pal, A., Kumar, A., Kumar, A., & Kumar, A. (2024). Chapter 08: Animal tribology. In A. Kumar, A. Kumar, & A. Kumar (Eds.), *Applications of biotribology in biomedical systems* (pp. 217–234). Springer Nature Switzerland. DOI: 10.1007/978-3-031-58327-8_8
43. A. K. Gupta, Choudhari, A., Kumar, A., Kumar, A., A. Gupta, S. Faisal, & A. Kumar (2024). Chapter 10: Composites for drug-eluting devices: Emerging biomedical applications. In A. Kumar, A. Kumar, A. Kumar (Eds.), *Applications of biotribology in biomedical systems* (pp. 251–311). Springer Nature Switzerland. DOI: 10.1007/978-3-031-58327-8_10
44. A. Choudhari, Gupta, A.K., Kumar, A., Kumar, A., Gupta, A., Chowdhury, N., & Kumar, A. (2024). Chapter 13: Wear and friction mechanism study in knee and hip replacement: A comprehensive review. In A. Kumar, A. Kumar, A. Kumar (Eds.), *Applications of biotribology in biomedical systems* (pp. 345–432). Springer Nature Switzerland. DOI: 10.1007/978-3-031-58327-8_13
45. Su, X., Wang, T., & Guo, S. (2021). Applications of 3D printed bone tissue engineering scaffolds in the stem cell field. *Regenerative Therapy*, 16, 63–72.
46. Haleem, A., Javaid, M., Khan, R. H., & Suman, R. (2020). 3D printing applications in bone tissue engineering. *Journal of Clinical Orthopaedics and Trauma*, 11, S118–S124.
47. Pavan Kalyan, B. G., & Kumar, L. (2022). 3D printing: Applications in tissue engineering, medical devices, and drug delivery. *Aaps Pharmscitech*, 23(4), 92.
48. Prasad, Arbind, Datta, Sudipto, Kumar, Ashwani, & Gupta, Manoj (2023). Chapter 01: Introduction to next-generation materials for biomedical applications. In Arbind Prasad, Ashwani Kumar, Manoj Gupta (Eds.), *Advanced materials and manufacturing techniques for biomedical applications* (pp. 01–24). John Wiley & Sons. DOI: 10.1002/9781394166985.ch1
49. De, Sriparna, Das, Dipankar, Prasad, Arbind, Kumar, Ashwani, & Chattopadhyay, Dipankar (2023). Chapter 03: Insights into multifunctional smart hydrogels in wound healing applications. In Arbind Prasad, Ashwani Kumar, Manoj Gupta (Eds.), *Advanced materials and manufacturing techniques for biomedical applications* (pp. 37–60). DOI: 10.1002/9781394166985.ch3
50. Kumar, Avinash, Byadwal, Mohit, Kumar¸ Abhishek, Kumar, Ashwani, Francis Luther King, M. (2023). Laser micromachining in biomedical industry. In Avinash Kumar, Ashwani Kumar, & Abhishek Kumar (Eds.), *Laser-based technologies for sustainable manufacturing* (pp. 169–206). CRC Press. DOI: 10.1201/9781003402398–8

51. Kumar, Avinash, Datta, Anka, Kumar, Ashwani, & Kumar, Abhishek (2022). Recent advancements and future trends in next-generation materials for biomedical applications. *Advanced Materials for Biomedical Applications*. CRC Press, Taylor & Francis, ISBN: 9781003344810. DOI: 10.1201/9781003344810-1
52. Datta, Anka, Kumar, Avinash, Kumar, Ashwani, Kumar, Abhishek, & Singh, Varun Pratap, (2022). Advanced materials in biological implants and surgical tools. *Advanced Materials for Biomedical Applications*. CRC Press, Taylor & Francis. ISBN: 9781003344810. DOI: 10.1201/9781003344810-2
53. Kumar, Ashwani, Gangwar, Arun Kumar Singh, Kumar, Avinash, Meena, Chandan Swaroop, Singh, Varun Pratap, Dutt, Nitesh, Prasad, Arbind, & Gori, Yatika (2022). Biomedical study of femur bone fracture and Healing. *Advanced Materials for Biomedical Applications*. CRC Press, Taylor & Francis. ISBN: 9781003344810, DOI: 10.1201/9781003344810-14
54. Alrashed, F. A., Alsubiheen, A. M., Alshammari, H., Mazi, S. I., Al-Saud, S. A., Alayoubi, S., ... & Dhiman, G. (2022). Stress, anxiety, and depression in pre-clinical medical students: Prevalence and association with sleep disorders. *Sustainability*, *14*(18), 11320. 10.3390/su141811320
55. Prasad, Arbind, Chakraborty, Gourhari, Kumar, Ashwani, & Gajrani, Kishor Kumar (2022). Introduction to biodegradable polymers. *Biodegradable composites for packaging applications*. CRC Press, Taylor & Francis. ISBN: 978103227908. DOI: 10.1201/9781003227908-1
56. Gupta, P., Gupta, H., Kairamkonda, M., Kumar, N., & Poluri, K. M. (2022). Elucidating the lactic acid tolerance mechanism in vaginal clinical isolates of Candida glabrata. *Medical Mycology*, *60*(6), myac042. DOI: 10.1093/mmy/myac042
57. Kumar, Ashwani, Gori, Yatika, Rana, Sachin, Sharma, Neelesh Kumar, & Yadav, Brijesh, (2022). FEA of humerus bone fracture and healing. *Advanced materials for biomechanical applications*. CRC Press (Taylor and Francis). ISBN: 9781032054490. DOI: 10.1201/9781003286806-14
58. Kumar, Ashwani, Mamgain, Deepak Prasad, Jaiswal, Himanshu, & Patil, Pravin P. (2015). Modal analysis of hand arm vibration (humerus bone) for biodynamic response using varying boundary conditions based on FEA. *Springer Book Series: Advances in Intelligent Systems and Computing*, 308, 169–176. DOI: 10.1007/978-81-322-2012-1_18
59. Kumar, Ashwani, Rana, Sachin, Gori, Yatika, & Sharma, Neelesh Kumar (2021). Thermal contact conductance prediction using FEM based computational techniques. In *Advanced computational methods in mechanical and materials engineering* (pp. 183–220). CRC Press (Taylor and Francis). DOI: 10.1201/9781003202233-13

Chapter 4

Natural biomaterials for tissue engineering and regenerative medicine

Shaik Arshid Banu and Subhash Singh

4.1 COLLAGEN

Collagen is the most prevalent protein found in the body, which makes up over one-third of the weight of the protein tissue in the body. It usually transfers load to tissues and provides a highly biocompatible environment for cells [1, 2]. Currently 28 types of collagens are known to exist. The primary types that comprise the key component of collagen found in bone, cartilage, tendon, skin and muscle are I, II, III and V [3].

4.1.1 Structure and properties of collagen

Collagen comprises a complex hierarchical structure which can be divided into four forms. The primary form, secondary form, tertiary form and the quaternary form [1] as shown in Figure 4.1 (a), (b), (c), (d).

(i) Primary form: amino acid triplet
The primary structure of the collagen protein can be identified by the presence of proline-rich Gly-X-Y polypeptide, where proline is represented as X and hydroxyproline as Y. Gly is present at every third position with the recurring $(Gly - X - Y)_n$ chain along the length of ~1000 amino acid chain.

(ii) Secondary form: α-helix
The α-helix structure is generated by the recurrence of $(Gly - X - Y)_n$ chain with the non-helical structures at the end of the chain. The two terminals of the α-helix structure are C-terminal and N-terminal. Terminal-C is responsible for the initiation of the tertiary structure and the primary fibril sizes are regulated by the N-terminal.

(iii) Tertiary form: triple helix
The triple helix is often produced as a heterotrimer comprising two identical $\alpha_1(\mathrm{I})$ and $\alpha_1(\mathrm{II})$-chains and one $\alpha_2(\mathrm{I})$-chain with roughly 1000 amino acids. It is approximately 1.5 nm in diameter and 300 nm in length (L). This is notably true for collagen type I. The three α-chains come together to create a left-handed, rod-shaped helix. The larger

DOI: 10.1201/9781003536352-4

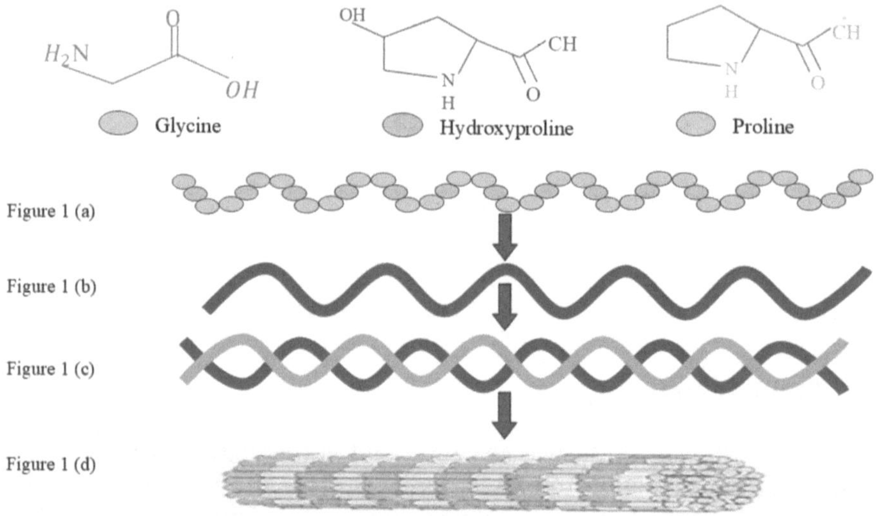

Figure 4.1 (a) Primary form, 1 (b): Secondary form, 1 (c): Tertiary form, 1 (d): quaternary form of collagen.

amino acids that make up the X and Y residues are positioned in the outer locations, while the glycine remnants are arranged around a central axis. The α-triple helical and β-sheet protein structures are stabilized primarily by the single interstrand Ca–H(Gly/Y)...O = C(X/Gly) and N-H(Gly)...O = C(X) hydrogen bonds that connect the α-chains.

(iv) Quaternary form: collagen fibrils
Collagen molecules form a supramolecular structure by self-assembling in a quarter-stagger unit structure of five triple-helical collagen molecules. These molecules are highly orientated and have D-periodic banding spaces (D = 67 nm). The telopeptides, which are non-helical sections with a length of roughly 20 amino acid residues, are crucial to fibrillogenesis because they help to stabilize mature collagen molecules by forming cross-links. Collagen cross-links are classified into two types: enzymatic cross-links, which are mediated by lysine hydroxylase and lysyl oxidase, and non-enzymatic cross-links, which are also referred to as glycation or oxidation-induced Advanced Glycation End Products (AGE) cross-links. Two forms of 3-hydroxypyridinium cross-linking are generated between the amine side group present in the lysine and hydroxy lysine residues in collagen telopeptides: hydroxyl lysyl pyridinoline (HP) and lysyl pyridoline (LP) cross-links.

Collagen, a key extracellular matrix protein plays a prominent role in upholding the structural and biological integrity of many connective tissues [3]. The following are the properties of collagen which makes it ideal for biological and clinical applications especially in tissue engineering [2]:

(i) Biocompatibility: Collagen's structure is highly biocompatible with human tissues, facilitating its use in medical implants and scaffolds.
(ii) Mechanical strength: The fibrous nature of collagen gives it the necessary strength and elasticity for tissue scaffolding and load bearing applications.
(iii) Thermal stability: Collagen's triple helix structure provides a stable form that denatures at body temperature, making it suitable for physiological applications.
(iv) Enzymatic degradation: Collagen's susceptibility to enzymatic degradation allows for controlled breakdown and integration within the body, aiding in healing and regeneration processes.

These properties collectively contribute to collagen's effectiveness in medical products like wound dressings, tissue repair, and organ transplantation scaffolds.

4.1.2 Applications of collagen in tissue engineering

The hydrogels of collagen are extensively used in tissue engineering and regenerative medicines because of its biocompatibility, biodegradability and structural similarity to the extracellular matrix [4]. Below are some of the crucial uses of collagen in tissue engineering and regenerative medicine as shown in Figure 4.2.

(i) Cartilage and bone repair: Collagen is well known for its biomimetic properties, which closely replicates the biological microenvironment of bone tissue. Collagen scaffolds are engineered to support cartilage and bone tissue regeneration, often combined with other bioactive materials to enhance performance. Collagen promotes osteogenesis by facilitating the proliferation and differentiation of bone mesenchymal stem cells (BMSCs). Collagen hydrogels support the growth and distribution of cells, aiding in the repair of bone defects [5].
(ii) Muscle tissue repair: Collagen scaffolds play a significant role in perfusion and muscle rebuilding processes, as well as they are crucial in differentiation of myoblasts in myotubes. Collagen-based hydrogels are found to be promising agents in cardiac muscle rebuilding in terms of viability of cardiomyocyte and syringe ability.
(iii) Nerve tissue regeneration: Biomaterials based on collagen have been widely used to address therapeutic problems in neural tissue engineering (NTE), such as neuro regeneration and neuro protection. They support nerve regeneration in various nerve cuffs (e.g., NeuroWrap and NeuroMend) and nerve scaffolds (e.g., NeuraGen and Neuromaix), with degradation times ranging from months to years. Additionally, collagen scaffolds can be enhanced with functional proteins or growth factors to improve nerve healing. For example, nerve growth factor

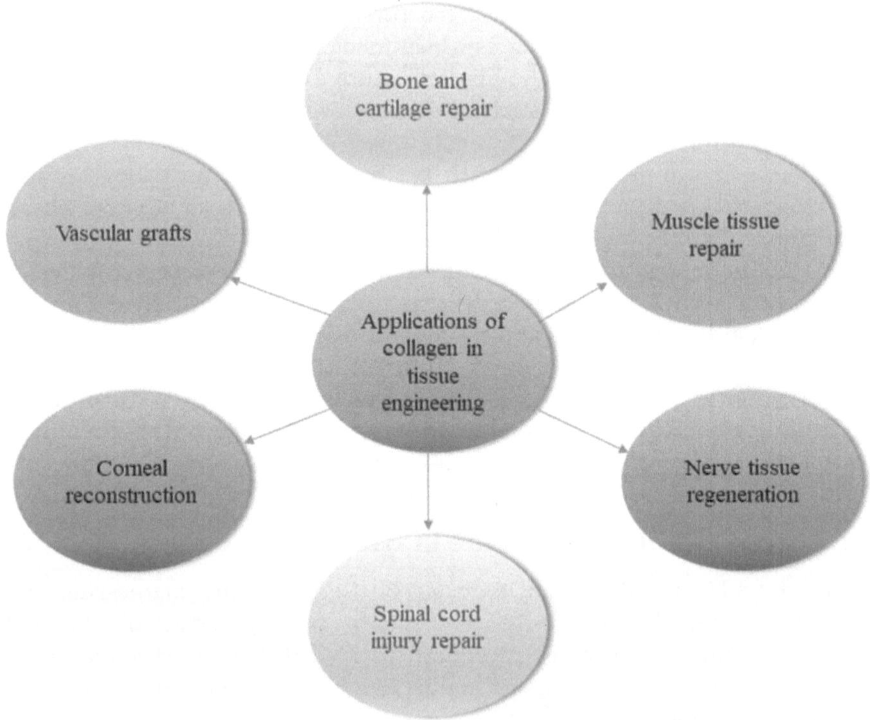

Figure 4.2 Various applications of collagen in tissue engineering.

coupled with collagen scaffolds has effectively reproduced nerve gaps of 5 to 35 mm in various animal models. The adaptability of collagen lies in its various forms, such as sponges, conduits, nano/microspheres, hydrogels, which can be tailored for specific peripheral nervous system and central nervous system [6].

(iv) Spinal cord injury repair: Collagen has been extensively used in spinal cord injury (SCI) repair due to its ability to create a neural-favorable microenvironment that enhances cell proliferation and differentiation. The reproducibility and applicability of collagen are obtained through a variety of processing techniques. As an example, collagen scaffolds enriched with neuro protective proteins have shown promise in SCI repair. A notable example is a collagen sponge loaded with basic fibroblast growth factor (bFGF) and encapsulating neural stem cells (NSCs), which significantly accelerates cell proliferation. This innovative platform could serve as a robust strategy for growth factor-functionalized collagen-scaffold-based SCI repair. Collagen scaffolds direct cell migration within the lesion cavity, aiding in recovery of motor functions. In addition, composite scaffolds such as collagen are tailored to enhance specific and effective binding with a wide range of bioactive and therapeutic agents like for example growth factors and neurotrophic agents. These scaffolds enhance axonal regeneration by increasing cell differentiation while decreasing glial scar formation and astrogliosis. Furthermore, functionalized collagen scaffolds support improved neuronal growth and neurite reconnection that led to considerably enhanced locomotor performance as indication of SCI recovery [6].

(v) Corneal reconstruction: Modern tissue engineering techniques recognized collagen hydrogels as promising materials for corneal regeneration. These hydrogels are engineered with a transparent core and an adjustable peripheral region designed to degrade at a relatively faster rate. The ability of collagen constructs to support the transparency, shape and integrity specific for corneal tissue has been demonstrated alongside their pro-growth effects on human epithelial cells. Furthermore, other cross-linking strategies were investigated to enhance the mechanical strength and enzymatic stability of these hydrogels. A recombinant human collagen was also used as a method to mitigate and evade immune responses while showing positive outcomes with regard to optimal transparency and corneal regeneration. Taken together, hydrogels composed of collagen are a suitable candidate for corneal reconstruction due to their excellent biocompatibility and superior structural properties.

(vi) Vascular grafts: Collagen-based hydrogels have been investigated for human vascular tissue engineering applications, owing to their biocompatibility and power of promoting cell proliferation. To generate 3D models, researchers seeded microfluidic tubes with endothelial cells and embedded the linear constructs in type I collagen hydrogels. These models have been designed to more accurately model the structure, mechanical environment and composition of natural blood vessels so as to study vascular biology such as pericyte migration, platelet adhesion and endothelial function. Additionally, in mice the formation of new vascular networks has been stimulated using injectable collagen-phenolic hydroxy gels [7]. When incorporated with endothelial and mesenchymal stem cells, these hydrogels facilitated large patent vascular structures that were anastomosed to the host tissue enhancing regeneration and reparative healing.

4.2 HYALURONIC ACID

In 1934, hyaluronic acid – along chain of repeating molecules known as glycosaminoglycans – is found in the vitreous fluid of cow's eye. This macromolecule, illustrated in Figure 4.3, is comprised of over 30,000 repeating units of D-glucuronic acid and N-acetyl-D-glucosamine that are connected

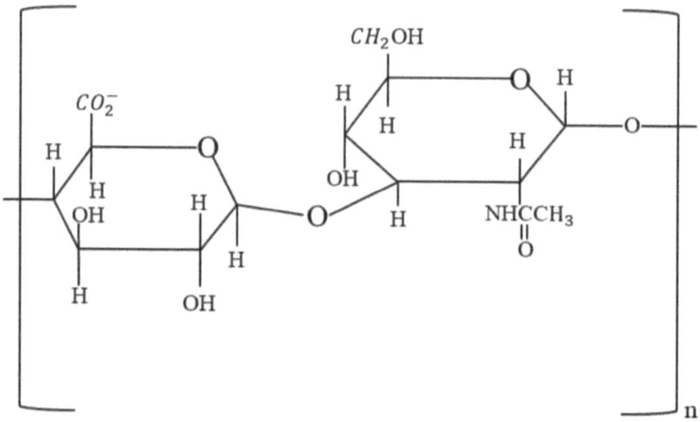

Figure 4.3 Molecular structure of hyaluronic acid.

by β1-3 and β1-4 linkages [8, 9]. The molecular weight of hyaluronic acid fluctuates, and this affects the stability, viscosity and viscoelasticity. A major constituent of the extracellular matrix (ECM), hyaluronic acid is found throughout epithelial, connective and neural tissues.

4.2.1 Properties and functions of hyaluronic acid

Hyaluronic acid plays an important role in cell differentiation, growth and wound healing, and its properties make it an ideal material in tissue engineering. Following are some properties of hyaluronic acid which significantly impacts its application in tissue engineering:

(i) Hydrophilicity: Hyaluronic acid is highly hydrophilic, which means that it retains water. This specific property makes it a perfect fit for hydration, as it can hold up to 1000 times its weight in water. This is the reason for hyaluronic acid being widely used in eye drops to maintain tear film stability and in skin products for keeping the skin moisturized.

(ii) Biocompatibility: A typical 70 kg human body contains 15 g of hyaluronic acid in synovial fluid, vitreous humor of the eye, skin, heart valves, umbilical cords and skeletal tissues [10]. As a naturally occurring substance in the body. Hyaluronic acid is generally well-tolerated with minimal adverse reactions. This biocompatibility makes it suitable for various medical applications, including dermal fillers, wound healing, and as a component in eye drops.

(iii) Viscoelasticity: Hyaluronic acid's large molecular weight allows it to act as a viscous liquid and elastic solid. This makes it excellent for lubricating joints and tissues, cushioning them and decreasing friction, which is very important in the treatment of osteoarthritis and other joint disorders.

(iv) Biodegradability: Hyaluronic acid is broken down by hyaluronidase enzymes (e.g., HYAL-1, HYAL-2) into smaller fragments that can be metabolized or eliminated from the body. This breakdown mechanism is critical to hyaluronic acid's function in cell signaling, wound healing and tissue engineering. Because of this property, it is commonly utilized in medical and cosmetic applications, including drug delivery systems and dermal fillers [11].

(v) Anti-inflammatory: Hyaluronic acid reduces inflammation by modulating the body's reactions. This feature is important in the treatment of illnesses such as osteoarthritis, where it reduces pain and improves joint function, as well as dry eye disease, where it soothes and protects the ocular surface.

All the above properties of hyaluronic acid make it a potential biomaterial to exhibit various functions in the human body from moisturizing the skin to filling the extracellular space [12]. Table 4.1 provides the list of functions performed by hyaluronic acid.

4.2.2 Hyaluronic acid-based scaffolds for tissue regeneration

Hyaluronic acid is having several applications in medical and cosmetic fields. It is a widely adopted biopolymer in tissue regeneration including dermatology, ophthalmology and orthopedics. Out of the various forms of hyaluronic acid, scaffolds are widely used in tissue regeneration. Scaffolds generally provide structural support for attachment of cell and tissue development [13]. The following are some key applications of hyaluronic acid-based scaffolds for tissue regeneration:

(i) Cardiovascular tissue engineering: Hyaluronic acid-based scaffolds are utilized to enhance regeneration of cardiovascular tissues, for instance, hyaluronic acid-coated biomaterials. These scaffolds improve left ventricular remodeling and cardiac repair, as well as support the growth and organization of smooth muscle cells, making them suitable for cardiovascular stents and heart valve tissue engineering. These scaffolds also improve blood circulation and terminated inflammation following infarction when implanted into the myocardial infarct region. Additionally, hyaluronic acid hydrogels enhance branching of vascular tube and seeding in endothelial colony-forming cells. These hydrogels also prevent cell restructuring and vascular development at the vacuole and lumen stages by generating kinetic chains. Overall, incorporating hyaluronic acid in copolymers and hydrogels shows promise for cardiovascular regeneration and therapies.

(ii) Brain and neural regeneration: Hyaluronic acid hydrogels are beneficial because of their capability to enhance penetration of blood vessel

Table 4.1 Functions of hyaluronic acid

Function	*Description*
Matrix structure maintenance	Hyaluronic acid helps in maintaining the structure of the extracellular matrix, particularly in cartilage and other connective tissues. In cartilage, hyaluronic acid binds specifically to proteoglycans like aggrecan with the help of link proteins, forming large aggregates that are essential for the tissue's structural integrity. These aggregates, which can weigh up to 100 MDa, are meticulously implanted within the collagen framework. This interaction is vital because the negatively charged polymers of the PGs bind water, which is necessary for the mechanical properties of cartilage. Without hyaluronic acid, the proteoglycans would not be retained within the cartilage, leading to water loss and, consequently, a loss of the tissue's mechanical properties. Thus, hyaluronic acid is indispensable for maintaining the matrix structure and ensuring the proper function of connective tissues.
Size-specific functions	Hyaluronic acid fragments perform a range of biological functions that are highly dependent on their size. Large hyaluronic acid polymers, with sizes ranging from 10^4 to 10^7 Da, are known for their space-filling, anti-angiogenic, and immunosuppressive properties. Intermediate-sized fragments, consisting of 25–50 disaccharide units, are associated with inflammatory and immunostimulatory activities, as well as being highly angiogenic. Smaller fragments, such as decasaccharides, can compete with larger fragments for receptor binding, while even smaller tetrasaccharides are known to be anti-apoptotic and induce heat shock proteins.
Lubrication	Concentrated hyaluronic acid solutions have remarkable rheological properties, showing viscoelastic behavior where their viscosity changes significantly with applied shear stress. Therefore, rotational viscometers are preferred for measuring the macroscopic properties of hyaluronic acid solutions. The primary shock-absorbing feature of synovial fluids is largely because of the viscoelastic nature of hyaluronic acid.
Steric Interactions	The steric interactions of hyaluronic acid play an important role in maintaining the structure and function of various tissues. At physiological concentrations, hyaluronic acid molecules form entangled networks that interact sterically with other macromolecular components in the tissue. These networks exclude larger molecules from the space they occupy, which helps to maintain the integrity and viscosity of the tissue.

(Continued)

Table 4.1 (Continued)

Function	*Description*
Signal Transduction	Hyaluronic acid plays a prominent role in signal transduction and cell-cell interaction. One of the most studied interactions is between hyaluronic acid and its receptor, CD44. This interaction initiates a variety of signal transduction pathways, influencing cell behavior. CD44 also interacts with the cytoskeleton, conferring motility upon cells, which is essential for processes like embryonic development and tumor cell movement. Another receptor, RHAMM, is involved in similar pathways and can substitute for CD44 when necessary. Hyaluronic acid's involvement at multiple levels, including opening tissue spaces and enabling cell movement, highlights its importance in cellular communication and function.

cells and nerve fibers. These can stimulate angiogenesis and neurite extension while preventing glial scar formation. Modified hyaluronic acid hydrogels also enhance neural stem/ progenitor cell proliferation and differentiation, supporting cell transplantation therapies in injured spinal cord and brain. In addition to this, these hydrogels when blended with other biomaterials like collagen improve cell adhesion and neural regeneration, making them ideal for various neural tissue engineering applications [14].

(iii) Cartilage repair: Hyaluronic acid-based scaffolds show significant promise in cartilage repair due to their unique biological and physicochemical properties. Hyaluronic acid-based scaffolds provide a suitable matrix for cartilage repair by enhancing the self-aggregation of mesenchymal stem cells (MSCs) and releasing bioactive components which foster MSC differentiation into cartilage cells. Additionally, hyaluronic acid-based scaffolds implanted with mesenchymal stem cells derived from bone marrow aspirate concentrate have demonstrated the capability to restore durable articular cartilage in knee. This approach offers better clinical outcomes and more durable cartilage repair compared to traditional methods like surgery.

(iv) Skin regeneration: The role of hyaluronic acid in promoting wound and burn healing is prominent. As it prevents tissue adhesion and scar formation, thiolated hyaluronic acid cross-linked scaffolds containing adipose-derived stem cells show promise as tissue-engineered adipose substitutes. Cross-linked hyaluronic acid-based biomaterials effectively treat wounds in various species, including rats, horses and dogs. Thiolated carboxymethyl hyaluronic acid enhances proliferation of keratinocyte, and cross-linked gels and films promote faster wound healing rates. Hyaluronic acid also aids in full-thickness skin wound healing, mitigating graft contracture and enhancing collagen expression. Composites of hyaluronic acid and adipose-derived tissue stem cells have shown complete healing of radiation-induced wounds. Hyaluronic acid scaffolds loaded with epidermal growth factor enhance dermis and epidermis formation, aiding in wound healing.

(v) Nanomedicines: The capacity to introduce minuscule amounts of medication, or nanoparticles, into the body holds the potential to enhance the efficiency and affordability of medications. These show promise as new and innovative biomaterial templates for the creation of hyaluronic acid-based nanogel particles that may find application in the encapsulation of drugs. Thus, a novel avenue for medication delivery is made possible by these nanocarrier-enhanced biomaterials. Gene delivery to the cornea and conjunctiva has been achieved by the development of hyaluronic acid and chitosan nanoparticles. They are ingested by CD44-mediated endocytosis and provide high transfection rates (up to 15%) without compromising cell viability. Paclitaxel (PTX), an insoluble anti-tumor drug, is delivered specifically to tumor cells with high levels of CD44 via lipid particles coated in hyaluronic acid. Furthermore, tumor-bearing animals administered PTX-hyaluronic acid systematically at dosages four times lower than those administered Taxol showed tumor shrinkage and a decrease in side effects. The targeted delivery of doxorubicin to tumors using hyaluronic acid-ceramide-based nanoparticles has also demonstrated a significant reduction in tumor growth in mice.

(vi) Drug delivery: The properties of hyaluronic acid such as viscoelastic, mucoadhesive and hydrophilicity make it highly suitable for drug delivery applications. It works well with the majority of excipients used in the treatment of cancer, rheumatoid arthritis and ophthalmology. It can be administered both topically and parentally. For instance, hyaluronic acid forms a protective film on the skin or cornea, creating a reservoir that releases drugs slowly, enhancing retention and efficiency. When administered intravenously, hyaluronic acid selectively transports medications to regions where these receptors are high by targeting particular receptors, such as CD44. Hyaluronic acid is effective in dermal delivery of drugs such as diclofenac, cyclosporine, ibuprofen and clindamycin phosphate, maintaining and localizing these drugs in the epidermis better than other gelling agents. Additionally, hyaluronic acid's mucoadhesive and viscoelastic properties make it an excellent vehicle for topical ophthalmic and nasal drug delivery, increasing the bioavailability of various drugs.

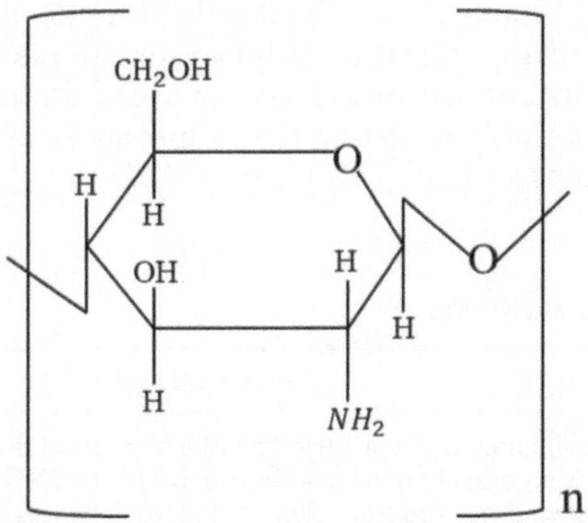

Figure 4.4 Structure of chitosan.

4.3 CHITOSAN

4.3.1 Chitosan: A versatile biomaterial for tissue engineering

Chitosan is a versatile biopolymer formed by the alkaline deacetylation of chitin, the earth's second most abundant natural biopolymer after cellulose. It is composed of N-acetyl-glucosamine and N-glucosamine linked by β-(1-4) glycosidic bonds as shown in Figure 4.4 in the existence of alkali. Higher the degree of deacetylation higher is the positive charge of the polymer, this makes chitosan cationic in nature. The cationic amino group of chitosan binds with anions on the bacterial cell wall, inhibiting biosynthesis. Additionally, chitosan disrupts mass transport across the cell wall, speeding up bacterial death. This ability of chitosan makes it antimicrobial against bacteria and fungi. Chitosan can also undergo various chemical modifications due to the presence of three functional groups namely primary, secondary hydroxyl groups and amino group at C-3, C-6, and C-2, respectively, which results in the useful derivatives of chitosan for tissue-specific applications [15, 16].

The versatility of chitosan results from its ability to be formulated in various forms such as gels, powders, films, sponges and nanofibers, and it also possesses certain characteristics such as biodegradability, biocompatibility and non-toxicity which make it a novel biomaterial scaffold in tissue engineering [17]. Because of these properties, chitosan is widely used in tissue regeneration, wound healing and in other applications listed in Table 4.2.

4.3.2 Surface modification strategies for chitosan

Even though chitosan possesses versatile chemical and biological properties, it can't be used in its pure form due to lack of bioactivity and mechanical strength, and poor solubility in neutral media. The surface chemistry of chitosan is crucial for cellular adhesion. Modifying the surface can increase its performance in certain applications such as medication delivery and tissue engineering [18]. Chitosan is subjected to several surface modifications such as:

Table 4.2 Applications of chitosan

Application	*Role of chitosan*
Wound healing	Chitosan's unique characteristics make it essential for wound healing. It is an organic, non-toxic, biocompatible and biodegradable polymer derived from chitin. Chitosan enhances wound healing by stimulating the actions of inflammatory and repairing cells. It helps in chemoattraction of macrophages and neutrophils leading to healing process. In addition, chitosan facilitates the development of granulation tissue and re-epithelization necessary for cutaneous wound healing process.
Bone	Biocompatible, biodegradable and bioactive features of chitosan that credit it as a critical component in bone tissue engineering. Chitosan, an organic biopolymer found in nature as a derivative of chitin, can be manipulated chemically and physically to modify its properties for special applications. Since it does not lead to significant adverse effects on the host, it is biocompatible and lends itself well in creating scaffolds. The fact that chitosan is biodegradable means it can break down inside the body, giving space for fresh bone growth as well as identity of the confinement at the time when new tissue shaped. The chitosan also has antibacterial properties which may help reduce the chances of infection in around implant area. Chitosan can also be combined with ceramics, synthetic polymers and natural polymer to improve mechanical and osteoconductive property; hence, it is true that chitosan has become a versatile material, where its incorporation of aforementioned materials interests many researches for bone tissue engineering.
Cartilage	Increased chondrocyte roundness by chitosan is also needed for maintenance of normal phenotypic characteristics and extracellular matrix molecule synthesis. The use of chitosan to coat substrates, poly (L-lactic acid) and alginate can promote the attachment enhance cell adhesion, proliferation and biosynthetic activity in bone. In addition, intra-articular injections of chitosan have proved to ameliorate epiphyseal cartilage in the joints and increase proliferation of chondrocytes. Chitosan is often combined with other materials, such as alginate and hyaluronic acid, to enhance cellular adhesion to form complexes that aid in the repair of cartilage. In addition, chitosan-based scaffolds enable sustained release of growth factors and enhance the chondrocyte ingrowth and biosynthetic activity, which postulates that chitosan-based scaffold is a type of "smart" biomaterial for cartilage tissue engineering.

(Continued)

Table 4.2 Continued

Application	*Role of chitosan*
Gene therapy	Chitosan and derivatives have been involved in gene therapy due to their good biocompatibility, biodegradability, low cytotoxicity. Its derivatives like nanoparticles, microspheres and gels have already been used as non-viral gene delivery vectors. These derivatives enhance the transfection efficiency while also protecting genes from nuclease breakdown in serum. The positive charge of chitosan allows it to form complexes with negatively charged DNA or RNA, facilitating the delivery of genetic material into cells. Additionally, chitosan derivatives can be modified to improve their solubility, stability and targeting capabilities, making them effective carriers for gene therapy. The ability to modify chitosan chemically enables the development of tailored delivery systems that can enhance the therapeutic efficacy of gene therapy by ensuring that the genetic material reaches the target cells efficiently and safely.

(i) Grafting onto chitosan: This includes connecting functional groups or polymers directly to the chitosan backbone. This technique takes use of chitosan's high functionality, which includes one primary amine and two hydroxyl groups per polysaccharide repeating unit. Various studies emphasize the grafting of vinyl monomers such as acrylonitrile, vinyl acetate, and methacrylate onto chitosan using initiators such as 2,2-azo-bisisobutyronitrile in aqueous acidic solutions. These approaches enable the manufacture of chitosan materials with specified functions, which improves their use in drug delivery systems, hydrogels, and porous scaffolds. This approach could provide routes in a plethora of patterns and the fusion of biological degradability with tunable properties afforded by synthetic polymers. This enhances the mechanical and biological functionalities of chitosan to a great extent. This provides an example, showing that chitosan revealed much improved application property when it was blended with polycaprolactone. The chitosan-polycaprolactone composite exhibited a swelling behavior upon drug loading and eluted drugs in PH-induced release profile. Moreover, chitosan has been altered with the aid of lactic acid which may act as a hydrogel for drug delivery systems.

(ii) Chitosan-based graft copolymerization: This procedure includes attaching side chains to the chitosan backbone, resulting in hybrid molecules containing both natural polysaccharides and synthetic polymers. This is an emerging field, and its growth is expected with the goal of its widespread applications such as pharmaceutical medication delivery systems, hydrogels and porous scaffolds. More importantly, graft copolymerization has twofold properties of low cost and biodegradability of the polysaccharide component.

Moreover, both the number of grafted side chains and degree-of-grafting (i.e., molecular structure) can be readily adjusted, enabling graft copolymers as an excellent technological tool for the preparation of functionalities and also rendering best performances on demand materials. This method considerably improves the mechanical, chemical and biological properties of chitosan for various biomedical applications. Polyacrylamide and poly(acrylic acid) will adhere to chitosan because of ceric ions. This allows the design of chitosan with certain properties.

(iii) Chitosan derivatives: As a nature-derived biopolymer, chitosan has been synthesized into various other derivatives (i.e., chitosan derivatives) with the introduction of functional groups to tailor materialistic properties for diverse applications. Alternatively, there may be addition of or substitution at the C-2 position by an amino group, hydroxyl groups to either (or both) the C-3 and C-6 places. The aim of this area is to enhance chitosan biodegradability, antibacterial property and hydrophilicity that bring them appropriate for pharmaceuticals and tissue engineering applications. For example, in a carboxylation reaction, the C6-OH or C2-NH2 groups of chitosan frequently reacted with glyoxylic acid or chloroalkanoic acid to create a COOH group. Carboxylated chitosan is extremely water soluble and may dissolve in both alkaline and neutral solutions. It also has superior thickening, heat retention, film formation, flocculation, and kneading properties than conventional chitosan. Furthermore, carboxylated chitosan has a broad range of uses in industry, agriculture, medicine, health and biochemical fields [19].

In summary, graft copolymers include side chains to create hybrid materials, chitosan derivatives modify specific functional groups to improve overall properties, and grafting onto chitosan attaches functional groups or polymers directly to the backbone to promote functionality.

4.4 DECELLULARIZED EXTRACELLULAR MATRIX (DECM)

The term "Decellularized Extracellular Matrix" refers to natural tissues or organs that have undergone a procedure known as decellularization to eliminate cells and antigenic components, leaving only the structural and functional proteins of the extracellular matrix [20]. The macromolecules found in this matrix forms a three-dimensional (3D) framework essential for tissue regeneration which includes collagen, elastin, fibronectin and also laminins. The extracellular matrix is a complex meshwork of proteins, glycoproteins and other chemicals that support tissue-based cells. ECM gives structural support, activity cell function and impact tissue integrity. Fundamentally, it is the scaffold that maintains and interconnects cells within a tissue. There are primarily two kinds of dECMs [21]:

(i) Organ/tissue-derived dECMs (O/T-dECMs): O/T-dECMs are sourced from specific organs or tissues. They produce a 3D porous environment that promotes cell infiltration and proliferation, essential for chondrogenesis. O/T-dECMs are non-cytotoxic and have good biocompatibility, making them suitable for supporting cell growth.

(ii) Cell-derived dECMs (C-dECMs): These are produced from chondrocytes or stem cells. The cells are cultured to form an extracellular matrix, which is then decellularized. This type of dECM supports cell proliferation and chondrogenic potential.

Both types are utilized to promote chondrogenesis by creating a scaffold that resembles the natural environment.

Decellularization strategies are widely classified into physical, chemical, biological and combinational procedures [20] as shown in Figure 4.5. Physical approaches modify tissue characteristics by temperature, stress and current interference, resulting in cell lysis and elimination. Freeze-thaw cycles, ultrasonic, pressure gradients, supercritical fluid dissolution and electroporation are some of the techniques used. These approaches are simple to use and prevent adverse effects, but they harm ECM structures and are

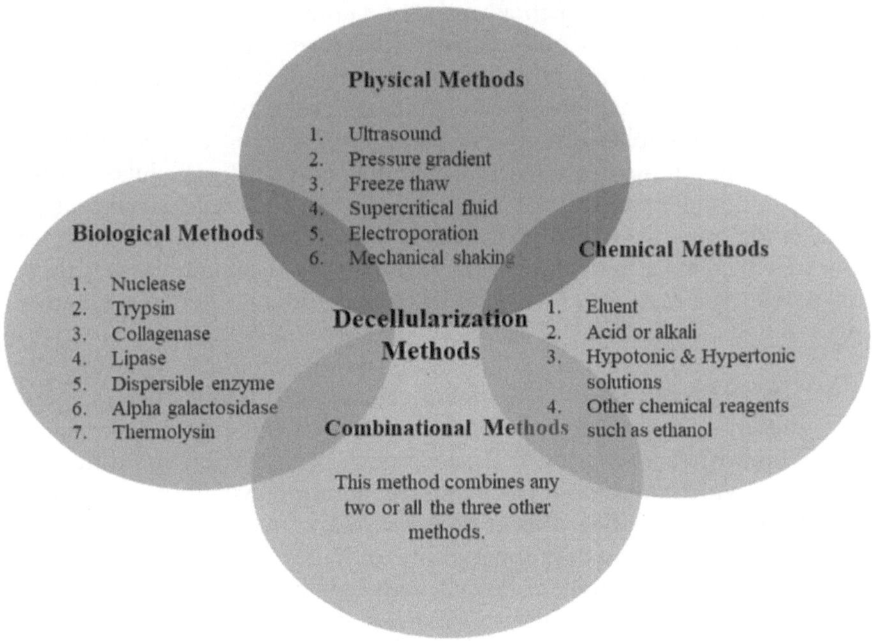

Figure 4.5 Various decellularization methods.

ineffective for thicker tissues. Chemical treatments, on the other hand, dissolve cells and other components while preserving the structure of the ECM by using chemicals such as acids, bases, detergents and solvents. Acetic acid, sodium hydroxide and Triton X-100 are all often used reagents. Chemical techniques eliminate cells effectively while causing minimum structural damage, although they may leave toxic residues and impair bioactivity.

However, biological approaches use enzymes like nucleases, trypsin and collagenase to selectively target and destroy cells. These approaches cause less harm to bioactive components but need precise control and longer processing durations. Residual enzymes can elicit immune responses. To address the shortcomings of existing approaches, a new method was developed which integrates physical, chemical and biological techniques to enhance decellularization efficiency and minimize ECM damage, so it is termed as combinational method. This procedure is targeted to specific tissues, using the advantages of two or more approaches to produce the best outcomes. For instance, complex tissues can be effectively decellularized while retaining mechanical qualities by combining freeze-thaw cycles with enzymatic digestion.

4.4.1 Decellularized extracellular matrix: Composition and advantages

Decellularized extracellular matrix scaffolds are composed mostly of extracellular macromolecules such as collagen, laminin, elastin, fibronectin and matricellular proteins. Collagen provides tensile strength and connects the framework of tissues and organs. Elastin offers elasticity and adjusts mechanical properties. Fibronectin regulates cell behavior and guides the formation of complex structures. Laminin promotes cell adhesion and migration, providing bioactive cross-linking sites. Matricellular proteins contain binding spots for cell surface receptors and ECM structural proteins, modulating the activities of specific growth factors. These components collectively create a three-dimensional framework that supports cell growth and tissue regeneration [21]. Due to its composition, it offers several advantages in tissue engineering [20]:

(i) Native Structure: dECMs retain the natural architecture of tissues, providing a scaffold that closely resembles the extracellular matrix. This structure supports cell attachment, proliferation and differentiation, which are crucial for tissue regeneration. Maintaining the structural integrity of dECMs at both micro and macro levels ensures that their tensile strength is comparable to that of native tissue scaffolds.

(ii) Good Biodegradability: dECMs with high biodegradability are essential for tissue engineering applications. dECMs are mostly made up of natural, degradable components. These compounds can be totally degraded into non-toxic metabolites that are safely eliminated from the body. To break down ECM components, inflammatory cells create oxidants and proteinases such as matrix metalloproteinases (MMPs) and metalloproteinase with thrombospodin motif families (ADAMTS). Such a fast prompt of newly forming and degenerating dECMs indicates the high biocompatibility and regeneration promoting action by these dECMs, without creating toxic remnants. For these reasons, dECMs are extremely well suited for regenerative medicine and tissue engineering applications.

(iii) Bioactive Substances: Several bioactive components present in dECMs that support regeneration of tissues. These include laminin, fibronectin (FN), collagen, elastin, glycosaminoglycans (GAGs), proteoglycans (PGs) and a range of growth factors, such as fibroblast growth factor (FGF), vascular endothelial growth factor (VGEF) and bone morphogenic protein (BMP-2). For instance, decellularized porcine brain has collagen, GAG and molecules like osteopontin, FGF-1 and FGF-2. Decellularized liver also contains type I and IV collagen, fibronectin, laminin and so on. These bioactive compounds are important key players for cell migration, differentiation and tissue construction in various tissue engineering applications, making dECMs highly useful.

(iv) Weak Immune Response: Due to their minimal immunological responses, dECMs are perfect for tissue engineering. Since most cells and antigenic components are removed during the decellularization process, the immunogenicity of dECMs – which are produced from natural tissues or organs – is significantly reduced. For instance, research indicates that DNA fragments with fewer than 200 base pairs do not significantly trigger inflammatory reactions. Additionally, by influencing the phenotypes of macrophages and T cells, dECMs can influence the immune response by promoting shift from pro-inflammatory (M1) to anti-inflammatory (M2) states. Its ability to modulate immunity is essential for creating the ideal conditions for tissue regeneration. For example, in models of spinal cord injuries, decellularized extracellular matrix from the porcine brain has been shown to promote M2 macrophage polarization and neurite outgrowth, suggesting that it may promote tissue regeneration without inducing undesirable immune reactions.

4.4.2 Applications of dECM in engineering different tissues

Because of the above advantages, dECMs can be widely employed in engineering different tissues such as:

(i) Heart: dECMs play an important role in cardiac tissue engineering by forming scaffolds that closely replicates the natural tissue environment.

Decellularization destroys cellular components from donor tissues but retains the structure properties and biochemical features of the ECM. This complete extracellular matrix contains vital proteins, growth factors and cytokines necessary for cellular responses such as adhesion, motility proliferation and differentiation. Decellularized ECM scaffolds are being explored for use within cardiac tissue engineering to provide a biocompatible and bioactive structure upon which cells such as cardiomyocytes or stem/progenitor cell can be re-implanted. These scaffolds have the potential to restore necessary mechanical integrity and elasticity of heart tissue, enabling complete regeneration and functional recovery that is not possible by non-bioengineered materials. Secondly, the decellularized ECM can be modified to better its properties whether simply by inclusion of anti-calcification treatments or vascularization approaches in order to enhance the incorporation as well as functionality of synthetic heart tissue. Together, the decellularized ECM scaffolds have shown exceptional potential for cardiac tissue engineering and regenerative medicine [22].

(ii) Tendon: Tendon dECMs have the ability to support tendon-like structures, emulating components in situ. Immature dECMs retain a structure that helps initiate cellular adhesion, migration and proliferation which is vital for biofunctional and biomechanical therapy of tendon injury since addition of cells would be done after the direct administration across sites. These matrices are manufactured from donated tissue that is processed to remove cells but retain the necessary structure and biochemistry of extracellular matrix. This preserves all of the critical proteins, growth factors and signaling molecules required for tissue regeneration. By shaping dECMs into thin sheets and multilayered constructs, the mechanical properties can be increased as well as promote cellular ingress. Previous studies reported dECM-based scaffolds could enhance cell homogeneity and alignment, promote upregulation of tendon-related genes expression in vivo, as well as improve the mechanical properties of repaired tissue. Additionally, dECMs can be combined with growth factors or utilized in dynamic culture systems to further enhance regenerative potential. Collectively, dECMs present an exciting avenue in the creation of biologically functional and structurally supportive tendon repair scaffolds that simulate normal tendon tissue [22].

(iii) Cartilage: dECMs formed from cartilage-forming cells and tissues can be biomaterials for cartilage regeneration using chemical, physical and enzymatic approaches. Both types of dECMs (T-dECMs and C-dECMs) are biocompatible and promote chondrogenesis by modulating cell proliferation and differentiation. Notably, cartilage T-dECMs are more successful at promoting chondrogenic differentiation, whereas C-dECMs increase chondrocyte/stem cell proliferation and chondrogenic abilities. Microarchitecture (mean pore size and fiber diameter), micromechanical qualities, insoluble components (collagen and GAGs), and soluble variables all play a role in these discrepancies. This indicates that C-dECMs and T-dECMs are both suitable to maintain the chondrogenic potential of cells when reseeded, giving these scaffolds as a new option for therapies in cartilage disorders [23].

(iv) Kidney: Both enzymatic digestion and a 1% SDS-based method successfully decellularized kidneys, with less than 10% residual DNA. This kidney dECM, which retains glomerulus, tubule and vasculature structure is then used to provide the scaffold for stem cells in renal regeneration. Embryonic stem cells adhered and displayed higher levels of renal marker production as well as capability to differentiate into endothelial and tubular cell while grown atop kidney dECM, whereas adipose tissue-derived stem cells also increased in secondary gene expression when cultured on liver dECM. Similarly, papillae-derived renal stem cells exhibited region-specific differentiation on kidney dECM. These findings suggest that kidney dECM retains renal-specific biochemical and biophysical cues that impact cell proliferation, differentiation and maturation. Hypoxia-inducible factor (HIF-1α) stimulates renal regeneration on dECM scaffolds by stimulating prominin-1 positive cells and expressing regeneration markers such as nephrin and nestin [24].

(v) Bone: dECMs are the excellent option to bone transplantation. It has been shown in many studies carried out in vitro as well as in vivo that decellularized bone extracellular matrix (dbECM) could be an effective bioactive scaffold for inducing osteogenesis and promoting the differentiation of mesenchymal stem cells into new bone. In addition, dbECM often mixed with collagen alone or other substances such as hydroxyapatite (HA), bone morphogenetic proteins (BMPs) and growth factor for enhancement of bone formation. A study illustrated that SDF-1α (stromal-derived factor) preconditioned decellularized bone scaffolds coated with collagen/hyaluronic acid and subcutaneously delivered stimulated MSC osteogenesis.

(vi) Liver: dECM has been tested in the field of tissue engineering. The perfusion-based decellularization can maintain the liver macro and micro architecture, rendering it a nearly ideal ECM scaffold for recellularization followed by implantation. Liver dECM was not only used to regenerate liver transplant variant but it also served as an in vitro model for the study of hepatic disease. For instance, their dECM was shown to promote differentiation and function of liver cells, revealing potential applications in experimental fibrosis models [25]. Besides, liver dECM-derived hydrogels can outperform collagen with regard to maintaining the function of liver cells under 3D bio-printing [26]. Nevertheless, several unproven questions surrounding the full endothelization of the vascular network and better cell-seeding techniques need to be addressed.

(vii) Lung: The methodologies commonly used for decellularizing of the lung ECM are vascular perfusion and airway decellularization. The real difficulty is holding onto that the ECM during the process. However, early approaches showed that the barrier-mediated cell injury led to subsequent blood leakage into airways at implantation. Newer protocols aim to improve this. Recellularization strategies focus on epithelial cells, with various cell types like fetal epithelial cells, alveolar progenitor cells and induced pluripotent stem cells showing growth or differentiation on acellular lung tissue. Preclinical research studies have shown that dECM lungs recellularized with airway and vascular cells can perform gas exchange in rodent models for up to 14 days [24–26].

(viii) Muscle: dECM demonstrates the ability to be used in various tissue repair and regeneration. Combining dECM with insulin-like growth factor-1 significantly enhances muscle tissue regeneration by supporting cell differentiation and proliferation [27–29]. The dECM-based scaffolds showed high cell viability and proliferation in vitro and improved muscle regeneration in a rabbit muscle defect model. This approach offers a promising alternative to cell-based tissue engineering strategies, potentially overcoming limitations such as donor tissue shortages and extensive cell expansion processes [30–33].

REFERENCES

[1] Ana Marina Ferreira, Piergiorgio Gentile et al., Collagen for bone tissue regeneration, *Acta Biomaterialia*, 8 (2012) 3191–3200.

[2] Michael Meyer, Processing of collagen based biomaterials and the resulting materials properties, *Biomedical Engineering Online*, 18 (2019) 24.

[3] Sharma, R., Kim, M., & Gupta, A. (2022). Motor imagery classification in brain-machine interface with machine learning algorithms: Classical approach to multi-layer perceptron model. *Biomedical Signal Processing and Control*, 71, 103101, 10.1016/j.bspc.2021.103101

[4] Jayaraman, R., Alshehri, M., Kumar, M., Abugabah, A., Samant, S. S., & Mohamed, A. A. (2023). Secure biomedical document protection framework to ensure privacy through blockchain. *Big Data*, 11(6), 437–451, 10.1089/big.2022.0170

[5] Youbin Li, Yuzhe Liu, Ronghang Li et al. (2021). Collagen-based biomaterials for bone tissue engineering, *Materials & Design*, 210, 110049.

[6] Wen-Hui Huang, Sheng-Long Ding et al. (2023). Collagen for neural tissue engineering: Materials, strategies, and challenges, *Materials Today Bio*, 20, 100639.

[7] KC Kuo, RZ Lin, HW Tien, PY Wu, YC Li, JM Melero-Martin, & YC Chen (2015) Bioengineering vascularized tissue constructs using an injectable cell-laden enzymatically crosslinked collagen hydrogel derived from dermal extracellular matrix, *Acta Biomaterialia*, 27, 151–166.

[8] S Zhang, J Dong, R Pan, Z Xu, M Li, & R Zang (2023). Structures, properties, and bioengineering applications of alginates and hyaluronic acid, *Polymers*, 15, 2149.

[9] NM Salwowska, KA Bebenek, DA Żądło, & DL Wcisło-Dziadecka (2016). Physiochemical properties and application of hyaluronic acid: A systematic review, *Journal of Cosmetic Dermatology*, 15(4), 520–526.

[10] Alexander Huynh, Ronny Priefer (2020). Hyaluronic acid applications in ophthalmology, rheumatology, and dermatology, *Carbohydrate Research*, 489, 107950.

[11] N Maurice (2013). Collins, Colin Birkinshaw, Hyaluronic acid based scaffolds for tissue engineering – A review, *Carbohydrate Polymers*, 92, 1262–1279.

[12] Grigorij Kogan, Ladislav Soltes et al. (2008). Hyaluronic acid: Its function and degradation in *in vivo* systems, *Studies in Natural Products Chemistry*, 34, 789–882.

[13] Santhosh Kumar, H.S., & Karibasappa, K. (2022). An effective hybrid deep learning with adaptive search and rescue for brain tumor detection. *Multimedia Tools and Applications*, 81(13), 17669–17701, 10.1007/s11042-022-12474-2

[14] Eun Ji Chung, Adam E Jakus, Ramille N Shah (2013). In situ forming collagen–hyaluronic acid membrane structures: Mechanism of self-assembly and applications in regenerative medicine, *Acta Biomaterialia*, 9, 5153–5161.

[15] Chunmeng Shi, Ying Zhu, Xinze Ran et al. (2006). Therapeutic potential of chitosan and its derivatives in regenerative medicine, *Journal of Surgical Research*, 133, 185–192.

[16] J Fourie, F Taute, L du Preez et al. (2022). Chitosan composite biomaterials for bone tissue engineering—A review. *Regenerative Engineering and Translational Medicine* 8, 1–21.

[17] Florence Croisier, Christine Jérôme (2013). Chitosan-based biomaterials for tissue engineering, *European Polymer Journal*, 49, 780–792.

[18] Dilip Depan, Raj Pal Singh (2015). Surface modification of chitosan and its implications in tissue engineering and drug delivery, *Surface Modification of Biopolymers*, first edition. Edited by Vijay Kumar Thakur and Amar Singh Singha. John Wiley & Sons. https://doi.org/10.1002/9781119044901.ch2

[19] W Wang, Q Meng, Q Li, J Liu, M Zhou, Z Jin, K Zhao (2020). Chitosan derivatives and their application in biomedicine, *International Journal of Molecular Sciences*, 21(2), 487.

[20] Jie Liao, Bo Xu et al. (2020). Applications of decellularized materials in tissue engineering: advantages, drawbacks and current improvements, and future perspectives, *Journal of Materials Chemistry B*, 8, 10023–10049.

[21] Xuewei Zhang, Xi Chen et al. (2022). Decellularized extracellular matrix scaffolds: Recent trends and emerging strategies in tissue engineering, *Bioactive Materials*, 10, 15–31.

[22] Aleksandra A. Golebiowska et al. (2024). Decellularized extracellular matrix biomaterials for regenerative therapies: Advances, challenges and clinical prospects, *Bioactive Materials*, 32, 98–123.

[23] Y Sun, Lianqi Yan, Song Chen, Ming Pei (2018). Functionality of decellularized matrix in cartilage regeneration: A comparison of tissue versus cell sources, *Acta Biomaterialia* https://doi.org/10.1016/j.actbio.2018.04.048

[24] DA Taylor et al. (2018). Decellularized matrices in regenerative medicine, *Acta Biomaterialia*. https://doi.org/10.1016/j.actbio.2018.04.044

[25] MA Karsdal, T Manon-Jensen, F Genovese, JH Kristensen, MJ Nielsen, JM Sand, NU Hansen, AC Bay-Jensen, CL Bager, A Krag, A Blanchard, H Krarup, DJ Leeming, & D Schuppan (2015). Novel insights into the function and dynamics of extracellular matrix in liver fibrosis, *American Journal of Physiology. Gastrointestinal and Liver Physiology*, 308, G807–G830.

[26] Swain, S., Bhushan, B., Dhiman, G., & Viriyasitavat, W. (2022). Appositeness of optimized and reliable machine learning for healthcare: a survey. *Archives of Computational Methods in Engineering*, 29(6), 3981–4003. 10.1007/s11831-022-09733-8

[27] Hyeongjin Lee et al. (2020). A novel decellularized skeletal muscle-derived ECM scaffolding system for in situ muscle regeneration, *Methods*, 171, 77–85.

[28] Thapliyal, S., Wazid, M., Singh, D. P., Das, A. K., Shetty, S., & Alqahtani, A. (2023). Design of robust Blockchain-envisioned authenticated key management mechanism for smart healthcare applications. *IEEE Access*, 10.1109/ACCESS.2023.3310264

[29] Pawar, D., Phansalkar, S., Sharma, A., Sahu, G. K., Ang, C. K., & Lim, W. H. (2023). Survey on the Biomedical Text Summarization Techniques with an Emphasis on Databases, Techniques, Semantic Approaches, Classification Techniques, and Similarity Measures. *Sustainability, 15*(5), 4216. 10.3390/su15054216

[30] Madan, P., Singh, V., Singh, D. P., Diwakar, M., & Kishor, A. (2022). Denoising of ECG signals using weighted stationary wavelet total variation. *Biomedical Signal Processing and Control*, *73*, 103478. 10.1016/j.bspc.2021.103478

[31] Wazid, M., Singh, J., Das, A. K., Shetty, S., Khan, M. K., & Rodrigues, J. J. (2022). ASCP-IoMT: AI-enabled lightweight secure communication protocol for internet of medical things. *IEEE Access*, *10*, 57990–58004, 10.1109/ACCESS.2022.3179418

[32] Alrashed, F. A., Alsubiheen, A. M., Alshammari, H., Mazi, S. I., Al-Saud, S. A., Alayoubi, S., ... & Dhiman, G. (2022). Stress, anxiety, and depression in pre-clinical medical students: Prevalence and association with sleep disorders. *Sustainability*, *14*(18), 11320. 10.3390/su141811320

[33] Gupta, P., Gupta, H., Kairamkonda, M., Kumar, N., & Poluri, K. M. (2022). Elucidating the lactic acid tolerance mechanism in vaginal clinical isolates of Candida glabrata. *Medical Mycology*, *60*(6), myac042. https://doi.org/10.1093/mmy/myac042

Chapter 5

Advanced synthetic biomaterials for tissue engineering and regenerative medicine

Pooja Bhati, Alok Srivastava, Pankaj Chauhan, and Aiman Zakir

5.1 INTRODUCTION

Synthetic biomaterials were developed by humans that are compatible with tissue, blood, and biological fluids. These biomaterials are the future in the medical field, finding various applications exhibiting multifunctionality, especially in pharmaceutical and bone tissue engineering [1]. These man-made biomaterials are used in medicine and almost all parts of the human body from eye lenses, catheters, stents, heart valves, pacemakers, dentistry, orthopedics, drug delivery, nanomedical applications, and wound healing. A wide range of applications of synthetic biomaterials are possible due to their tailored properties, low cost, and ease of manufacturing [2, 3]. Based on applications and requirements, synthetic biomaterials can be classified into three groups: polymers, metals, and ceramics. These groups are further subdivided into degradable and non-degradable biomaterials, as shown in Figure 5.1.

However, synthetic biomaterials have a few disadvantages, including their structure, composition, impurities, and addition of inhibitors/compatibilizers, which was used to improve physicomechanical properties. This may negatively affect the interaction with native tissues/organs, causing tissue inflammation, biocompatibility, stress shielding, and low tissue remodeling.

Hence, developing synthetic biomaterials has many challenges to overcome. They require state-of-the-art materials science and bioengineering combined with the latest manufacturing technologies.

5.2 POLYMERIC BIOMATERIALS

Today, polymeric biomaterials are essential in stimulating healing, tissue regeneration, drug delivery, and other biofunctional activities. Polymeric biomaterials have been used for various applications, including tissue engineering scaffolds, mimicking specific cellular functions, medical implants, and devices [4, 5]. Polymeric biomaterials derived naturally or synthetically have been successfully exploited for different uses in the biomedical domain

DOI: 10.1201/9781003536352-5

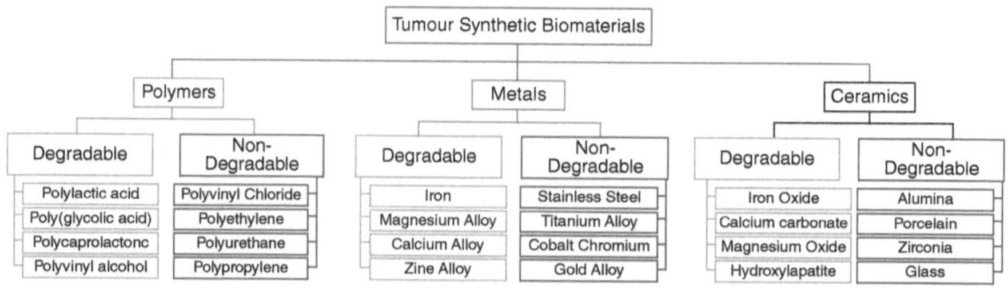

Figure 5.1 Classification of synthetic biomaterials.

owing to their excellent biocompatibility, mechanical stability, and biodegradability. However, as the complexity of these applications increases, the demand for new materials with sophisticated characteristics also increases, particularly adjustable or customizable materials with enhanced bioactivity.

Hence, polymers can be classified into two main groups based on their source: natural and synthetic biopolymers.

Naturally derived biopolymers demonstrate high biocompatibility, biodegradability, and tissue remodeling. Therefore, these are applied to repair or replace damaged human tissues or organs or mimic the biological and mechanical function. Natural biopolymers can be categorized into chitin/chitosan, cellulose, and glucose which are polysaccharide-based, protein-based biopolymers: silk, collagen, and gelatin; glycosaminoglycan-derived and tissue/organ-derived biopolymers: livers, blood vessels, and decellularized heart valves [6–8].

On the other side, synthetic biopolymers have several other advantages, such as their application in regenerative medicine and achieving sustained drug release [9]. The most widely used synthetic polymers for biomedical applications are polyanhydrides (PA), saturated aliphatic polyesters (SAP), and polyurethanes (PU). These polymers can be mass-producible, attain high quality, and address desired bulk and surface properties. Moreover, they show good processibility in a wide range of shapes, high toughness, low specific weight, low frictional properties, and cost-effectiveness [10]. This makes them suitable for cardiovascular, breast implants, eye lenses, orthopedic, orthodontic, soft tissue scaffolds, and artificial tendons [11]. Hence, these materials were preferred over metals and ceramics due to the following benefits, as follows:

- Easy to fabricate: Polymers can easily be fabricated into many shapes and sizes depending on the clinical application [12–14].
- Compatible with tissues: Many bioresorbable polymers have a very close resemblance to natural tissues, such as PLLA, PLGA, and PCL.
- Available with a choice: A wide variety of polymers are available with different properties, such as transparent, degradable, non-degradable, high-strength and brittle [15, 16].

- Non-corrosive: Unlike many metals, polymers are less corrosive.
- Low density: The densities of polymeric implants are closer to natural tissues.

However, still, a few limitations must be overcome, such as low mechanical strength, brittleness, slower degradation rate, high deformability, residual initiators, and other residual compounds or present impurities that can compromise cellular response [17].

Thus, researchers are developing advanced and novel polymeric materials by forming newer compositions using natural and/or synthetic polymer blends by incorporating compatibilizers/nanoparticles/metals/ceramics. Furthermore, to enhance biocompatibility, the blends can be surface treated [18, 19] and coated with bioactive materials while, at the same time, possessing good thermomechanical properties. Thus, polymeric biomaterials can be further characterized based on degradability into biodegradable and non-biodegradable polymers.

5.2.1 Biodegradable polymers

Many biodegradable polymeric materials have been investigated for biomedical engineering applications. These biodegradable polymers, after restoring the natural state of the tissue/organs, are absorbed *in vivo* or degraded over time without traumatizing the tissues. Thus, the major advantage of degradation is to eliminate the need for a second surgery, reduce long-term inflammation, and shorten prolonged medication over other permanent biomaterials.

Commonly categorized as polyesters, polyanhydrides, or polyorthoesters, bioabsorbable polymers each have a different degradation rate. In addition to lowering the risk of immunological reactions or the spread of bacteria or viruses, synthetic biodegradable polymers can be engineered to improve mechanical and chemical properties [12]. New generations of biodegradable polymers are free from toxic and mutagenic effects [20].

Nevertheless, these implants have several issues, including an unstable degradation rate that can release a high amount of by-products near the tissue and biopolymer interface, leading to failure of implants for long-term use and tissue necrosis. Additionally, high mechanical stiffness, unfavorable tissue responses, hydrophobicity, strength restrictions, foreign body reactions, and infection are a few other limitations [14, 21, 22].

5.2.2 Non-degradable polymers

Non-degradable polymers are used in biomedicine and as a permanent scaffold. It is resistant to physiological fluid over time, delivers excellent mechanical performance, and remains bioinert throughout the patient's life span. They are easily manufactured in various desirable shapes and can be combined with different types of materials. Similarly, surface coatings improve the tolerance and acceptance of tissue [23].

Non-degradable polymers are used in manufacturing orthopedic implants, heart valves, vascular grafts, artificial hips, bone cement, drug delivery systems, ocular lenses, and bone and cartilage substitutes. For example, electrically simulating devices such as pacemakers are provided with protective coatings.

High-density polyethylene, polyesters, and silicone rubber were investigated for a variety of devices and implants for various clinical uses as given in Table 5.1 [24].

These polymers with chemical linkages provide resistance to hydrolytic degradation and oxidation in biological environments. Furthermore, poly(olefins), PUs, poly(carbonates), poly-siloxanes, poly(amides), poly(ethers), poly(sulphones), and specific varieties of poly(esters) are among the other primary classes of non-biodegradable synthetic polymers.

There are significant drawbacks of non-degradable biopolymers, as they stay useless for their whole life. As a result, it leads to chronic stress and imposes unnecessary strains at the implant site, long endothelial dysfunction, thrombogenicity, permanent physical irritation, and mismatches in

Table 5.1 General properties and major biomedical applications of non-degradable synthetic polymers

Non-degradable polymers	*Properties*	*Biomedical applications*
Poly(propylene)-(PP)	Linear thermoplastic, high toughness and good resistance to fatigue, and flexible	Medical pouches, non-absorbable sutures, and mesh manufacturing for hernia application
Poly(ethylene)-(PE)	Linear thermoplastic, excellent chemical resistance, low and high-density grades	Total hip, knee, and spine implants
Poly(dimethyl siloxane)-(PDMS)	Excellent viscoelastic properties, Transparent, high elasticity, non-toxic, bioinert, non-flammable	Prosthesis, contact lens, breast implant
Polyurethane-PU)	Depending on crosslinking, it can become biostable or biodegradable.	Pacemaker, vascular grafts, catheters
Poly(methyl methacrylate)-(PMMA)	Transparent thermoplastic with higher impact strength and poor chemical resistance and also lighter in weight	Encapsulation device for cells, orthopedic, dental, controlled release of peptide and protein drug
Poly(ether ether ketone)-(PEEK)	Superior mechanical properties and chemically resistant	Spinal fusion, disc arthroplasty, interspinous spacers

mechanical behavior between implant and tissue. Furthermore, causing chronic inflammation, local reactions, and inability to adapt in young patients' growth leads to re-surgery.

5.2.3 Bioceramics

Ceramics, in general, can be defined as oxides, nitrides, sulfides, or carbides of metals and metalloids. Bioceramics are any ceramic, glass, or glass-ceramic materials that are used as a biomaterial. They form an important subset of biomaterials and due to advancements in processing technology, their applications in the medical field have increased many fold since the 20th century. Reconstructive surgeons first used ceramic implant biomaterials. In 1964, alumina was used to make dental implants; in 1970, alumina (Al_2O_3), zirconia (ZrO_2), and bioglass bioceramics were further developed for clinical application [25].

Bioceramics can be classified based on origin synthetic or natural. Bioceramic materials have excellent biocompatibility and better mechanical properties than metallic biomaterials. They also have high melting temperatures and are non-corrosive. However, bioceramics have low fracture toughness and low elastic modulus, and are harder and more fragile compared to bone. Their applications include making implants for hard and soft tissues, as a drug delivery carrier, in dentistry for teeth restoration, stents, and heart valves fabrication, etc. Based on the needs for the particular application in body parts, these material's properties like mechanical, physical, and biological properties can be further modified [26].

Synthetic ceramic materials are classified as bioactive, bioinert, and bioresorbable based on the interaction of the implant material and body tissues.

5.2.4 Bioactive ceramics

The term "bioactive" is used along with the material or surface that exhibits active interactions with the tissues where they are implanted and shows biocompatibility properties somewhat between bioinert and bioresorbable materials. These materials in contact with bone/tissues generate an artificial hydroxyl apatite layer which has a composition similar to natural hydroxyapatite found in the bone and can bind with the bone. This ability of bone bonding is termed "osteoconductivity" or "bioactivity." Osteoconductive properties along with the high corrosion resistance of bioactive ceramics make them the material of choice for coating the bone graft implants. They act as scaffolds by enhancing bone formation on the implant and bone graft surfaces. Tissue engineering applications of bioactive materials include dental (regeneration of bone and dental tissue), repair of craniofacial structures like skull and face bones in trauma, graft materials in chronic osteomyelitis, etc. The commonly used bioceramics in this category are bioglasses (BG) and bioactive glass ceramics.

5.2.4.1 Bioglasses/glass ceramics

The term bioactive glass was first coined by Larry Hench in 1969. Bioglass (BG) was first used in bone replacement in the 1970s. The bioactivity of bioglasses can be explained based on two mechanisms: (i) the ability to bond with bone by forming an apatite layer on its surface when it comes in contact with body fluids/ similar environments and (ii) the release of ions that are biologically active to stimulate the particular process of integration or regeneration [27, 28].

The main compositions of bioglass are CaO and P_2O_5. The bioactivity of bioglasses is attributed to Ca and P present as the main constituents similar to the natural bone. Other constituents like MgO, Na_2O, or CaF_2 can also be added to the bioglass to modify or tailor their bioactivity as per specific applications. Bioglasses can be further classified based on their compositions: i) silicate based, ii) borate based, and iii) phosphate based. 45S5 Bioglass is the first original bioglass synthesized by Hench. Borate glasses have higher reactivity compared to silicate materials, and phosphate glasses come in the resorbable category as their dissolution rate is high and can be tuned by adjusting the oxide content [27].

The application of bioglasses for soft tissue regeneration and replacement includes peripheral nerve regeneration, heart valves, lung parts, and ophthalmology applications. The hard tissue applications include mainly bones and dental tissues and the material properties can be tailored based on the distribution of pore and morphology, surface area, and glass composition and fabrication methodology. Different application requirements can be achieved by changing the fabrication methods (like sol-gel method can be used instead of the melt-quench method to improve the osteoconductivity), altering the process parameters, composition, and so on. The newer emerging applications and research directions of bioactive glasses are neuromuscular repair (it consists of fibrous constructs for muscle repair and regeneration as well as neural/nerve regeneration), orbital implants and artificial cornea in ophthalmology, engineering of cardiac tissue engineering, and cancer therapy [29].

Bioactive glass ceramics are another class of bioactive ceramics that are polycrystalline unlike bioglass (amorphous). They are fabricated by a process where first glass is formed by quenching melt followed by pouring the molten glass into mold resulting in controlled polycrystalline materials. It exhibits higher mechanical properties, but lesser bioactivity compared to bioglass. Their main applications include dental restorations like onlays, crowns, and bridges where moderate to high strength is required. The commercial example of glass ceramic for coating of implants and bone fillers includes cerabone. It is composed of apatite (38 wt%) and wollastonite (34 wt%), and the remaining is glass phase [30, 31].

5.2.4.2 *Bioresorbable ceramics*

Bioresorbable ceramics are completely resorbed and replaced by the new tissues inside the body. They are degraded by either chemical or biological processes, and the degradation products are also biocompatible. These are used as an alternative to polymeric biomaterials as the major drawback of polymeric biomaterials like polylactic acid is that they release acidic by-products which cause inflammation to local tissues inside the human body. This class of bioceramics includes calcium and sulphate and calcium phosphate-based ceramics. Synthetic and porous hydroxyapatite (Hap) are similar to natural hydroxyapatite that exists inside the body [32, 33].

Synthetic hydroxyapatite ($Ca_{10}(PO4)_6(OH)_2$) has a composition similar to that found in natural bones and is widely used in bone repair. It is an alloplastic material, crystalline in nature and biocompatible. The Ca/P ratio is 1:67 which has a similar chemistry as found in the mineralized bone and thus has an osteoconductive property and ability to bond with the bone. The major drawbacks of this class of materials are the poor mechanical properties (low fracture toughness, brittle, and low Young's modulus) of the scaffold. Recent research in nanohydroxyapatite powder has led to improvement in its mechanical properties. Various methods are being investigated to fabricate nanohydroxyapatite and scaffold constructs like the sol-gel method, microemulsion, hydrothermal, etc. At the nanoscale, hydroxyapatite power has become the main attraction to improve biological and mechanical properties. Further hydroxyapatite can carry growth factors and drugs, thus significantly enhancing the osteogenic ability of the scaffold. This capacity paves a carrier for these materials in drug delivery applications. HA is brittle with lower Young's modulus and fracture toughness [34].

5.2.4.3 *Calcium sulphate*

Naturally occurring calcium sulphate is an inorganic crystalline material and has osteoconductive properties. It is used as a hemihydrate and dihydrate form and applications include dentistry and orthopedics. Although its compressive strength is similar to cancellous bone, the material is very brittle. It can be used in powder form, as pellets, or as an injectable suspension. The α-hemihydrate form is advocated as a component of bone graft material due to better handling with regard to injectability, appropriate resorption rate, good biocompatibility, and ability to induce hemostasis and angiogenesis. Also, it is used nowadays as an antibiotic carrier to prevent surgical site infections [35].

5.2.4.4 *Calcium phosphate (CaP)*

Calcium phosphate-based ceramics have a slower degradation rate as compared to calcium sulphate. Different forms of calcium phosphates like tricalcium phosphate (TCP), dicalcium phosphate (DCP), biphasic calcium phosphate (BCP), fluorapatite (FAp), amorphous hydroxyapatite (ACp), etc. are used in bone tissue engineering. These different forms have different bioactivities based on differences in degradation and solubility as well as based on different Ca/P ratio [36]. Biodegradation or resorption rate further depends on several factors like composition of the material, surface area and porosity, and crystal structure. For example, materials having body-centered cubic crystal structures are less stable due to open structure, so, they dissolve at a faster rate than face-canter crystal structures. The most commonly used CaP ceramics in bone tissue engineering are beta-tricalcium phosphate, synthetic hydroxyapatite, and biphasic calcium phosphate.

5.2.5 Bioinert ceramics

5.2.5.1 Alumina

Alumina was first used to fabricate femur head implants in the 1970s. Alumina forms stable oxide due to the strong ionic and covalent bond between aluminum and oxygen, thus making it resistant to galvanic reactions or corrosion. Alumina possesses high surface smoothness and energy. The other properties of alumina, like high corrosion resistance, abrasion resistance, chemical inertness, and good mechanical strength, make it suitable for applications in hard tissue replacement/repair (orthopedic and dental implants).

The high standard of quality assurance during the manufacturing of Al_2O_3 implants is mandatory if the implants are to be used for making orthopedic prostheses, especially in younger patients as these prostheses are to be used in the long run. Due to aging and fatigue, there is degradation in the mechanical properties of alumina which leads to failure of implants in long-term use if not fabricated by strict protocols. Other clinical applications of alumina include orthopedic applications like prosthetic knee, bone replacement, maxillofacial reconstruction, bone screws, and dental implants.

Porous alumina is also used as a scaffold material for bone tissues. It can also be used for coating the implant materials making porous ceramic prosthetic devices. For success as a porous scaffold, there should be a functional balance between porosity and mechanical strength as the size of pores, their interconnectivity, and distribution affect the osteoconductive properties of the resultant material [37].

5.2.5.2 Zirconia

Zirconia oxide occurs in three crystal phases/structures i) monoclinic, ii) tetragonal, and iii) cubic based on the processing temperature. There is a reduction in the mechanical properties of zirconia due to phase transformation (from tetragonal to monoclinic). This can lead to cracking so various oxides are added to zirconia as zirconia stabilizers, like yttria (Y_2O_3), MgO, CaO, and CeO_2. These stabilizers prevent phase transformation and thus show enhanced mechanical performance [38]. The better mechanical properties of zirconia make it a superior ceramic compared to alumina. This material also possesses color/shades matching the natural teeth and has good mechanical properties. Hence it is the most preferred in dentistry for the fabrication of veneers, crowns, multiunit bridges, and orthodontic brackets [39].

The aging of zirconia (degradation over the time inside human body) is the major shortcoming. The presence of water leads to phase transformation, resulting in surface roughness and further proceeding to the crack and fractures. Hence, despite the superior mechanical properties of zirconia, alumina is still used in weight-bearing implants. To overcome this problem, partially stabilized zirconia was introduced. Yttria-stabilized zirconia is an example of this and is widely used nowadays in clinical applications [40].

Additionally, alumina-zirconia composites are also introduced to reduce the phase transformation in zirconia with better mechanical properties. Titania (TiO_2) is also added to these composites to enhance the sintering process. These composites showed good bioactivity, are non-corrosive, and can be used as implants in bone tissues [41].

5.2.5.2.1 Non-oxide bioinert ceramics

Nitrides and carbon are classified as non-oxide based bioinert ceramic materials. Although carbon is a good biomaterial, it is not useful or has gained success for strength-bearing orthopedic device applications. Carbon also can inhibit blood clotting at its interface with the tissues. So, these materials also have applications in cardiac valve prostheses as well as a coating material on implants. Advancement in the fabrication of carbon nanotubes (CNT) results in excellent mechanical properties like improved fracture toughness and strength. Carbon nanotubes also have applications in nerve tissue engineering. Nitrides are used as a coating material on metallic components of prostheses. They improve the surface hardness and increase the wettability of the metallic surface of the prosthesis or implants.

5.3 HYDROGELS

Hydrogels are a group of polymeric materials that are predominantly useful for different biological and various biomedical applications. Hydrogels possess a remarkable ability to both absorb and hold vast quantities of water [42, 43]. They are networks of crosslinked polymers which have a three-dimensional structure that could mimic soft tissue properties like softness porosity and high moisture content [44].

The diverse properties of hydrogels, including their biocompatibility, biodegradability, and precise drug release profile, make them a suitable and popular candidate for the delivery of drugs [45]. In addition to their drug delivery applications, hydrogels have found use in other biomedical fields, such as tissue engineering, wound management, and regenerative medicine [44]. As hydrogels are porous, nutrients, oxygen, and other tiny molecules can diffuse through them and into the material, promoting the development and multiplication of cells [46].

Creating novel and new hydrogels has been an area of active research, with ongoing efforts to improve their synthesis, characterization, and administration [46]. Current innovations in the field of hydrogels have led to the advancement of stimuli-responsive hydrogels. These hydrogels can be activated by many factors, like changes in temperature, changes in pH, or magnetic fields [47, 48].

While regenerative medicine has made extensive use of a variety of hydrogel types, polymeric hydrogels have also been employed in clinical settings. Two major classes of hydrogels based on their source are natural hydrogels and synthetic hydrogels.

5.3.1 Natural hydrogels

Natural hydrogels are exclusive materials with unique properties and versatility, making them highly relevant in biomedical engineering. The key classifications of natural hydrogels are polysaccharide-based hydrogels, hydrogels based on proteins, and hybrid hydrogels. Hydrogels based on polysaccharides are derived from alginate, chitosan, and hyaluronic acid, imitate the cellular environment, and provide conducive surroundings for tissue regeneration and cell growth. However, protein-based hydrogels are derived from natural proteins like collagen, gelatin, and another one is fibrin, and exhibit superior biocompatibility and cell-adhesive properties, making these hydrogels potential candidates for tissue engineering and wound healing applications. Hybrid hydrogels, which combine natural and synthetic polymers, offer the benefits of both components, allowing for tailoring specific properties to meet various biomedical applications.

5.3.1.1 Cellulose and cellulose-based hydrogels

The most abundant natural polymer on the earth is cellulose, which is a plant-based polymer, and is a polysaccharide made of β-1,4-linked glucose units [49]. Cellulose-based hydrogels are typically manufactured by crosslinking cellulose or its derivatives, such as carboxymethylcellulose, with various crosslinking agents [50]. The primary benefit of hydrogels based on cellulose is their superior mechanical performance, which is essential for uses in drug delivery and regenerative medicine.

The extensive network of hydrogen bonds results in the molecular cohesion of the cellulose molecules, which is further enhanced by the dissolution process of intramolecular hydrogen bonds. This disintegration enhances the activity of the hydroxyl groups in cellulose and allows it to mix with different polymers. This makes cellulose an ideal candidate for hydrogel preparation, offering specific properties such as biodegradability, better renewability, tailored flexibility, and higher molar strength [51].

Cellulose can be further categorized based on its sources, such as plant cellulose or bacterial cellulose [52]. Plant cellulose, as the name suggests, is present in various plants such as wood, cotton, and phloem fiber to name a few [53]. However, specific species of microorganisms such as pseudomonas and acetobacter synthesize bacterial cellulose [54].

Cellulose and cellulose-based hydrogels have been exhaustively employed in various biomedical applications, including scaffold fabrication, regenerative application, and drug delivery [55, 56]. Guamba et al. used the plant cellulose extracted from various sources in Ecuador for the fabrication of antifouling hydrogel and found that cellulose derived from pitaya has better wound healing ability when applied to porcine skin [57]. Deng et al. modified bacterial cellulose with quaternized chitosan and developed a hydrogel with improved antibacterial properties and enhanced wound healing with no scarring [58].

For drug delivery, cellulose-based hydrogels have emerged as a potential material [59]. Hu et al. fabricated a novel double-layered hydrogel-based sustained drug release system by employing an inner and outer hydrogel of different types. Using different hydrogels for different layers leads to sustained release of the drug using this bilayer approach [60]. Cellulose-based hydrogel has been used in film form for the delivery of sulfadiazine drugs [61].

Cellulose and its based hydrogels have been extensively used for the fabrication of scaffolds such as nerve conduits and bone tissue [62]. Bacterial cellulose functionalized with phosphate has shown apatite-like bone formation in the research studies carried out by Suneetha et al. [63]. Huang et al. fabricated and incorporated PEGylated gold nanoparticles in bacterial cellulose hydrogel to enhance the properties of the hydrogel. It has been observed that PEGylated gold nanoparticle-enriched hydrogel has enhanced mechanical properties, improved biocompatibility, and superior osteogenic properties [64].

5.3.1.2 Chitosan and chitosan-based hydrogels

Natural biomaterial chitosan is made up of repeating units of N-acetyl-D-glucosamine and D-glucosamine [65]. It comes from both plant and animal sources and is the second most prevalent natural polymer. It is prepared by chitin's partial deacetylation in an alkaline medium [66]. The properties of chitosan and chitosan-based hydrogel can be improved by chemical modification for better performance, lower inflammatory response, and flexibility [67]. Chitosan and chitosan-based hydrogels have been exhaustively used for wound healing [68, 69] tissue engineering [70, 71], and dentistry [72, 73] to name a few. Wang et al. used chitosan and hyaluronic acid-based hydrogel as a vitreous substitute [74]. The developed hydrogel has a self-healing and controllable swelling ratio.

5.3.1.3 Alginate

Alginate is an anionic natural polymer that is majorly extracted from brown algae, but bacteria like *Azotobacter* and *Pseudomonas* are also used for the extraction of alginate [75].

Alginate hydrogels are created by crosslinking of alginate chains that consist of both mannuronic (M) and guluronic (G) acid groups [76]. Also, these hydrogels can be tailored as per the applications by varying the alginate concentration or the molecular weight, rheological properties and also by controlling the degree of crosslinking [77, 78].

Alginate is biocompatible, its mechanical properties can be altered and it supports the majority of the cell types. These are degradable and their degradation rate depends on the degree of crosslinking [79].

Moreover, alginate hydrogels have been used in dental and other medical fields comprising drug delivery systems, bone grafts, hemostatic bandages, and in the formation of organ bioprinting matrices [80, 81]. The characteristic of tunability of these hydrogels also enables the immobilization of diverse biological signals including growth factors and signaling molecules, optimizing the wanted cell response and tissue formation [82].

Although alginate hydrogels have many useful characteristics, the following shortcomings have to be taken into consideration [77]. Alginates' intrinsic biophysical and chemical properties compromise the diffusion of nutrients and wastes across alginate-based hydrogels, which complicates the long-term culture and vitality of cells encapsulated in alginate [83, 84]. To overcome these issues, the researchers try to optimize certain characteristics of alginate hydrogels by carrying out different approaches connected to the addition of extra biomaterials or usage of dynamic culture models [84].

Additionally, current studies aim at improving the biomechanical properties of alginate hydrogels for better matches of the characteristics of targeted tissues and the strategies for controlling the cell behavior in the hydrogels at the spatiotemporal level [79].

Therefore, alginate hydrogels are very potential and widely used biomaterials for tissue engineering and regenerative research studies. Thus, researchers are constantly discovering novel applications of these hydrogels based on their structural, mechanical, and biological characteristics to further enhance biomedical applications and patients' quality of life.

5.3.2 Synthetic hydrogel

Generally, to prevent hydrogel dissolution in an aqueous environment, the materials of the hydrogel are chemically crosslinked. The polymers mentioned below are frequently used clinically.

5.3.2.1 Polyacrylamide

Polyacrylamide (PAAM) is made up of entangled polymer chains which are connected through crosslinkers [85]. It forms hydrogels that are soft, non-degradable, and cationic. Due to their hydrophilic nature, they swell to a greater extent and tend to support cell adhesion, migration, fibrosis, and granuloma formation in vivo [86]. Despite being composed of 99% water, PAAM maintains great mechanical, physical, and chemical stability. By adjusting the degree of crosslinking or copolymerizing various synthetic or biological monomers, the physical properties of PAAM can be modified, affecting the swelling capacity, charge, stiffness, and surface characteristics [87]. PAAM requires proper purification to remove acrylamide monomers before clinical use, as it degrades into the genotoxic compound glycidaminde [88].

PAAM hydrogels find biomedical applications, particularly in tissue bulking processes by injecting the hydrogel to treat conditions like urinary incontinence and providing volumes and structural help to tissues [89]. Used as dermal fillers, the hydrogel enables the enhancement of facial contours through the filling of wrinkles due to its high-water content and stability [90]. The PAAM hydrogel also allows for the regeneration of muscles by providing a supporting matrix that promotes cell adhesion, migration, and proliferation, thus enabling growth and repair of the muscle [87].

5.3.2.2 Poly(2-hydroxyethylmethacrylate)

Poly(2-hydroxyethylmethacrylate) (pHEMA) is a non-degradable and extremely transparent inert hydrogel that is water soluble in nature [91]. By varying the crosslinking density, introducing mesoscopic pores, and adding different chemistries through copolymerization, we can tune the physical properties of pHEMA such as swelling, rheology, stiffness, etc. [92]. By reducing the crosslinking density, it leads to a softer and a malleable hydrogel that is ideal for regeneration of soft tissues. Copolymerizing pHEMA with acetic acid, dextran, and methacrylate can lead to modification in its hydrophilicity, permanence, and cellular adhesion in vivo [91]. Additionally, the incorporation of mesoscopic porogens helps in vascular ingrowth that improves cellular affinity and restricted permeability.

pHEMA has been available under various generic names like etafilcon A and vifilcon A, and has been used for ophthalmic applications because of its exceptional optical properties [93]. It has also been examined for the release of drugs and proteins at a controlled rate, regeneration of heart tissue, neural regeneration in the situation of a spinal cord injury, and as an alternative for intervertebral discs [94, 95].

5.3.2.3 Polyvinyl alcohol

Polyvinyl alcohol (PVA) is a biocompatible and biodegradable polymer that is protein-resistant. It spontaneously gels when it is kept in an aqueous media [96]. Upon freeze-thawing, improved stability has been noticed and the same could be attained by covalent crosslinking. Crosslinked PVA can be fabricated in different forms, like solutions, pellets, sponges, foam, sheets, meshes, coatings, and microspheres both chemically and physically [97, 98]. Its degradation rate can be tailored by varying the molecular weight of the polymer, its concentration, and the physical and chemical crosslink combinations [99].

Polyvinyl alcohol (PVA) hydrogels have found widespread use, attracting significant interest in a variety of biomedical and sensor applications [100]. In the medical field, they are used as soft contact lens materials (because of their great water-holding and comfortability) [101]. They are also investigated for cardiovascular purposes as they have anisotropic behavior and are capable of mimicking natural tissue response [102]. Furthermore, the PVA hydrogels also play a key role in aspects of environmentally friendly sensing devices including ionic conductive sensors [103] and photonic crystal-based sensors that use these materials as biosensors to sense environmental variation and monitor physiological signals [104]. PVA's nature of resistance toward cell adhesion and protein absorption enables it prevent to bacterial infection, postoperative adhesions, and granuloma formation. Hence, regenerative medicine has seen the widespread use of PVA-based biomaterials.

5.3.2.4 Polyethylene glycol

Polyethylene glycol or (PEG) materials are mainly considered biodegradable and biocompatible, thus making them a desirable candidate for use in various medical applications [105–107]. PEG hydrogels are biodegradable in situ via the process of hydrolysis, and PEG oligomers having low molecular weights are excreted in urine. PEGs are considered to be "stealth materials" as they lack side chains and also their overall hydrophilicity is poor. A dense layer of water surrounds PEG in vivo and allows diffusion, inhibiting cell adhesion and also adsorption of protein and thus leading to a reduction in both the formation of biofilms on PEG-coated devices and the degradation of PEG-encapsulated drug particles in vivo [108].

PEG is widely used in medicine as adhesion barriers, surgical sealants, osmotic laxatives, dressings, and an antibacterial, low-fouling coating on medical equipment [109]. PEG-based transparent liquids serve as efficient aids in pulmonary tissue closure, in neurological surgeries, and vascular surgery [97, 110]. It is used for a stable structure during conservation and underwater bonding, to remove delicate wooden artifacts [111]. In addition, PEG-based hydrogels are used as antifouling membranes because they can avoid biofouling and also be traced for monitoring membrane performance [112]. Moreover, the development of tunable PEG-based hydrogels is often utilized to investigate cell mechanosensing in tissue engineering and research where the mechanical environment can be precisely controlled [113].

5.4 BIOCOMPOSITES

Composite combines two or more distinct compounds to enhance each material's unique qualities, including biocompatibility, mechanical strength, and surface features. Biocomposites, a novel class of materials, have shown an increased interest in biomedicine applications for various uses like targeted drug delivery, tissue engineering, regenerative medicine, wound dressings, surgical operations, medical imaging in cancer detection, and dental composites [114]. Biocomposites demonstrate design flexibility and a high strength-to-weight ratio. Also, it can be molded in desired properties, unlike polymeric, metallic, and ceramic biomaterials [115]. Apart from this, high X-ray visibility, electrical conductivity, magnetic characteristics, and thermal properties of polymer/metal or ceramic are additional benefits of biocomposite. However, in some cases, it may also result in an undesirable X-ray radiography artifact, increasing degradation rate and compromising thermal stability [114].

5.4.1 Polymer/metal biocomposite

Biopolymers can be reinforced with metal particulates like Al, Mg, Zn, Ca, Sn, and Fe or their alloy, making them suitable for bone-tissue applications [116, 117]. The reinforcing agent imparts strengthening effects, which nucleate and grow in an appropriate size, shape, and distribution in the matrix [118] It improves ductility, increases toughness, low weight, and high fatigue strength. The role of metal reinforcement can overcome the shortcomings of polymeric implants like high strength, neutralizing acid inflammation, control the degradation process, and stabilize local pH at the implant site. It also shows a few shortcomings, like inorganic fillers can act as catalysts, which break the polymeric chains, resulting in an accelerated corrosion rate. Thus, it becomes important to stabilize metal in the body fluid to control the rate of hydrolytic degradation of polymers [114, 119, 120].

5.4.2 Polymer/ceramics biocomposite

Ceramics as reinforcement enhance osteoconductivity and compressive strength, while polymers introduce ductility and bioresorbability. Hence, polymer/ceramics can be a suitable biocomposite for bone implants and tissue engineering applications. Also, polymer/ceramic composites induce superior mechanical properties and corrosion resistance toward the body fluid than either ceramics or polymers. However, it negatively impacts thermal stability and degradation of biocomposite [121, 122]. The reason can be the presence of metal cations Ca^{2+}, Mg^{2+}, Zn^{2+}, and Fe^{3+} that lead to the ionic interaction with the matrix, ultimately causing chain scissoring of the polymer. It was observed that during the in vivo degradation of polymer/ceramics, the inflammatory reactions were significantly reduced. Presently, polymer/ceramics biocomposites are gaining attention to treating bone-related diseases or disorders like bone-fracture fixations, sutures, and interference screws [123, 124].

5.4.3 Polymer/Nanoparticle biocomposite

Nanoparticles have been actively interacting directly with cells. It can deliver targeted drugs at a desired rate that enhances the therapeutic effect and develops antimicrobial features in wound dressing. Nanoparticles include silver complexes, hydroxyapatite, titanium dioxide, silicate, nanoclays, gold, zinc oxide, smectite, and carbon nanotubes. However, their nanosize, shape, morphology, and surface charge limit their amount as a reinforcement. Also, it can directly enter the cells, disrupting cell membranes and leading to genotoxic effects, or even causing damage to DNA [125–127].

In contrast, polymer/nanoparticle biocomposites are gaining attention in nanomedicine, drug delivery, bone tissue formation, cancer immunotherapy, and imaging purposes [128]. The preparation of these nanocomposites includes solvent casting, melt blending, and electrospinning techniques. The results have indicated that blending nanoparticles with polymers yields higher strength, improves thermal properties, and provides barriers to water vapor or gases. Biocomposites were also extensively explored, making them suitable for nanocarriers to deliver drugs, biosensing, cell targeting, exploit magnetic resonance imaging, artificial organs, and anticancer drug-controlled release devices [129–131]. Still, nanoparticle-based biocomposites require detailed investigations and clinical validation to be accepted by the market.

5.4.4 Polymer ceramic composite

Polymer ceramic composites are an emerging, advanced, and newer class of materials that has shown considerable promise in various biomedical applications or uses [118]. As the name suggests, they are made up of polymer and ceramics, and thus these composites therefore have some of the favorable qualities of polymers and ceramics as they can be used effectively in medical implants and devices due to better biocompatibility and mechanical characteristics. Many polymers of both biodegradable and non-biodegradable categories have been used for the fabrication of polymer-ceramic composite materials. Among them, biodegradable ones have attracted attention since they can be eliminated safely from the body once they have served their function of repairing the tissue, thus obviating the need for removal with subsequent surgery and eliminating long-term problems associated with non-resorbable materials [132]. Furthermore, the application of different ceramics like hydroxyapatite and tricalcium phosphate in the formation of these composites improves the mechanical characteristics and bioactivity to allow for the load-bearing application and osseointegration for bone interaction in therapy and treatment [132–134]. A selection of manufacturing methods that can be used to produce polymer–ceramic composites includes particle leaching, electrospinning, and additive manufacturing They also help in fabrication of structures that can support cellular attachment, deposition and tissue regeneration because they include features of natural extracellular matrix. Also, the recent developments in the synthesis of these composites in the scope of tissue engineering underlined their possibilities not only as structural elements to build up the scaffolds but also as agents to deliver drugs that stimulate the healing process.

5.4.5 Polymer hydrogel composite

Based on the growing market interest for medical products and tissue engineering, the biomedical study has expanded significantly in terms of research area of focus, including polymer-based composites [133]. This is mainly because they contain superior characteristics like biocompatibility, non-toxicity, and degradability, in correlation with the fact that most applications involve contact with biological tissues [135]. Furthermore, the typification of composites is that the application of nanoparticles can improve the mechanical and physical properties of these composites [136]. In this regard, the field of biomedical applications of these composites ranges from wound dressings to scaffolds for tissue engineering [135]. In addition, the polymer hydrogel composites can be subdivided into several categories: natural hydrogels, synthetic hydrogels, and hybrid hydrogels each of which has distinct features that meet unique biomedical applications including drug delivery methods, tissue engineering, and soft tissue prosthetic devices [134, 135, 137].

Therefore, one of the most important uses of polymer hydrogel composites is that it can closely replicate the environment of the body's extracellular matrix in which cells may develop and multiply. These types of materials can be designed to display certain mechanical characteristics desirable for degradation rates and porosity and hence their application for solving different biomedical demands. Furthermore, these hydrogels contain bioactive components which can stimulate the behavior of cells and facilitate better integration with the tissue, and hence can be useful in applications such as bone and cartilage tissue engineering or for wound healing [118, 138–141].

Furthermore, due to the flexibility of the polymer hydrogel composites, they can possibly be applied in numerous professional fields of biomedicine, for example as a center for the controlled release of therapeutic substances and biodegradable scaffolds to support cell attachment and proliferation, and soft tissue implants with characteristics similar to the human tissues [142–146].

5.5 CONCLUSION

Synthetic polymeric biomaterials have advanced the domain of biomaterials and have been used in a very widespread manner in this field due to their biocompatibility and other conducive properties. These polymeric biomaterials can be tailored as per the need of the applications and thus are apt materials for these special and focused applications. Novel and current researchers are focused on the development of newer materials and manufacturing methods for the fabrication of these synthetic biomaterials. Recent advancements in technologies have given much required momentum in these directions and researchers have come up with advanced and precise fabrication methods.

REFERENCES

[1] M. Chelu and A. M. Musuc, "Advanced Biomedical Applications of Multifunctional Natural and Synthetic Biomaterials," *Processes*, vol. 11, no. 9, p. 2696, Sep. 2023, doi: 10.3390/pr11092696

[2] E. Insuasti-Cruz et al., "Natural Biomaterials from Biodiversity for Healthcare Applications," *Adv Healthc Mater*, vol. 11, no. 1, Jan. 2022, doi: 10.1002/adhm.202101389

[3] S. Prete, M. Dattilo, F. Patitucci, G. Pezzi, O. I. Parisi, and F. Puoci, "Natural and Synthetic Polymeric Biomaterials for Application in Wound Management," *J Funct Biomater*, vol. 14, no. 9, p. 455, Sep. 2023, doi: 10.3390/jfb14090455

[4] M. J. Austin and A. M. Rosales, "Tunable biomaterials from synthetic, sequence-controlled polymers," *Biomater Sci*, vol. 7, no. 2, pp. 490–505, 2019, doi: 10.1039/C8BM01215F

[5] J. Kurowiak, T. Klekiel, and R. Będziński, "Biodegradable Polymers in Biomedical Applications: A Review—Developments, Perspectives and Future Challenges," *Int J Mol Sci*, vol. 24, no. 23, p. 16952, Nov. 2023, doi: 10.3390/ijms242316952

[6] G. Mazza et al., "Decellularized Human Liver as a Natural 3D-Scaffold for Liver Bioengineering and Transplantation," *Sci Rep*, vol. 5, no. 1, p. 13079, Aug. 2015, doi: 10.1038/srep13079

[7] M. Brovold et al., "Naturally-Derived Biomaterials for Tissue Engineering Applications," in *Advances in Experimental Medicine and Biology*, vol. 1077, 2018, pp. 421–449. doi: 10.1007/978-981-13-0947-2_23

[8] P. Gunatillake, "Biodegradable Synthetic Polymers for Tissue Engineering," *Eur Cell Mater*, vol. 5, pp. 1–16, Oct. 2003, doi: 10.22203/eCM.v005a01

[9] K. J. Rambhia and P. X. Ma, "Controlled Drug Release for Tissue Engineering," *J Control Release*, vol. 219, pp. 119–128, Dec. 2015, doi: 10.1016/j.jconrel.2015.08.049
[10] T. H. Mourey and T. C. Schunk, "Chapter 22 Synthetic Polymers," 1992, pp. B475–B512. doi: 10.1016/S0301-4770(08)61515-8
[11] S. Todros, M. Todesco, and A. Bagno, "Biomaterials and Their Biomedical Applications: From Replacement to Regeneration," *Processes*, vol. 9, no. 11, p. 1949, Oct. 2021, doi: 10.3390/pr9111949
[12] J. K. Arora and P. Bhati, "Fabrication and Characterization of 3D Printed PLA Scaffolds," *AIP Conf Proc*, vol. 2205, Dec., 2020, doi: 10.1063/1.5142980
[13] P. Netti, *Biomedical Foams for Tissue Engineering Applications*. Woodhead Publishing, 2014.
[14] P. Bhati et al., "Physicochemical Characterization and Mechanical Performance Analysis of Biaxially Oriented PLA/PCL Tubular Scaffolds for Intended Stent Application," *SN Appl Sci*, vol. 2, no. 12, 2020, doi: 10.1007/s42452-020-03795-8
[15] P. Bhati, A. Kumar, R. Ahuja, and N. Bhatnagar, "Evaluating the Effect of Manufacturing Method on the Radial Compressive Force of the Bioresorbable Tubes," *Mater Lett*, vol. 235, pp. 23–26, Jan. 2019, doi: 10.1016/J.MATLET.2018.09.136
[16] S. Krishnan, P. Pandey, S. Mohanty, and S. K. Nayak, *Toughening of Polylactic Acid: An Overview of Research Progress*. Oct. 12, 2016, Taylor and Francis Inc doi: 10.1080/03602559.2015.1098698
[17] E. Leclerc, K. S. Furukawa, F. Miyata, Y. Sakai, T. Ushida, and T. Fujii, "Fabrication of Microstructures in Photosensitive Biodegradable Polymers for Tissue Engineering Applications," *Biomaterials*, vol. 25, no. 19, pp. 4683–4690, Aug. 2004, doi: 10.1016/j.biomaterials.2003.10.060
[18] P. Bhati, A. Srivastava, R. Ahuja, P. Chauhan, P. Vashisth, and N. Bhatnagar, "Physicochemical Properties of UV-Irradiated, Biaxially Oriented PLA Tubular Scaffolds," *Polymers (Basel)*, vol. 15, no. 5, p. 1097, Feb. 2023, doi: 10.3390/polym15051097
[19] P. Bhati and N. Bhatnagar, "Effect of Processing Parameters on Surface Hydrophilicity of Porous PLA Tubes Prepared by Gas Assisted Microcellular Extrusion Foaming Technique," *Mater Lett*, Aug. 2017, doi: 10.1016/j.matlet.2017.08.076
[20] A. Srivastava et al., "Fabrication and Characterization of PLLA/Mg Composite Tube as the Potential Bioresorbable/Biodegradable Stent(BRS)," *Materialia (Oxf)*, p. 100661, Mar. 2020, doi: 10.1016/J.MTLA.2020.100661
[21] R. Ahuja et al., "Biocompatibility Analysis of PLA Based Candidate materials for Cardiovascular Stents in a Rat Subcutaneous Implant Model," *Acta Histochem*, vol. 122, no. 7, p. 151615, 2020, doi: https://doi.org/10.1016/j.acthis.2020.151615
[22] F. D. Al-Shalawi et al., "Biodegradable Synthetic Polymer in Orthopaedic Application: A Review," *Mater Today Proc*, vol. 74, pp. 540–546, 2023, doi: 10.1016/j.matpr.2022.12.254
[23] R. Liu, Q. Zhang, Q. Zhou, P. Zhang, and H. Dai, "Nondegradable Magnetic Poly (Carbonate Urethane) Microspheres With Good Shape Memory as a Proposed Material for Vascular Embolization," *J Mech Behav Biomed Mater*, vol. 82, pp. 9–17, Jun. 2018, doi: 10.1016/j.jmbbm.2018.02.010

[24] P.A.Gunatillake and R.Adhikari, "Nondegradable Synthetic Polymers for Medical Devices and Implants," in *Biosynthetic Polymers for Medical Applications*, Elsevier, 2016, pp. 33–62. doi: 10.1016/B978-1-78242-105-4.00002-X
[25] M. M. Subedi, "Ceramics and Its Importance," *Himalayan Physics*, vol. 4, pp. 80–82, Dec. 2013, doi: 10.3126/hj.v4i0.9433
[26] J. Chevalier and L. Gremillard, "Ceramics for Medical Applications: A Picture for the Next 20 Years," *J Eur Ceram Soc*, vol. 29, no. 7, pp. 1245–1255, Apr. 2009, doi: 10.1016/j.jeurceramsoc.2008.08.025
[27] J. R. Jones, D. S. Brauer, L. Hupa, and D. C. Greenspan, "Bioglass and Bioactive Glasses and Their Impact on Healthcare," *Int J Appl Glass Sci*, vol. 7, no. 4, pp. 423–434, Dec. 2016, doi: 10.1111/ijag.12252
[28] M. Cannio, D. Bellucci, J. A. Roether, Dino N. Boccaccini, and V. Cannillo, "Bioactive Glass Applications: A Literature Review of Human Clinical Trials," *Materials*, vol. 14, no. 18, p. 5440, Sep. 2021, doi: 10.3390/ma14185440
[29] A.-L. Mîrţ, D. Ficai, O.-C. Oprea, G. Vasilievici, and A. Ficai, "Current and Future Perspectives of Bioactive Glasses as Injectable Material," *Nanomaterials*, vol. 14, no. 14, p. 1196, Jul. 2024, doi: 10.3390/nano14141196
[30] A. Kumar, S. Murugavel, A. Aditya, and A. R. Boccaccini, "Mesoporous 45S5 Bioactive Glass: Synthesis, In Vitro Dissolution and Biomineralization Behavior," *J Mater Chem B*, vol. 5, no. 44, pp. 8786–8798, 2017, doi: 10.1039/C7TB01738C
[31] F. Baino, S. Hamzehlou, and S. Kargozar, "Bioactive Glasses: Where Are We and Where Are We Going?," *J Funct Biomater*, vol. 9, no. 1, p. 25, Mar. 2018, doi: 10.3390/jfb9010025
[32] L. Vaiani et al., "Ceramic Materials for Biomedical Applications: An Overview on Properties and Fabrication Processes," *J Funct Biomater*, vol. 14, no. 3, p. 146, Mar. 2023, doi: 10.3390/jfb14030146
[33] R. Kumar, I. Pattanayak, P. A. Dash, and S. Mohanty, "Bioceramics: A Review on Design Concepts Toward Tailor-Made (Multi)-Functional Materials for Tissue Engineering Applications," *J Mater Sci*, vol. 58, no. 8, pp. 3460–3484, Feb. 2023, doi: 10.1007/s10853-023-08226-8
[34] M. Sadat-Shojai, M.-T. Khorasani, E. Dinpanah-Khoshdargi, and A. Jamshidi, "Synthesis Methods for Nanosized Hydroxyapatite With Diverse Structures," *Acta Biomater*, vol. 9, no. 8, pp. 7591–7621, Aug. 2013, doi: 10.1016/j.actbio.2013.04.012
[35] H. Hsu, R. A. Waris, M. Ruslin, Y. Lin, C. Chen, and K. Ou, "An Innovative α-Calcium Sulfate Hemihydrate Bioceramic as a Potential Bone Graft Substitute," *J Am Ceram Soc*, vol. 101, no. 1, pp. 419–427, Jan. 2018, doi: 10.1111/jace.15181
[36] R. Narayanan, S. K. Seshadri, T. Y. Kwon, and K. H. Kim, "Calcium Phosphate-Based Coatings on Titanium and Its Alloys," *J Biomed Mater Res B Appl Biomater*, vol. 85B, no. 1, pp. 279–299, Apr. 2008, doi: 10.1002/jbm.b.30932
[37] C. Piconi and A. A. Porporati, "Bioinert Ceramics: Zirconia and Alumina," in *Handbook of Bioceramics and Biocomposites*, Springer International Publishing, 2016, pp. 59–89. doi: 10.1007/978-3-319-12460-5_4
[38] T. K. Gupta, J. H. Bechtold, R. C. Kuznicki, L. H. Cadoff, and B. R. Rossing, "Stabilization of Tetragonal Phase in Polycrystalline Zirconia," *J Mater Sci*, vol. 12, no. 12, pp. 2421–2426, Dec. 1977, doi: 10.1007/BF00553928

[39] C. Piconi and G. Maccauro, "Zirconia as a Ceramic Biomaterial," *Biomaterials*, vol. 20, no. 1, pp. 1–25, Jan. 1999, doi: 10.1016/S0142-9612(98)00010-6
[40] C. Sanon et al., "Low Temperature Degradation and Reliability of One-Piece Ceramic Oral Implants With a Porous Surface," *Dent Mater*, vol. 29, no. 4, pp. 389–397, Apr. 2013, doi: 10.1016/j.dental.2013.01.007
[41] A. Khaskhoussi, L. Calabrese, J. Bouaziz, and E. Proverbio, "Effect of TiO2 Addition on Microstructure of Zirconia/Alumina Sintered Ceramics," *Ceram Int*, vol. 43, no. 13, pp. 10392–10402, Sep. 2017, doi: 10.1016/j.ceramint.2017.05.074
[42] T.-C. Ho et al., "Hydrogels: Properties and Applications in Biomedicine," *Molecules*, vol. 27, no. 9, p. 2902, May 2022, doi: 10.3390/molecules27092902
[43] A. Chyzy, M. Tomczykowa, and M. E. Plonska-Brzezinska, "Hydrogels as Potential Nano-, Micro- and Macro-Scale Systems for Controlled Drug Delivery," *Materials*, vol. 13, no. 1, p. 188, Jan. 2020, doi: 10.3390/ma13010188
[44] A. Onaciu, R. A. Munteanu, A. I. Moldovan, C. S. Moldovan, and I. Berindan-Neagoe, "Hydrogels Based Drug Delivery Synthesis, Characterization and Administration," *Pharmaceutics*, vol. 11, no. 9, p. 432, Aug. 2019, doi: 10.3390/pharmaceutics11090432
[45] K. Pal, A. K. Banthia, and D. K. Majumdar, "Polymeric Hydrogels: Characterization and Biomedical Applications," *Des Monomers Polym*, vol. 12, no. 3, pp. 197–220, Jan. 2009, doi: 10.1163/156855509X436030
[46] A. Sosnik and K. Seremeta, "Polymeric Hydrogels as Technology Platform for Drug Delivery Applications," *Gels*, vol. 3, no. 3, p. 25, Jul. 2017, doi: 10.3390/gels3030025
[47] C. Chen et al., "Photothermal-Promoted Multi-Functional Dual Network Polysaccharide Hydrogel Adhesive for Infected and Susceptible Wound Healing," *Carbohydr Polym*, vol. 273, p. 118557, Dec. 2021, doi: 10.1016/j.carbpol.2021.118557
[48] I. Gholamali, M. Asnaashariisfahani, and E. Alipour, "Silver Nanoparticles Incorporated in pH-Sensitive Nanocomposite Hydrogels Based on Carboxymethyl Chitosan-Poly (Vinyl Alcohol) for Use in a Drug Delivery System," *Regen Eng Transl Med*, vol. 6, no. 2, pp. 138–153, Jun. 2020, doi: 10.1007/s40883-019-00120-7
[49] M. C. Catoira, L. Fusaro, D. Di Francesco, M. Ramella, and F. Boccafoschi, "Overview of natural hydrogels for regenerative medicine applications," *J Mater Sci Mater Med*, vol. 30, no. 10, 2019, doi: 10.1007/s10856-019-6318-7
[50] F. Camponeschi, A. Atrei, G. Rocchigiani, L. Mencuccini, M. Uva, and R. Barbucci, "New Formulations of Polysaccharide-Based Hydrogels for Drug Release and Tissue Engineering," Gels, vol. 1, no. 1, pp. 3–23, Jan. 2015, doi: 10.3390/gels1010003
[51] Mitra, S., Anjum, J., Muni, M., Das, R., Rauf, A., Islam, F., ... & Wilairatana, P. (2022). Exploring the journey of emodin as a potential neuroprotective agent: novel therapeutic insights with molecular mechanism of action. *Biomedicine & Pharmacotherapy*, *149*, 112877. https://doi.org/10.1016/j.biopha.2022.112877
[52] P. Zou, et al., "Citation: Advances in Cellulose-Based Hydrogels for Biomedical Engineering: A Review Summary," 2022, doi: 10.3390/gels8060364

[53] U. Ray, S. Zhu, Z. Pang, and T. Li, "Mechanics Design in Cellulose-Enabled High-Performance Functional Materials," *Adv Mater*, vol. 33, no. 28, Jul. 2021, doi: 10.1002/adma.202002504
[54] G. F. Picheth et al., "Bacterial Cellulose in Biomedical Applications: A Review," *Int J Biol Macromol*, vol. 104, pp. 97–106, Nov. 2017, doi: 10.1016/j.ijbiomac.2017.05.171
[55] Diwakar, M., Singh, P., Ravi, V., & Maurya, A. (2023). A non-conventional review on Multi-modality-based Medical Image Fusion. *Diagnostics*, *13*(5), 820. 10.3390/s23063287
[56] R. J. Hickey and A. E. Pelling, "Cellulose Biomaterials for Tissue Engineering," *Front Bioeng Biotechnol*, vol. 7, Mar. 2019, doi: 10.3389/fbioe.2019.00045
[57] E. Guamba et al., "Cellulose-based hydrogels towards an antibacterial wound dressing," *Biomater Sci*, vol. 11, no. 10, pp. 3461–3468, 2023, doi: 10.1039/D2BM01369J
[58] L. Deng et al., "Bacterial Cellulose-Based Hydrogel With Regulated Rehydration and Enhanced Antibacterial Activity for Wound Healing," *Int J Biol Macromol*, vol. 267, p. 131291, May 2024, doi: 10.1016/j.ijbiomac.2024.131291
[59] M. Dattilo, F. Patitucci, S. Prete, O. I. Parisi, and F. Puoci, "Polysaccharide-Based Hydrogels and Their Application as Drug Delivery Systems in Cancer Treatment: A Review," *J Funct Biomater*, vol. 14, no. 2, p. 55, Jan. 2023, doi: 10.3390/jfb14020055
[60] Y. Hu et al., "A Double-Layer Hydrogel Based on Alginate-Carboxymethyl Cellulose and Synthetic Polymer as Sustained Drug Delivery System," *Sci Rep*, vol. 11, no. 1, p. 9142, Apr. 2021, doi: 10.1038/s41598-021-88503-1
[61] M. Sultan, O. A. Mohamed, H. M. El-Masry, and G. Taha, "Fabrication and Evaluation of Antimicrobial Cellulose/Arabic Gum Hydrogels as Potential Drug Delivery Vehicle," *Int J Biol Macromol*, vol. 242, p. 125083, Jul. 2023, doi: 10.1016/j.ijbiomac.2023.125083
[62] T. R. Stumpf, X. Yang, J. Zhang, and X. Cao, "In Situ and Ex Situ Modifications of Bacterial Cellulose for Applications in Tissue Engineering," *Mater Sci Eng C*, vol. 82, pp. 372–383, Jan. 2018, doi: 10.1016/j.msec.2016.11.121
[63] M. Suneetha, H. Kim, and S. S. Han, "Bone-Like Apatite Formation in Biocompatible Phosphate-Crosslinked Bacterial Cellulose-Based Hydrogels for Bone Tissue Engineering Applications," *Int J Biol Macromol*, vol. 256, p. 128364, Jan. 2024, doi: 10.1016/j.ijbiomac.2023.128364
[64] C. Huang et al., "Biofabrication of Natural Au/Bacterial Cellulose Hydrogel for Bone Tissue Regeneration via In-Situ Fermentation," *Smart Mater Med*, vol. 4, pp. 1–14, 2023, doi: 10.1016/j.smaim.2022.06.001
[65] L. Zhao, Y. Zhou, J. Zhang, H. Liang, X. Chen, and H. Tan, "Natural Polymer-Based Hydrogels: From Polymer to Biomedical Applications," *Pharmaceutics*, vol. 15, no. 10, p. 2514, Oct. 2023, doi: 10.3390/pharmaceutics15102514
[66] M. Rajabi, M. McConnell, J. Cabral, and M. A. Ali, "Chitosan Hydrogels in 3D Printing for Biomedical Applications," *Carbohydr Polym*, vol. 260, p. 117768, May 2021, doi: 10.1016/j.carbpol.2021.117768
[67] L. Racine, I. Texier, and R. Auzély-Velty, "Chitosan-Based Hydrogels: Recent Design Concepts to Tailor Properties and Functions," *Polym Int*, vol. 66, no. 7, pp. 981–998, Jul. 2017, doi: 10.1002/pi.5331
[68] X. Wang et al., "Chitosan-Based Hydrogels for Infected Wound Treatment," *Macromol Biosci*, vol. 23, no. 9, Sep. 2023, doi: 10.1002/mabi.202300094

[69] Q. Yu et al., "A Multifunctional Chitosan-Based Hydrogel With Self-Healing, Antibacterial, and Immunomodulatory Effects as Wound Dressing," *Int J Biol Macromol*, vol. 231, p. 123149, Mar. 2023, doi: 10.1016/j.ijbiomac.2023.123149
[70] Y. Kim et al., "Chitosan-Based Biomaterials for Tissue Regeneration," *Pharmaceutics*, vol. 15, no. 3, p. 807, Mar. 2023, doi: 10.3390/pharmaceutics15030807
[71] T. Tolstova et al., "Preparation and In Vitro Evaluation of Chitosan-g-Oligolactide Based Films and Macroporous Hydrogels for Tissue Engineering," *Polymers (Basel)*, vol. 15, no. 4, p. 907, Feb. 2023, doi: 10.3390/polym15040907
[72] J. Andrade del Olmo et al., "Multifunctional Antibacterial Chitosan-Based Hydrogel Coatings on Ti6Al4V Biomaterial for Biomedical Implant Applications," *Int J Biol Macromol*, vol. 231, p. 123328, Mar. 2023, doi: 10.1016/j.ijbiomac.2023.123328
[73] E. Fakhri et al., "Chitosan Biomaterials Application in Dentistry," *Int J Biol Macromol*, vol. 162, pp. 956–974, Nov. 2020, doi: 10.1016/j.ijbiomac.2020.06.211
[74] S. Wang et al., "A Self-Healing and Injectable Hydrogel Based on Water-Soluble Chitosan and Hyaluronic Acid for Vitreous Substitute," *Carbohydr Polym*, vol. 256, p. 117519, Mar. 2021, doi: 10.1016/j.carbpol.2020.117519
[75] D. R. Sahoo and T. Biswal, "Alginate and its Application to Tissue Engineering," *SN Appl Sci*, vol. 3, no. 1, p. 30, Jan. 2021, doi: 10.1007/s42452-020-04096-w
[76] A. D. Augst, H. J. Kong, and D. J. Mooney, "Alginate Hydrogels as Biomaterials," *Macromol Biosci*, vol. 6, no. 8, pp. 623–633, Aug. 2006, doi: 10.1002/mabi.200600069
[77] S.-M. Kang, J.-H. Lee, Y. S. Huh, and S. Takayama, "Alginate Microencapsulation for Three-Dimensional In Vitro Cell Culture," *ACS Biomater Sci Eng*, vol. 7, no. 7, pp. 2864–2879, Jul. 2021, doi: 10.1021/acsbiomaterials.0c00457
[78] K. Enoch, C.S. Rakavi, and A. A. Somasundaram, "Tuning the Rheological Properties of Chitosan/Alginate Hydrogels for Tissue Engineering Application," *Colloids Surf A Physicochem Eng Asp*, vol. 697, p. 134434, Sep. 2024, doi: 10.1016/j.colsurfa.2024.134434
[79] Q. Chen, X. Tian, J. Fan, H. Tong, Q. Ao, and X. Wang, "An Interpenetrating Alginate/Gelatin Network for Three-Dimensional (3D) Cell Cultures and Organ Bioprinting," *Molecules*, vol. 25, no. 3, p. 756, Feb. 2020, doi: 10.3390/molecules25030756
[80] Q. Gu et al., "Functional 3D Neural Mini-Tissues from Printed Gel-Based Bioink and Human Neural Stem Cells," *Adv Healthc Mater*, vol. 5, no. 12, pp. 1429–1438, Jun. 2016, doi: 10.1002/adhm.201600095
[81] T. Gonzalez-Fernandez, A. J. Tenorio, K. T. Campbell, E. A. Silva, and J. K. Leach, "Alginate-Based Bioinks for 3D Bioprinting and Fabrication of Anatomically Accurate Bone Grafts," *Tissue Eng Part A*, vol. 27, no. 17–18, pp. 1168–1181, Sep. 2021, doi: 10.1089/ten.tea.2020.0305
[82] F. Charbonier, D. Indana, and O. Chaudhuri, "Tuning Viscoelasticity in Alginate Hydrogels for 3D Cell Culture Studies," *Curr Protoc*, vol. 1, no. 5, May 2021, doi: 10.1002/cpz1.124
[83] L. Yao, K. L. Billiar, A. J. Windebank, and A. Pandit, "Multichanneled Collagen Conduits for Peripheral Nerve Regeneration: Design, Fabrication, and Characterization," *Tissue Eng Part C Methods*, vol. 16, no. 6, pp. 1585–1596, 2010, doi: 10.1089/ten.tec.2010.0152

[84] Z. Gan, X. Qin, H. Liu, J. Liu, and J. Qin, "Recent advances in defined hydrogels in organoid research," *Bioact Mater*, vol. 28, pp. 386–401, Oct. 2023, doi: 10.1016/j.bioactmat.2023.06.004

[85] L. Bromberg, A. Y. Grosberg, E. S. Matsuo, Y. Suzuki, and T. Tanaka, "Dependency of Swelling on the Length of Subchain in Poly(N,N-Dimethyl acrylamide)-Based Gels," *J Chem Phys*, vol. 106, no. 7, pp. 2906–2910, Feb. 1997, doi: 10.1063/1.474084

[86] B. A. Baker, R. L. Murff, and V. T. Milam, "Tailoring the Mechanical Properties of Polyacrylamide-Based Hydrogels," *Polymer (Guildf)*, vol. 51, no. 10, pp. 2207–2214, 2010, doi: https://doi.org/10.1016/j.polymer.2010.02.022

[87] M. Bassil, J. Davenas, and M. E. L. Tahchi, "Electrochemical Properties and Actuation Mechanisms of Polyacrylamide Hydrogel for Artificial Muscle Application," *Sens Actuators B Chem*, vol. 134, no. 2, pp. 496–501, Sep. 2008, doi: 10.1016/J.SNB.2008.05.025

[88] J. M. Rice, "The Carcinogenicity of Acrylamide," *Mutat Res Genet Toxicol Environ Mutagen*, vol. 580, no. 1–2, pp. 3–20, Feb. 2005, doi: 10.1016/J.MRGENTOX.2004.09.008

[89] P. Toozs-Hobson, W. Al-Singary, M. Fynes, G. Tegerstedt, and G. Lose, "Two-Year Follow-Up of an Open-Label Multicenter Study of Polyacrylamide Hydrogel (Bulkamid®) for Female Stress and Stress-Predominant Mixed Incontinence," *Int Urogynecol J*, vol. 23, no. 10, pp. 1373–1378, 2012, doi: 10.1007/s00192-012-1761-8

[90] K. Gupta, N. Bhari, K. K. Verma, and S. Gupta, "Permanent Injectable Polyacrylamide Hydrogel Dermal Filler for a Large Subcutaneous Defect Secondary to Lupus Panniculitis," *Dermatol Surg*, vol. 43, no. 1, 2017, [Online]. https://journals.lww.com/dermatologicsurgery/fulltext/2017/01000/permanent_injectable_polyacrylamide_hydrogel.25.aspx

[91] B. V. Slaughter, S. S. Khurshid, O. Z. Fisher, A. Khademhosseini, and N. A. Peppas, "Hydrogels in Regenerative Medicine," *Adv Mater*, vol. 21, no. 32–33, pp. 3307–3329, Sep. 2009, doi: https://doi.org/10.1002/adma.200802106

[92] W. Zhao, C. Lenardi, P. Webb, C. Liu, T. Santaniello, and F. Gassa, "A Methodology to Analyse and Simulate Mechanical Characteristics of Poly(2-Hydroxyethyl Methacrylate) Hydrogel," *Polym Int*, vol. 62, no. 7, pp. 1059–1067, Jul. 2013, doi: https://doi.org/10.1002/pi.4392

[93] H. Gupta and M. Aqil, "Contact Lenses in Ocular Therapeutics," *Drug Discov Today*, vol. 17, no. 9–10, pp. 522–527, May 2012, doi: 10.1016/J.DRUDIS.2012.01.014

[94] A. Hejčl et al., "Macroporous Hydrogels Based on 2-Hydroxyethyl Methacrylate. Part 6: 3D Hydrogels With Positive and Negative Surface Charges and Polyelectrolyte Complexes in Spinal Cord Injury Repair," *J Mater Sci Mater Med*, vol. 20, no. 7, pp. 1571–1577, 2009, doi: 10.1007/s10856-009-3714-4

[95] L. R. Madden et al., "Proangiogenic Scaffolds as Functional Templates for Cardiac Tissue Engineering," *Proc Natl Acad Sci*, vol. 107, no. 34, pp. 15211–15216, Aug. 2010, doi: 10.1073/pnas.1006442107

[96] L. Zeng, B. Liu, L. Duan, and G. Gao, "Tough, Recyclable and Biocompatible Carrageenan-Modified Polyvinyl Alcohol Ionic Hydrogel With Physical Cross-Linked for Multimodal Sensing," *Int J Biol Macromol*, vol. 253, p. 126954, Dec. 2023, doi: 10.1016/J.IJBIOMAC.2023.126954

[97] S. Samavedi, L. K. Poindexter, M. Van Dyke, and A. S. Goldstein, "Synthetic Biomaterials for Regenerative Medicine Applications," in *Regenerative Medicine Applications in Organ Transplantation*, Elsevier Inc., 2014, pp. 81–99. doi: 10.1016/B978-0-12-398523-1.00007-0

[98] M. I. Baker, S. P. Walsh, Z. Schwartz, and B. D. Boyan, "A Review of Polyvinyl Alcohol and Its Uses in Cartilage and Orthopedic Applications," *J Biomed Mater Res B Appl Biomater*, vol. 100B, no. 5, pp. 1451–1457, Jul. 2012, doi: https://doi.org/10.1002/jbm.b.32694

[99] K. Yan Zhang, D. Li, Y. Wang, and L. Jun Wang, "Carboxymethyl Chitosan/Polyvinyl Alcohol Double Network Hydrogels Prepared by Freeze-Thawing and Calcium Chloride Cross-Linking for Efficient Dye Adsorption," *Int J Biol Macromol*, vol. 253, p. 126897, Dec. 2023, doi: 10.1016/J.IJBIOMAC.2023.126897

[100] S. Jiang, S. Liu, and W. Feng, "PVA Hydrogel Properties for Biomedical Application," *J Mech Behav Biomed Mater*, vol. 4, no. 7, pp. 1228–1233, Oct. 2011, doi: 10.1016/J.JMBBM.2011.04.005

[101] M. Kita, Y. Ogura, Y. Honda, S.-H. Hyon, W.-I. Cha, and Y. Ikada, "Evaluation of Polyvinyl Alcohol Hydrogel as a Soft Contact Lens Material," *Graefes Arch Clin Exp Ophthalmol*, vol. 228, no. 6, pp. 533–537, 1990, doi: 10.1007/BF00918486

[102] L. E. Millon, H. Mohammadi, and W. K. Wan, "Anisotropic Polyvinyl Alcohol Hydrogel for Cardiovascular Applications," *J Biomed Mater Res B Appl Biomater*, vol. 79B, no. 2, pp. 305–311, Nov. 2006, doi: https://doi.org/10.1002/jbm.b.30543

[103] Z. Li et al., "Design Strategies for Environmentally Friendly Polyvinyl Alcohol Hydrogel Sensors: Research Progress and Perspectives," *Mater Today Commun*, vol. 39, p. 109401, Jun. 2024, doi: 10.1016/J.MTCOMM.2024.109401

[104] H. Adelnia, R. Ensandoost, S. Shebbrin Moonshi, J. N. Gavgani, E. I. Vasafi, and H. T. Ta, "Freeze/Thawed Polyvinyl Alcohol Hydrogels: Present, Past and Future," *Eur Polym J*, vol. 164, p. 110974, Feb. 2022, doi: 10.1016/J.EURPOLYMJ.2021.110974

[105] S. R. Caliari and J. A. Burdick, "A Practical Guide to Hydrogels for Cell Culture," *Nat Methods*, vol. 13, no. 5, pp. 405–414, 2016, doi: 10.1038/nmeth.3839

[106] J. Dai, H. Zhang, C. Huang, Z. Chen, and A. Han, "A Gel-Based Separation-Free Point-of-Care Device for Whole Blood Glucose Detection," *Anal Chem*, vol. 92, no. 24, pp. 16122–16129, Dec. 2020, doi: 10.1021/acs.analchem.0c03801

[107] M. J. Webber and E. T. Pashuck, "(Macro)Molecular Self-Assembly for Hydrogel Drug Delivery," *Adv Drug Deliv Rev*, vol. 172, pp. 275–295, May 2021, doi: 10.1016/J.ADDR.2021.01.006

[108] J. H. Lee, H. B. Lee, and J. D. Andrade, "Blood Compatibility of Polyethylene Oxide Surfaces," *Prog Polym Sci*, vol. 20, no. 6, pp. 1043–1079, Jan. 1995, doi: 10.1016/0079-6700(95)00011-4

[109] K. F. Güenaga, D. Matos, and P. Wille-Jørgensen, "Mechanical Bowel Preparation for Elective Colorectal Surgery," *Cochrane Database Syst Rev*, vol. 9, 2011, doi: 10.1002/14651858.CD001544.pub4

[110] R. P. G. Ten Broek, N. Kok-Krant, H. R. Verhoeve, H. van Goor, and E. A. Bakkum, "Efficacy of Polyethylene Glycol Adhesion Barrier After Gynecological Laparoscopic Surgery," *Gynecol Surg*, vol. 9, no. 1, pp. 29–35, 2012, doi: 10.1007/s10397-011-0698-0

[111] Y. Wang, X. Wang, W. Chen, L. Zhu, and B. Zhang, "Environmental Stimulant-Responsive Hydrogels Based on Polyethylene Glycol-Derived Polymer for Underwater Bonding and Extraction of Fragile Wooden Relics: Synthesis, Characterization, and Preliminary Application," *Int J Adhes Adhes*, vol. 131, p. 103651, May 2024, doi: 10.1016/J.IJADHADH.2024.103651

[112] M. Ma, Y. Qi, Q. Chen, and Z. Zhang, "Robust Fluorescent Silica/Polyethylene Glycol Hydrogel Membrane for Tracking and Antifouling," *ACS Appl Polym Mater*, vol. 6, no. 6, pp. 3534–3543, Mar. 2024, doi: 10.1021/acsapm.4c00377

[113] E. Ferchichi, S. Stealey, P. Bogert, and S. P. Zustiak, "Tunable Gelatin Methacrylate Polyethylene Glycol Diacrylate Hydrogels for Cell Mechanosensing Applications," *Front Biomater Sci*, vol. 3, Jul. 2024, doi: 10.3389/fbiom.2024.1408748

[114] A. Srivastava and N. Bhatnagar, "Production and Characterisation of New Bioresorbable Radiopaque Mg–Zn–Y Alloy to Improve X-ray Visibility of Polymeric Scaffolds," *J Magnes Alloy*, vol. 10, no. 6, pp. 1694–1703, Jun. 2022, doi: 10.1016/j.jma.2020.11.010

[115] M. K. Egbo, "A Fundamental Review on Composite Materials and Some of Their Applications in Biomedical Engineering," *J King Saud Univ Eng Sci*, vol. 33, no. 8, pp. 557–568, Dec. 2021, doi: 10.1016/j.jksues.2020.07.007

[116] A. Srivastava, N. Kumari, M. Agarwal, P. Bhati, and N. Bhatnagar, "Fabrication and Characterization of Bioresorbable Radiopaque PLLA/PCL/Mg Alloy Composite Tubes for Cardiovascular Stent Application," *Int J Polym Mater Polym Biomater*, pp. 1–17, Mar. 2023, doi: 10.1080/00914037.2023.2182783

[117] A. Srivastava et al., "Fabrication and Characterization of PLLA/PCL/Mg-Zn-Y Alloy Composite Stent," *Polym Eng Sci*, vol. 64, no. 1, pp. 243–253, Jan. 2024, doi: 10.1002/pen.26543

[118] S. Ramakrishna, J. Mayer, E. Wintermantel, and K. W. Leong, "Biomedical Applications of Polymer-Composite Materials: A Review," *Compos Sci Technol*, vol. 61, no. 9, pp. 1189–1224, Jul. 2001, doi: 10.1016/S0266-3538(00)00241-4

[119] M. Bednarek, E. Wojtczak, and M. Pluta, "Spontaneous Formation of Polylactide Stereocomplex Microspheres Containing Metal Ions," *Polym Int*, vol. 66, no. 1, pp. 108–118, Jan. 2017, doi: 10.1002/pi.5251

[120] V. Lassalle and M. L. Ferreira, "PLA Nano- and Microparticles for Drug Delivery: An Overview of the Methods of Preparation," *Macromol Biosci*, vol. 7, no. 6, pp. 767–783, Jun. 2007, doi: 10.1002/mabi.200700022

[121] D. G. Morales-Hernandez, D. C. Genetos, D. M. Working, K. C. Murphy, and J. K. Leach, "Ceramic Identity Contributes to Mechanical Properties and Osteoblast Behavior on Macroporous Composite Scaffolds," *J Funct Biomater*, vol. 3, no. 2, pp. 382–397, May 2012, doi: 10.3390/jfb3020382

[122] Madan, P., Singh, V., Singh, D. P., Diwakar, M., & Kishor, A. (2022). Denoising of ECG signals using weighted stationary wavelet total variation. *Biomedical Signal Processing and Control*, *73*, 103478. 10.1016/j.bspc.2021.103478

[123] O. Fraile-Martínez et al., "Applications of Polymeric Composites in Bone Tissue Engineering and Jawbone Regeneration," *Polymers (Basel)*, vol. 13, no. 19, p. 3429, Oct. 2021, doi: 10.3390/polym13193429

[124] S. V. Dorozhkin, "Biocomposites and Hybrid Biomaterials Based on Calcium Orthophosphates," *Biomatter*, vol. 1, no. 1, pp. 3–56, Jul. 2011, doi: 10.4161/biom.1.1.16782

[125] A. Diez-Pascual, "Tissue Engineering Bionanocomposites Based on Poly(propylene fumarate)," *Polymers (Basel)*, vol. 9, no. 7, p. 260, Jun. 2017, doi: 10.3390/polym9070260
[126] J. Radwan-Pragłowska, Ł. Janus, M. Piątkowski, D. Bogdał, and D. Matýsek, "Hybrid Bilayer PLA/Chitosan Nanofibrous Scaffolds Doped With ZnO, Fe3O4, and Au Nanoparticles With Bioactive Properties for Skin Tissue Engineering," *Polymers (Basel)*, vol. 12, no. 1, p. 159, Jan. 2020, doi: 10.3390/polym12010159
[127] W. Shen, G. Zhang, Y. Li, and G. Fan, "Research on Electrospinning Three-Branched-Chain PLA Porous Microspheres and Adsorption for Silver Ions," *J Appl Polym Sci*, vol. 135, no. 45, Dec. 2018, doi: 10.1002/app.46735
[128] A. M. Al-Enizi, M. M. Zagho, and A. A. Elzatahry, "Polymer-Based Electrospun Nanofibers for Biomedical Applications," *Nanomaterials*, vol. 8, no. 4, p. 259, Apr. 2018, doi: 10.3390/nano8040259
[129] P. Vashisth and J. R. Bellare, "Development of Hybrid Scaffold With Biomimetic 3D Architecture for Bone Regeneration," Nanomedicine, vol. 14, no. 4, pp. 1325–1336, Jun. 2018, doi: 10.1016/j.nano.2018.03.011
[130] D. D. Deligianni, "Nanotubes Reinforcement of Degradable Polymers for Orthopedic Applications," *Adv Tissue Eng Regen Med Open Access*, vol. 2, no. 6, Aug. 2017, doi: 10.15406/atroa.2017.02.00047
[131] M. Rahim, M. R. H. Mas Haris, and N. U. Saqib, "An Overview of Polymeric Nano-Biocomposites as Targeted and Controlled-Release Devices," *Biophys Rev*, vol. 12, no. 5, pp. 1223–1231, Oct. 2020, doi: 10.1007/s12551-020-00750-0
[132] M. Alizadeh-Osgouei, Y. Li, and C. Wen, "A Comprehensive Review of Biodegradable Synthetic Polymer-Ceramic Composites and Their Manufacture for Biomedical Applications," *Bioact Mater*, vol. 4, no. 1, pp. 22–36, Dec. 2019, doi: 10.1016/J.BIOACTMAT.2018.11.003
[133] Z. Guo, A. A. Poot, and D. W. Grijpma, "Advanced Polymer-Based Composites and Structures for Biomedical Applications," *Eur Polym J*, vol. 149, p. 110388, Apr. 2021, doi: 10.1016/J.EURPOLYMJ.2021.110388
[134] T. Biswal, S. K. BadJena, and D. Pradhan, "Synthesis of Polymer Composite Materials and Their Biomedical Applications," *Mater Today Proc*, vol. 30, pp. 305–315, Jan. 2020, doi: 10.1016/J.MATPR.2020.01.567
[135] I. Id, "Applications of Polymers in the Biomedical Field," *Curr Trends Biomed Eng Biosci*, vol. 4, no. 5, May 2017, doi: 10.19080/ctbeb.2017.04.555650
[136] J. Li et al., "Promoting Tissue Repair Using Deferoxamine Nanoparticles Loaded Biomimetic Gelatin/HA Composite Hydrogel," *Biomed Mater*, vol. 19, no. 4, p. 045009, 2024, doi: 10.1088/1748-605X/ad46ba
[137] C. Belda Marín et al., "Gold, Silver, and Iron Oxide Nanoparticle Incorporation Into Silk Hydrogels for Biomedical Applications: Elaboration, Structure, and Properties," *ACS Biomater Sci Eng*, vol. 7, no. 6, pp. 2358–2371, Jun. 2021, doi: 10.1021/acsbiomaterials.1c00441
[138] N. H. Thang, T. B. Chien, and D. X. Cuong, "Polymer-Based Hydrogels Applied in Drug Delivery: An Overview," *Gels*, vol. 9, no. 7, 2023, doi: 10.3390/gels9070523
[139] Yadav, S., Chamoli, S., Kumar, P., & Maurya, P. K. (2023). Structural and functional insights in polysaccharides coated cerium oxide nanoparticles and their potential biomedical applications: A review. *International*

Journal of Biological Macromolecules, 125673, https://doi.org/10.1016/j.ijbiomac.2023.12567
[140] Gupta, P., Gupta, H., Kairamkonda, M., Kumar, N., & Poluri, K. M. (2022). Elucidating the lactic acid tolerance mechanism in vaginal clinical isolates of Candida glabrata. *Medical Mycology*, *60*(6), myac042. https://doi.org/10.1093/mmy/myac042
[141] Ahmad, W., & Kumar, S. (2024). T axus wallichiana leaf extract-mediated microwave-assisted one-pot biosynthesis of MgO NPs for biomedical and photocatalytic applications. *Emergent Materials*, *7*(3), 1081–1090. https://doi.org/10.1007/s42247-023-00612-x
[142] Alrashed, F. A., Alsubiheen, A. M., Alshammari, H., Mazi, S. I., Al-Saud, S. A., Alayoubi, S., ... & Dhiman, G. (2022). Stress, anxiety, and depression in pre-clinical medical students: Prevalence and association with sleep disorders. *Sustainability*, *14*(18), 11320. 10.3390/su141811320
[143] Elashiri, M. A., Rajesh, A., Pandey, S. N., Shukla, S. K., & Urooj, S. (2022). Ensemble of weighted deep concatenated features for the skin disease classification model using modified long short term memory. *Biomedical Signal Processing and Control*, *76*, 103729. 10.1016/j.bspc.2022.103729
[144] Wazid, M., Singh, J., Das, A. K., Shetty, S., Khan, M. K., & Rodrigues, J. J. (2022). ASCP-IoMT: AI-enabled lightweight secure communication protocol for internet of medical things. *IEEE Access*, *10*, 57990–58004, 10.1109/ACCESS.2022.3179418
[145] Sharma, R., Kim, M., & Gupta, A. (2022). Motor imagery classification in brain-machine interface with machine learning algorithms: Classical approach to multi-layer perceptron model. *Biomedical Signal Processing and Control*, *71*, 103101, 10.1016/j.bspc.2021.103101
[146] Pawar, D., Phansalkar, S., Sharma, A., Sahu, G. K., Ang, C. K., & Lim, W. H. (2023). Survey on the Biomedical Text Summarization Techniques with an Emphasis on Databases, Techniques, Semantic Approaches, Classification Techniques, and Similarity Measures. *Sustainability*, *15*(5), 4216. 10.3390/su15054216

Chapter 6

Study to analyze the efficacy of three types of polishing techniques on two commercially available denture base acrylic resins

Pronob Sanyal and Deepika Khanna

6.1 INTRODUCTION

For the development of different dental prostheses, as well as orthodontic appliances, acrylic resin is a substance that is often utilized in dentistry. It is used to replace missing tissues and transmit chewing pressures to remaining ridges when making removable partial or full dentures, as well as overdentures that are implant-supported or implant-retained. Acrylic resin is used extensively in dentistry, which emphasizes how significant it is [1, 2].

Clinical restoration methods must include the polishing and finishing of dental components as a critical component. The paste can easily be drawn naturally to the rough surface in the mouth, which can be especially difficult for long-term usage. Only microorganisms that can cling to non-shedding surfaces may live in the mouth, including those that cause periodontal disease, caries, as well as stomatitis associated with dentures. Plaque accumulation results from bacterial adhesion [3].

The adherence of bacteria to hard tooth surfaces is greatly affected by free surface energy and surface roughness. The adherence and retaining may be significantly affected by variations in these important factors. A tiny coating of obtained salivary pellicle may dramatically lower free surface energy on rough oral surfaces. The surface free energy of various dental materials varies. According to studies, compared to smooth surfaces, plaque and bacterial growth are more likely to occur on surfaces made of abrasive acrylic resin.

Since dental clinics are rarely close to dental labs including remedial sanding of the acrylic resin components of removable dentures is essential in daily dental practice, numerous polishing kits such as chairside have already been developed to be used right away after grinding operational processes on the denture base as well as orthodontic or occlusal devices. The producers of chairside polish kits claim that these methods result in surfaces made of acrylic resin that are sufficiently smooth. The polished surfaces of acrylic sealers of two chairside polishing tools were significantly more smooth than

DOI: 10.1201/9781003536352-6

tungsten carbide burs, though less smoothly than conventional polishing in a dental office, according to research on these polishing methods that had been documented in the literature [4, 5].

Studies have revealed that in supragingival regions, surface free energy has less impact on microbial adhesion than surface roughness. There is a surface roughness threshold (Ra = 0.2 m), according to some in vivo studies, beyond which plaque deposition cannot be inhibited any more. The buildup of plaque will, however, rise concurrently with a higher surface roughness if it exceeds this threshold.

Microorganisms that stick to the acrylic surface of dentures produce denture plaque. This plaque may cause periodontal disease, tooth and root caries, and denture-related stomatitis. The plaque on the basis of dentures often contains yeast from *Candida* spp. Numerous additional bacteria may thrive in denture plaque, proving in studies that *Candida* spp. are not the sole pathogens in it. Numerous investigations have shown that *Streptococcus oralis* and *Candida albicans* adhere more readily to rough acrylic resin surfaces [6].

Acrylic resin that has been polished using abrasive stones, rubber polishers, prophylaxis pastes, and pumices may still have surface roughness that is more than Ra = 0.2 m. Surface roughness of an acrylic resin that is smooth is 0.12 m. The roughness of polished acrylic resin, however, may vary from 0.03 to 0.75 microns. Due to the frequent need for corrective grinding of acrylic resin dentures and the fact that dentist offices are not usually close to dental labs, chairside polishing kits have been created for use in routine dental practice [4]. These kits claim to produce acrylic resin surfaces that are sufficiently smooth, but a study found that they were smoother than those made by tungsten carbide burs, the surfaces formed by two chairside polishing devices (Kenda Queen and Shofu) were still not as smooth as those made by traditional polishing in a dental lab [7].

In a dental laboratory, the standard mechanical polishing process involves primary finishing, pre-polishing with freshwater and finer pumice or silicon polishers, as well as fine polishing with the use of a polishing solution or liquid polish containing fine aluminum oxide particles. Although time-consuming, this approach is effective since each step must be carried out in order.

6.2 AIM AND OBJECTIVES

6.2.1 Aim

The aim of the study is to assess and contrast the performance of three polishing methods in creating smooth surfaces when used on two different acrylic denture base resins that are available on the market.

6.2.2 Objectives

1. To assess the performance of two different widely available acrylic denture base resins using the mechanical polishing technique.
2. To examine how well two available on the market acrylic denture base resins may be polished using both mechanical and chemical approaches.
3. To assess the efficiency of integrating chairside with chemical polishing techniques on two different acrylic denture base resins that are readily accessible in the marketplace.
4. To assess the performance of the aforementioned three polishing processes on two separate acrylic denture base resins that are readily accessible on the market.

6.3 LITERATURE REVIEW

In a research, Schwindling et al. [8] assessed the heat-cured acrylic resin's surface roughness after they had been polished using three distinct chairside kits, traditional sandpaper, and laboratory polishing. The findings revealed that the chairside kits were in the middle and that chairside polishing provided the smoothest surfaces, with the sandpaper producing the roughest. If laboratory polishing is not achievable, the researchers found that chairside polishing kits may be employed as an alternate polishing technique.

After polishing, the denture bases' and repair materials' surface roughness was determined using chairside polishing kits and traditional laboratory procedures, and it was compared in a research by Gungor et al. [9]. According to the findings, traditional laboratory polishing remained the most efficient technique, and even though the Ra value was still higher than what was considered acceptable, the chairside polishing kits produced a smoother surface than that of the placebo group. The researchers proposed that chairside silicone polishing kits would be an effective alternative in dental offices when traditional polishing is not accessible, and standard laboratory polishing can be utilized for the denture base as well as repair materials.

Jeyapalan et al. [10] performed a research to examine the average surface roughness values of denture base acrylic resins that had undergone mechanical polishing (MP) versus chemical polishing (CP) after being heat-cured and light-cured. The results demonstrated that MP generated the smoothest surface as well as that the kind of acrylic resin had no impact on the values of mean roughness of the surface.

In a study by Elnailia and Patrickb, 25 disks of each kind of acrylic resin, each sized 11 mm in diameter as well as 3 mm in thickness, were molded [11]. The samples were polished using 1200 and 600 surface polishers to achieve various roughness characteristics. A profilometer was used to assess the average surface roughness (Ra), and the average mean was computed. Additionally, a scanning electron microscope (SEM) was used to study the surface features (SEM). The average means of surface roughness for the 600 surface polishers of all kinds (HC, HIHC, CC, and HCC) were greater than those for the 1200 surface polishers. The average surface roughness of each kind of acrylic denture between 1200 and 600 grit surface polishers had a significant P value between 0.018, 0.006, and 0.013 in HIHC, CC, and HCC, respectively. It was determined that different kinds of resin materials had different surface textures, but HIHC had by far the greatest average surface roughness.

According to several studies, a reduction in the friction caused by the denture's surface roughness lessens the effect of abrasion on the patient's soft tissue [12]. Also, according to other research, a high degree of surface roughness increases surface stains and microbe adherence. Biofilm adhesion will be hampered if the denture base is chemically polished to a surface roughness of less than 0.2 m. To prevent microbial aggregation, strict oral hygiene and potential surface changes to modify the surface properties have been advised [12–15].

6.4 MATERIALS AND METHODS

After receiving proper clearance from the Institutional Ethical Committee, the current research was carried out at the Department of Prosthodontics, Crown and Bridge, School of Dental Sciences, KIMS (Deemed University), Karad, Maharashtra.

6.4.1 Materials and equipment used during the course of study

- Custom-made stainless steel mold
- Heat-cured denture base resin (Trevalon and Trevalon HI)
- Vaseline petroleum jelly
- Hydraulic press
- Acrylizer
- Tungsten carbide burs
- Sand paper
- Cotton wheel buff
- Pumice slurry
- Pumice cake
- Thermocycling unit
- Methyl methacrylate monomer
- Chairside acrylic adjusting and polishing kit

- Universal polishing paste
- Scanning electron microscope
- Contact profilometer

6.4.2 Methods followed during the course of study

6.4.2.1 Preparation of stainless steel mold

Two rectangular stainless steel plates with a thickness of 2 mm and 3 mm were purchased out of a collection of three rectangular stainless steel plates. The plate with a thickness of 3 mm was constructed with 12 circular holes, each measuring 20 mm in diameter. To help in the manufacturing of acrylic specimens, this was done. The circular-holed plates were positioned among the other two rectangular plates, each of which had a thickness of 2 mm. Four nuts and bolts that were positioned at each of the rectangular plates' four corners helped to tighten and hold this arrangement in place.

6.4.2.2 Preparation of acrylic denture base resin specimens

The acrylic orthodontic resin composites specimens were manufactured, replicated, and standardized with the aid of the stainless steel mold. Two varieties of commercial products heat-cured acrylic denture base material, namely high-impact denture base (Trevalon HI, Dentsply International, USA) and traditional denture base (Trevalon, Dentsply International, USA) were used to create a total of 60 specimens (20 mm diameter × 3 mm thickness). The 60 specimens were divided into 30 high-impact acrylic denture base resin specimens (Trevalon HI) and the remaining 30 into standard acrylic denture base resin specimens (Trevalon). The manufacturer's instructions were followed while working with the acrylic denture base resin material.

The stainless steel molds were coated with a separating agent (Vaseline, Unilever, UK), and the denture-based material was packed using a hydraulic press (Hydraulic Press P 400, Sirio Dental division, Italy) at a pressure of 3500 psi. The assembly was then given 120 minutes to cure on a bench before being given another 120 minutes to cure in an acrylizing machine at 740C. After that, the assembly was given another 60 minutes to cure before being subjected to a second processing step at 1000 C. This assembly underwent curing, bench cooling, specimen removal, and trimming of any extra material.

6.4.2.3 Finishing and polishing of acrylic resin specimens

6.4.2.3.1 Mechanical laboratory polishing

A force sensor (Samyak SMIT-3016, Samyak Instrumentation Pvt Ltd. Ahmedabad India) of load cell variety was used to standardize the procedure.

For this, a suggested force of 4N was applied using the counter-balanced load weight system (0 to 500 gm). One experimenter carried out every step of the polishing and finishing process.

The following steps were carried out in the specified order:

Step 1: With their shanks color labelled as white (Ultra Fine), yellow (Extra Fine), red (Fine), blue (Medium coarse), green (Coarse), and black (Extra coarse), tungsten carbide burs of six grits were used to polish specimen surfaces. Each bur was spun for 15 seconds at 15,000 rpm.

Step 2: Next, sandpaper with grit sizes 400 (fine), 320 (medium), and 220 (coarse) was used to complete the specimens. Both dry and wet sand papers were used for 15 seconds each for all the specimens.

Step 3: Polishing of specimens was carried out using a cotton wheel buff as a carrier medium at 2800 rpm. During this procedure, we used wet buff with pumice slurry for 15 seconds followed by dry buff with pumice cake for 15 seconds.

6.4.2.3.2 Chemical polishing

Using tweezers, the specimens were submerged in methyl-methacrylate monomer (Trevalon) that had been heated to 75°C ±1°C for 10 seconds to perform chemical polishing. The samples were taken out of the solution, dried at 30°C for 15 seconds, and then washed under running water for approximately one minute to eliminate extra fluid. Prior to examination, the samples were given 10 minutes to dry at room temperature (30°C). One researcher handled all of the procedures.

6.4.2.3.3 Chairside polishing

To make the process more consistent, a pressure transducer was employed. With the counter-balanced load weight system (0–500 gm), a suggested force of 4 N was employed for this. One investigator carried out every step of the polishing and finishing process.

The following steps were carried out in specific order: Acrylic adjusting and polishing kit (Shofu Dental Corporation, USA) was used for performing the final procedure. The kit provides tungsten carbide burs and silicone points which were color coded brown, gray, and light gray suggesting decreasing order of coarseness [2]. Each of these burs and silicone points was used in the sequential order as per manufacturer's instructions for 15 seconds each unidirectionally.

To carry out the polishing procedure, universal polishing paste (Ivoclar Vivadent Inc. New York, USA) was used by directly dispensing from the tubes, as per manufacturer's instructions multidirectionally for 15 seconds each using cotton buff as a carrier medium.

6.4.2.4 *Surface roughness measurements*

Using a contact profilometer, the acrylic resin samples' surface roughness was evaluated (Mitutoyo SJ-210, USA). The device's diamond stylus was moved over the surface of the specimen to measure surface roughness (Ra), which is expressed in micrometers. The path of the diamond stylus was parallel to the finishing and polishing plane. Each tracing's cut-off length was 2 mm. Each specimen had its surface roughness measured twice, and the statistical analysis employed mean average Ra values.

For the convenience of analysis, the surface roughness values obtained were tabulated into six groups as per the type of polishing method employed.

- Group 1: Mechanical Laboratory Polishing (Conventional Heat Cured Denture Base Resin – Trevalon)
- Group 2: Mechanical Laboratory Polishing (High Impact Heat Cured Denture Base Resin – Trevalon HI)
- Group 3: Mechanical Laboratory + Chemical Polishing (Conventional Heat Cured Denture Base Resin – Trevalon)
- Group 4: Mechanical Laboratory + Chemical Polishing (High Impact Heat Cured Denture Base Resin – Trevalon HI)
- Group 5: Chairside + Chemical Polishing (Conventional Heat Cured Denture Base Resin – Trevalon)
- Group 6: Chairside + Chemical Polishing (High-Impact Heat Cured Denture Base Resin – Trevalon HI).

6.4.2.5 *Scanning electron microscopy (SEM)*

Following the process of polishing of acrylic resin, a 2.5 mm ×2.5 mm fragment was cut-off (Marathon N3S handpiece S07 Micromotor, South Korea. SSW HP 701L bur, SS White, Lakewood. New Jersey, USA) from each specimen and prepared for scanning electron microscopy (SEM) analysis.

Subsequently, all the samples were treated in an ultrasonicator with 70% alcohol before being sputter-coated with gold.

6.5 STATISTICAL ANALYSIS

SPSS for Windows version 17.0 was used to do the statistical computations. The current research used the following statistical techniques:

- Analysis of Variance (ANOVA) – one way.
- Independent samples 't' test
- Tukey's multiple post hoc

Tukey's test for post hoc comparisons (= 0.05) and one-way ANOVA were used to examine the average mean surface roughness data. The values of surface roughness of one polishing group were contrasted to five other groups in the Tukey's test for post hoc comparisons, using the I and J groups to carry out multiple comparisons.

6.6 RESULTS

6.6.1 One-way ANOVA

The one-way ANOVA test generates a one-way analysis of variance for a measurable variable of interest by a single element (independent) variable. The hypothesis is tested using analysis of variance when all means are equal. This technique extends the two-sample t-test.

We may need to determine which means are different in addition to confirming the existence of differences between them. Preconceived contrasts as well as post hoc tests are the two sorts of tests being utilized to establish the means. A priori tests, those that were set up before the experiment, contrasts, and post hoc tests, which were conducted after the trial, were all carried out. To contrast the surface roughness variations among the three polishing processes used with two different heat-cure acrylic denture base resins that are commercially available, one-way ANOVA was used in the current investigation.

6.6.2 Tukey's multiple post hoc tests

Should it be observed that the other means vary, pairwise multiple comparisons and post hoc range tests may be used to pinpoint the specific means that differ. Range studies identify identically grouped means that are homogeneous in nature. Pairwise significance of differences, which examine the differences between each pair of means, resulted in a matrix with asterisks designating group means that are significantly different from one another at an alpha level of 0.05. Tukey's HSD is one of the often used post hoc tests (honestly significant difference). In the present investigation, paired t-tests were performed to compare each pair of mean values across the six study groups using Tukey's HSD post hoc test.

6.6.3 Test for independent samples

The independent t-test determines if the means of two independent groups based on the same dependent continuous variable differ statistically substantially from one another. It is often referred to as the student's t-test or the two-sample t-test. Only quantitative data may be evaluated with this test. To compare the differences in the polishing capabilities of the two commonly available heat-cured acrylic denture base resins, in the present study, Independent Samples 't' test has been used. Samples of acrylic denture base resin were heated to cure and a contact profilometer was used to assess the surface roughness (Ra). The average mean values of the acrylic resin's surface roughness were examined using the one-way ANOVA outcomes.

6.7 DISCUSSION

A well-polished but smooth surface is one of the essential components of a good dental prosthesis. The traditional technique for polishing dental materials involves gently scraping the rough surface's outermost layers. The goal of the procedure is to create a surface that is sufficiently bright and smooth enough to prevent the proliferation of bacterial plaque. Surface roughness is a severe issue, according to in-vivo study [1, 3–10] since it either has an indirect or direct impact on the development of bacterial plaque, tooth health, staining, as well as patient comfort. The surfaces of dental restorations should be as smooth as possible in order to achieve maximum aesthetic appeal as well as oral health since roughness may facilitate microbe adhesion regardless of whether the patient performs adequate dental implant care [7, 9, 11]. Denture base material roughness is chiefly impacted by the characteristics of the raw material, the polishing method, and the physical dexterity of the operator [16].

Rough acrylic surfaces have been linked to bacterial growth and plaque development, according to many researchers [2, 7, 12]. Smooth acrylic resin is described as having a 0.12-m value. The surface roughness of polished acrylic resin, though, may vary from 0.03 mm to 0.75 mm [17]. There would be substantial bacterial colonization if somehow the surface roughness was more than 2 mm. A considerable concentration of microbial colonization occurs once the value of surface roughness is more than 2.0 mm, according to the authors of [5, 8, 10] and [18]. The thickness of a smooth acrylic resin surface, according to the authors, might vary from 0.03 mm to 0.75 mm, depending on the finishing and polishing process [10].

The objective of the current study was to assess and contrast how well three polishing procedures worked on two distinct commercial products, acrylic denture base resins, to produce smooth surfaces.

The initial null hypothesis stated that the polishing method had no impact on the denture base resin materials' surface roughness. The second null hypothesis was that the values of surface roughness after polishing would be comparable for both traditional and high-performance heat-polymerized acrylic resins that are available [19].

The investigation's results led to the rejection of the original null hypothesis. The data demonstrated that the surface roughness value of heat-cured acrylic dental composite resins was significantly influenced by polishing techniques ($P = 0.000$). The surface roughness varied significantly across the chairside + chemical polishing technique, mechanical laboratory, and mechanical laboratory + chemical polishing methods (P = 0.000).

Additionally, there were significant variations in the surface roughness values of the Trevalon traditional heat-cured acrylic resin and the Trevalon HI high-impact heat-cured acrylic resin samples (P>0.001).

The study's findings revealed that the average mean values of surface roughness for mechanical laboratory polishing of heat-cured acrylic resin (Trevalon) were 0.301 mm and 0.257 mm, respectively (Trevalon HI). In terms of mechanical laboratory + chemical polishing of heat-cured acrylic resin (Trevalon), the average values of mean surface roughness were 0.466 mm and 0.409 mm, respectively (Trevalon HI). While the average values of mean surface roughness for chairside + chemical polishing of heat-cured acrylic resin were 0.58 mm (Trevalon) and 0.3 mm (Trevalon HI). The range reported by several other researchers and the mean values discovered in this study are in agreement.

Trevalon and Trevalon HI denture base resin materials showed a significant difference (P = 0.001) on comparison based on the kind of materials utilized, which explains the improved polishability of Trevalon HI denture base resin.

Furthermore, the post hoc Tukey's test findings of this research showed that the surface roughness of mechanical laboratory + chemical polishing of heat-cured acrylic denture basis resin, regardless of the kind of heat-cured denture base resin employed, was not substantially different from chairside + chemical polishing of heat-cured acrylic denture base resin (P = 0.994), but there was a significant difference among the mechanical laboratory polishing versus chemical polishing + mechanical laboratory polishing [20].

Regardless of the material employed, mechanical laboratory polishing provided the lowest surface roughness values of all the others, Ra = 0.257. This discovery is consistent with previous research' findings [19–21]. These outcomes were anticipated because during polishing, the mechanical action of the abrasive gradually eliminates surface notches.

The polishing performance of the surface with chemical polishing technology can very well be demonstrated by the ability of the polishing liquid to permeate the polymeric surface of the acrylic resin as well as to disrupt the secondary bonds that bind them, resulting in a final impact of plasticity on the acrylic resin surface [21, 22]. Molecules of the methyl-methylacrylate monomer were also present in the polishing solution. The underlying imperfections brought on by the finishing operations 29, 36, and 39 are unaffected by this surface layer. In the current investigation, chairside polishing and mechanical laboratory polishing procedures were coupled with chemical polishing. However, there were no discernible differences between the mechanical laboratory + chemical polishing method as well as the chairside + chemical polishing method. The surface roughness values obtained for the mechanical laboratory + chemical polishing mechanism were significantly different from those obtained for the mechanical laboratory polishing method. This meant that, regardless of the subject matter, both strategies are equivalent to one another.

The silicone polishers in the Shofu chairside polishing kit come in a variety of shapes and abrasiveness levels. The silicone abrasive particle size determines how abrasive a polisher is and how smooth the polished surface is. In the current investigation, the samples of both Trevalon and Trevalon HI thermal cure acrylic denture base resins were finished and polished using a Shofu chairside polishing kit. The final polishing step was then completed using universal polishing paste. The chairside technique of polishing was subsequently merged with the chemical polishing process. The findings of the surface roughness study showed that there was no difference between the chairside + chemical polishing technique (Trevalon HI) and mechanical laboratory polishing (Trevalon HI) (P = 0.950).

The average value of surface roughness of the chairside + chemical polishing method (Trevalon HI) (Ra = 0.3) was marginally lower than that of the mechanical laboratory polishing method (Trevalon HI) (Ra = 0.257), which indicates that, when the material being polished has a high polishability, the two methods are comparable. The results of the current research correspond in many ways with those published by the researchers of other comparable studies [12, 18–22].

6.8 CONCLUSION

Surface roughness (Ra) measurements were taken for each sample, as well as the results for mechanical laboratory polishing of heat-cured acrylic resin (Trevalon) were 0.301 µm and 0.257 µm, respectively (Trevalon HI). For mechanical laboratory + chemical polishing of heat-cured acrylic resin (Trevalon), the mean surface roughness values were 0.466 µm, and for mechanical laboratory polishing + chemical polishing of heat-cured acrylic resin, they were 0.409 µm (Trevalon HI). The mean average values of surface roughness for chairside + chemical polishing of heat-cured acrylic resin (Trevalon) were 0.58 pm and 0.3 µm, respectively. However, comparing the two heat-curable denture base resin types, Trevalon HI performed significantly better than Trevalon as a material for the purpose of polishability. A comparison of the three various polishing methods reveals that classic mechanical laboratory polishing remains the most effective and has maintained the accepted practice, irrespective of the material. Depending upon the polishing method and the kinds of materials, the denture base's surface varies. As a result, using 1200 grit as the last step for a surface polisher before using a polishing paste should be advised based on the findings of the present research rather than 600 grit. Given that the effect of chemical polishing on the values of surface roughness depends upon the type of acrylic resin, chairside + chemical polishing might be the best alternative when conventional polishing is not an approach at a dental laboratory.

REFERENCES

1. Al-Dulaijan YA, Alsulaimi L, Alotaibi R, Alboainain A, Alalawi H, Alshehri S, Khan SQ, Alsaloum M, AlRumaih HS, Alhumaidan AA, Gad MM. Comparative Evaluation of Surface Roughness and Hardness of 3D Printed Resins. *Materials*. 2022 Oct 1;15(19):6822.
2. Alammari MR. The influence of polishing techniques on pre-polymerized CAD\CAM acrylic resin denture bases. *Electronic physician*. 2017 Oct;9(10):5452.
3. Porwal A, Khandelwal M, Punia V, Sharma V. Effect of denture cleansers on color stability, surface roughness, and hardness of different denture base resins. *The Journal of the Indian Prosthodontic Society*. 2017 Jan;17(1):61.
4. Quassem MA, Mahross HZ. Comparative Evaluation of Porosities and Solubility for Different Non-Metallic Denture Base Material. *Journal of Clinical & Diagnostic Research*. 2018 Oct 1;12(10).
5. Freitas-Pontes KM, Silva-Lovato CH, Paranhos HF. Mass loss of four commercially available heat-polymerized acrylic resins after toothbrushing with three different dentifrices. *Journal of Applied Oral Science*. 2009;17:116–121.
6. Melo CB, Feitosa MD, Maia SD, Barreto JO, Peixoto RF, Regis RR. Effect of a continuous mechanical polishing protocol on the color stainability, microhardness, mass, and surface roughness of denture base acrylic resin. *The Journal of Prosthetic Dentistry*. 2021 Dec 1;126(6):796–802.
7. Al-Saleh S, Alshahrani A, Albaqawi AH, Alqarawi FK, Alzahrani KM, Tanveer SA, Siddiqui S, Naseem M, Vohra F, Abduljabbar T. Use of Photosensitizer, Glutaraldehyde, alcohol and Ultrasonics in disinfection of polished and rough surfaces of self-curing polymethyl methacrylate denture base material. *Photodiagnosis and Photodynamic Therapy*. 2022 Mar 1;37:102566.
8. Schwindling FS, Rammelsberg P, Stober T. Effect of chemical disinfection on the surface roughness of hard denture base materials: a systematic literature review. *International Journal of Prosthodontics*. 2014 May 1;27(3).
9. Gungor H, Gundogdu M, Duymus ZY. Investigation of the effect of different polishing techniques on the surface roughness of denture base and repair materials. *The Journal of Prosthetic Dentistry*. 2014 Nov 1;112(5):1271–1277.
10. Jeyapalan K, Kumar JK, Azhagarasan NS. Comparative evaluation of the effect of denture cleansers on the surface topography of denture base materials: An in-vitro study. *Journal of Pharmacy & Bioallied Sciences*. 2015 Aug;7(Suppl 2):S548.
11. Mitra, S., Anjum, J., Muni, M., Das, R., Rauf, A., Islam, F., ... & Wilairatana, P. (2022). Exploring the journey of emodin as a potential neuroprotective agent: novel therapeutic insights with molecular mechanism of action. *Biomedicine & Pharmacotherapy*, *149*, 112877. https://doi.org/10.1016/j.biopha.2022.112877
12. Batak B, Çakmak G, Johnston WM, Yilmaz B. Surface roughness of high-performance polymers used for fixed implant-supported prostheses. *The Journal of Prosthetic Dentistry*. 2021 Aug 1;126(2):254-e1.
13. Rapone B, Pedone S, Carnevale A, Plantamura P, Scarano A, Demelio A, Demelio GP, Corsalini M. Profilometer Comparison of the Surface Roughness of Four Denture Base Resins: An In Vitro Study. *Applied Sciences*. 2022 Feb 10;12(4):1837.

14. El-Din MS, Badr AM, Agamy EM, Mohamed GF. Effect of two polishing techniques on surface roughness of three different denture base materials (an in vitro study). Alexandria *Dental Journal*. 2018 Dec 1;43(3):34–40.
15. Darwish M, Nassani MZ. Evaluation of the effect of denture adhesives on surface roughness of two chemically different denture base resins. *European Journal of Dentistry*. 2016 Jul;10(03):321–326.
16. Rahaman Ali AA, John J, Mani SA, El-Seedi HR. Effect of Thermal Cycling on Flexural Properties of Microcrystalline Cellulose-Reinforced Denture Base Acrylic Resins. *Journal of Prosthodontics*. 2020 Aug;29(7):611–616.
17. Onwubu SC, Mdluli PS. Comparative analysis of abrasive materials and polishing system on the surface roughness of heat-polymerized acrylic resins. *European Journal of Dentistry*. 2022 Jul;16(03):573–579.
18. Choi JJ, Uy CE, Ramani RS, Waddell JN. Evaluation of surface roughness, hardness and elastic modulus of nanoparticle containing light-polymerized denture glaze materials. *Journal of the Mechanical Behavior of Biomedical Materials*. 2020 Mar 1;103:103601.
19. Gandhi N, Daniel S, Benjamin S, Kurian N, Varghese VS. Evaluation of surface microhardness following chemical and microwave disinfection of commercially available acrylic resin denture teeth. *Journal of Clinical and Diagnostic Research: JCDR*. 2017 May;11(5):ZC87.
20. Kumar MN, Thippeswamy HM, Swamy KR, Gujjari AK. Efficacy of commercial and household denture cleansers against Candida albicans adherent to acrylic denture base resin: An in vitro study. *Indian Journal of Dental Research*. 2012 Jan 1;23(1):39.
21. Degirmenci K, Hayati Atala M, Sabak C. Effect of different denture base cleansers on surface roughness of heat polymerised acrylic materials with different curing process. *Odovtos International Journal of Dental Sciences*. 2020 Dec;22(3):145–153.
22. Pradhan S, Mathuriya S, Sonkesriya S, Maheshwari A, Gaur G, Choubey A. Evaluation of surface topography of heat cure acrylic denture-base resin before and after reinforcement with different fibers using stylus-based profilometer. *The Journal of Contemporary Dental Practice*. 2022 Jul 11;23(4):415–418.

Chapter 7

Detecting the accuracy of cancer stem cell in brain tumour

R. Suganya, Akash Kumar Barik, Keerthana Balakrishnan, and Aditya Raj

7.1 INTRODUCTION

The spectrum of Artificial Intelligence (Al) is debatable: as robots become more capable, occupations seen as requiring "power" are usually removed from this description, a process known as the Al effect, giving rise to the adage, "Al is whatever hasn't been done yet." For example, visual character recognition is frequently removed from AI, despite the fact that it has become a common application [1–3]. Modern machine skills widely classed as Al includes successfully comprehending human language, competing at the highest level in key play organizations, driving autonomously, and intelligent routing in content delivery networks and war simulations. Deep learning has been utilized in the medical field to discover novel information and techniques for identifying tumours and malignancies, such as cervical cancer, breast cancer, liver tumours, and brain tumours. A brain tumour becomes one of the most serious infectious diseases in contemporary medicine. Brain tumours are fibrous structures that are formed uncontrollably as a result of aberrant brain tissue proliferation. According to a 2022 research by the American Society of Clinical Oncology (ASCO), an estimated 25,050 people in the United States have now been diagnosed with brain tumours, comprising 10,880 women and 14,170 men [4–6]. The most frequent primary tumour of the central nervous system is glioma, which has a high mortality rate. As a result, gliomas are the primary targets of brain tumour segmentation. It is classified as high-grade glioma (HGG) or low-grade glioma (LGG) based on the degree of tumour malignancy [7–9]. LGG grows slowly, and patients have a better outlook for survival. HGG patients have a high death rate and a dismal prognosis. MRI scans have already been used to diagnose brain malignancies in several earlier investigations. To detect brain cancers, the researchers used a convolutional neural network model. The suggested model is a convolutional network with 50 fully connected nodes that employs the activation functions of ReLU, Sigmoid, and SoftMax. The findings suggest that the built model was 75.42% accurate. M. D. Gowda et al. suggested a deep learning model for detection and classification utilizing VGG-16 and mask RCNN. The VGG-16 model was suggested to divide

DOI: 10.1201/9781003536352-7

brain cancers into two categories using MRI images: no tumour and existent tumour. According to the research, the suggested model has 90% accuracy. A transfer learning technique has been developed in further study. In this investigation, feature extraction was performed using pre-trained deep network models, Inception-v3, MobileNetV2, and VGG19. The findings indicated that the accuracy of the model trained with MobileNetV2 was 92%, that of the model trained with Inception-v3 was 91%, and that of the model trained with VGG-19 was only 88%.The prototype in the prior study still showed low precision and had room for improvement [10, 11].

This study made the following contributions:

1) Create a deep learning algorithm to determine brain cancers using MRI images.
2) Recommending a hybrid multi-layer perceptron based on the Inception-v3 model.
3) Improve performance matrices for detecting brain cancers, such as precision, accuracy, recall, and F1 score models.

7.2 METHODOLOGY FOLLOWED

I) Dataset and Cleaning

This study made use of a public dataset including 3,160 brain MRI scans. This data came from the Kaggle's pool. There are 937 meningioma tumour photos, 926 glioma tumour images, 901 pituitary tumour images, and 396 non-tumour images in the collection. Figure 7.1 depicts a frequency histogram of species from the dataset, and Figure 7.2 depicts a representative picture from the collection that shows different types of brain tumour, glioma, which affect the central nervous system. There are different other types of tumours such as acoustic neuromas, medulloblastomas, germ cell tumours and craniopharyngiomas.

II) Standard VGG-16

Any of the network setups considers the input to be a 224 × 224 picture with three channels – R, G, and B. Condoning the RGB values for each pixel is the only pre-processing carried out. This is accomplished by removing the mean value from each pixel. The image is sent via the initial stack of two convolution layers with very small receptive sizes of 3 x 3, followed by ReLU activations. There are 64 filters in each of these two levels. The convolution stride is set at one pixel and also the padding is one pixel. The spatial resolution is preserved in this arrangement, and the resultant activation map is the same size as the input picture dimensions. Figure 7.3. Structure of VGG-16 model.

From Figure 7.2 we see that how every pixel of the image given as input is being extracted to several filters. These filters are passed on to the convolutional layers in order to identify as many feature maps as

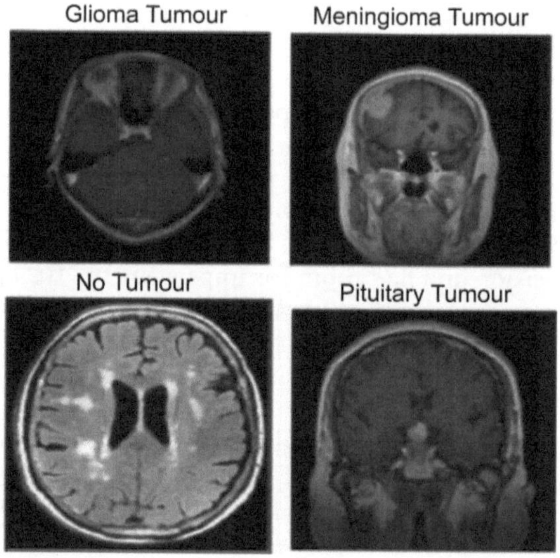

Figure 7.1 Sample image of the dataset.

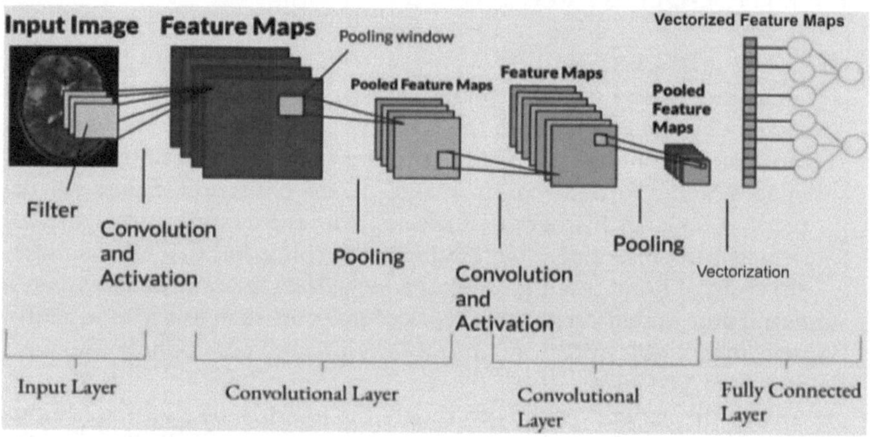

Figure 7.2 Structure of VGG-16.

possible to help break down the problem into simpler terms. Pooling helps in dimensionality reduction which enhances the models speed and memory.

The VGG-16 model's accuracy was evaluated throughout training and validation. AUC was shown to vary throughout training and became more non-linear as the number of repetitions raised. AUC in VGG 16's validation remained constant at 98.15%. We used two classes to examine the accuracy of the preceding method. Our model's F1 score was 92.6%, and its recall was 94.4%. The more training

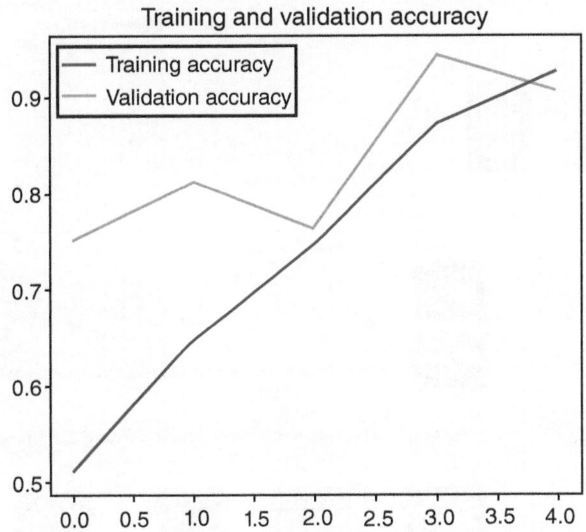

Figure 7.3 Accuracy of VGG-16.

photos and hyperparameters we had, the better our algorithm did. Figure 7.3 displays the VGG 16's training and validation accuracy.

III) Modified Inception-v3
It is the third iteration of a Deep Learning Convolutional Architectures series. The original ImageNet dataset, which was trained using more than 1 million training pictures, yielded 1,000 classes for Inception-v3; however, the Tensor flow version contains 1,001 classes since it includes a "background" class that was not included in the original ImageNet.

As shown in Figure 7.4, the proposed technique consists of four main steps: (1) enhancement, (2) classification, (3) localization, and (4) segmentation. Input pictures are improved using homomorphic wavelet filters, and classification is done using deep feature extraction from Inception-v3. The classified pictures are segmented based on Kapur entropy and localized using the suggested YOLOv2-Inception-v3 method.

IV) Transfer Learning and Fine Tuning
Pre-trained models are stored networks that have already undergone training on a sizable dataset, generally for a sizable image-classification job. You may either utilize the pre-trained model as is or apply transfer learning to tailor it to a specific job. The premise behind transfer learning for image analysis is that if a model is trained on a big and diverse dataset, it may successfully serve as a baseline model of the visual world. You may then use these learnt feature maps instead of reinventing the wheel by training a huge model on a large dataset.

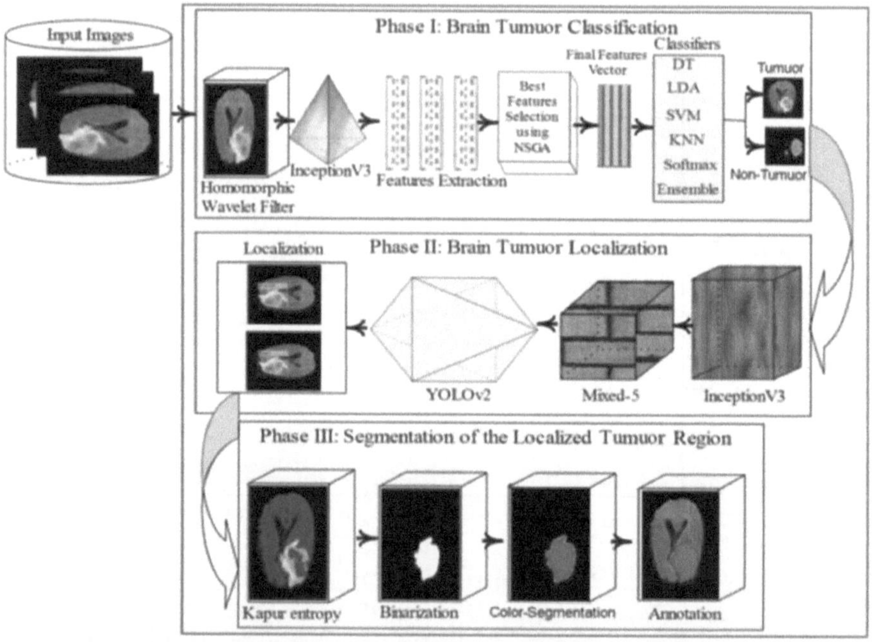

Figure 7.4 Inception work flow.

Transfer learning is the method of training a new machine how to solve a problem that has already been solved by another machine. This model can assist in eliminating a certain possibility from the outcomes by using pertinent data from the earlier model. As a result, the model may locate the answer more quickly and can reduce the number of possible answers. The objective of transfer learning is to reduce the processing time required for the model to arrive at its solution. When a network is being fine-tuned, its weights are used as the initial values for training a new network. Figures 7.5 and 7.6 show transfer learning and fine tuning, respectively.

V) Performance Evaluation Criteria

Model assessment metrics are used to assess the created model's correctness and performance. The model may be evaluated using a variety of measures. The suggested model is evaluated in this study using a classification measure that includes a confusion matrix, accuracy, recall (sensitivity), and F1 score. The confusion matrix comprises the test phase predictions and is used to describe the model's performance. Accuracy is the degree to which the forecast results match the valid values, both positive and negative, given global data. The difference between the projected result and the true number is used to determine accuracy.

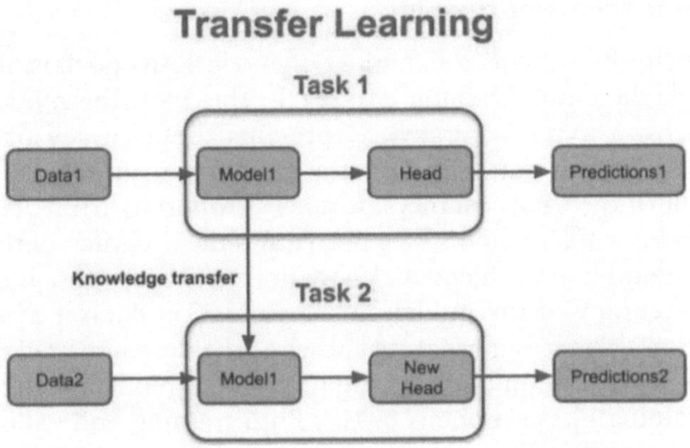

Figure 7.5 Transfer learning.

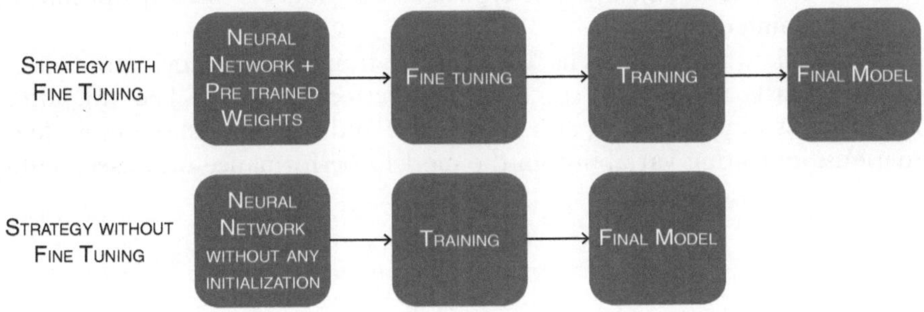

Figure 7.6 Fine tuning.

$$\text{Accuracy}(\%) = \frac{(\text{TP} + \text{TN})}{(\text{TP} + \text{FP} + \text{FN} + \text{TN})} \times 100$$

$$\text{Precision}(\%) = \frac{(\text{TP})}{(\text{TP} + \text{FP})} \times 100$$

$$\text{Recall}(\%) = \frac{(\text{TP})}{(\text{TP} + \text{FP})} \times 100$$

$$F1 - \text{Score} = 2 \times \frac{\text{Peecision} \times \text{Recall}}{\text{Peecision} + \text{Recall}} \times 100$$

Evaluation Metrics

7.3 RESULT AND ANALYSIS

7.3.1 Performance of VGG-16 model

Figure 7.7 illustrates the plot showing the accuracy of a VGG-16 model over 50 epochs for both training and validation datasets.

7.3.1.1 Components of the plot

X-axis (Epoch): Represents the number of epochs. An epoch is one complete pass through the entire training dataset. In this plot, the model is trained for 50 epochs. Y-axis (Accuracy): Represents the accuracy of the model. Accuracy is a metric that indicates the proportion of correctly predicted instances out of the total instances. It ranges from 0 to 1 (or 0% to 100%).

Train Accuracy (black line): This line shows the accuracy of the model on the training dataset at each epoch. Validation Accuracy (grey line): This line shows the accuracy of the model on the validation dataset at each epoch. The validation dataset is a separate subset of the data not used for training, intended to provide an unbiased evaluation of the model during training.

Initial Training Phase (Epochs 0–10): Both training and validation accuracy increase rapidly, indicating that the model is learning and improving its performance on both datasets. The training accuracy increases faster than the validation accuracy, which is typical as the model is directly optimizing on the training data.

Intermediate Phase (Epochs 10–20): The training accuracy continues to rise and starts to plateau, reaching near-perfect accuracy. The validation accuracy also increases but at a slower rate and begins to show more fluctuations, indicating variability in the model's performance on unseen data.

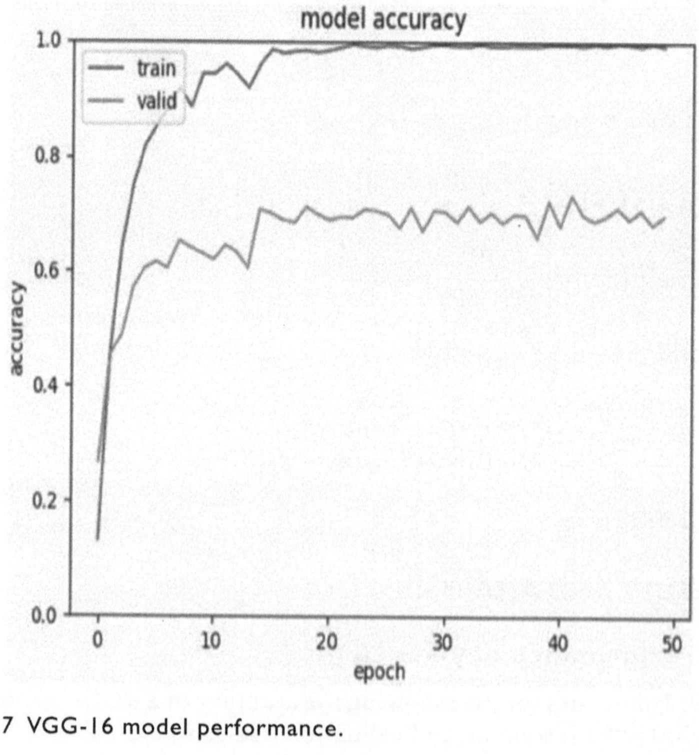

Figure 7.7 VGG-16 model performance.

Later Training Phase (Epochs 20–50): The training accuracy reaches a very high value, close to 1 (or 100%), indicating that the model is almost perfectly predicting the training data. The validation accuracy, however, stabilizes at a lower value (around 0.7 to 0.75 or 70–75%) and does not improve further. It also shows some fluctuations, which is a sign that the model's performance on unseen data is not as stable or consistent.

7.3.1.2 Observations and possible issues

Overfitting: The most apparent observation is the gap between training accuracy and validation accuracy after around 10 epochs. The training accuracy is very high, while the validation accuracy is significantly lower and fluctuating. This indicates that the model might be overfitting the training data. Overfitting occurs when the model learns the training data too well, including its noise and outliers, leading to poor generalization to new, unseen data.

Stabilization: The validation accuracy stabilizes early (around epoch 20) and does not improve much beyond that, suggesting that further training does not benefit the model in terms of generalization. This stabilization indicates that the model has reached its capacity to generalize from the given training data and further epochs do not help.

7.3.2 Performance of modified Inception-v3

This set of plots (Figure 7.8) shows the training and validation accuracy and loss over 100 epochs for a machine learning model.

7.3.2.1 Left plot: Training and validation accuracy

X-axis (Epoch): Represents the number of epochs. Each epoch is a complete pass through the entire training dataset. Y-axis (Accuracy): Represents the accuracy of the model, ranging from 0 to 1 (or 0% to 100%). Training Accuracy (black line): Shows the accuracy on the training dataset at each epoch. Validation Accuracy (grey line): Shows the accuracy on the validation dataset at each epoch.

Initial Phase (Epochs 0–20): Both training and validation accuracy increase rapidly, indicating the model is learning effectively from the training data and generalizing well to the validation data. There is some fluctuation in the validation accuracy, which is common as the model adapts to the data.

Intermediate Phase (Epochs 20–80): Training accuracy continues to improve and begins to plateau around 90%. Validation accuracy also improves and stabilizes around 80–90%, but with noticeable fluctuations.

Later Phase (Epochs 80–100): Training accuracy remains high, slightly below 100%, indicating the model is performing very well on the training data. Validation accuracy remains stable but fluctuates between 85 and

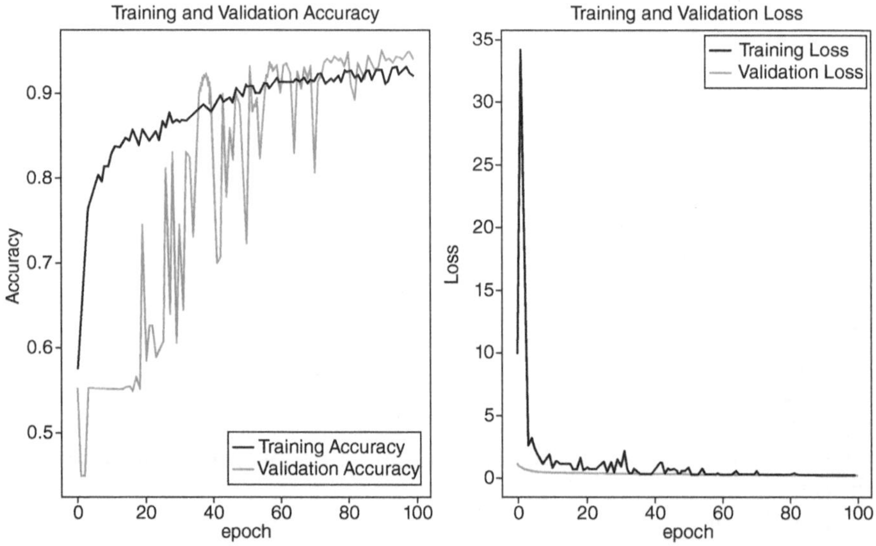

Figure 7.8 Inception accuracy.

90%. These fluctuations suggest variability in the model's performance on the validation set, potentially due to overfitting.

7.3.2.2 Right plot: Training and validation loss

X-axis (Epoch): Represents the number of epochs. Y-axis (Loss): Represents the loss value. Loss is a measure of model error, with lower values indicating better model performance. Training Loss (black line): Shows the loss on the training dataset at each epoch. Validation Loss (grey line): Shows the loss on the validation dataset at each epoch.

Initial Phase (Epochs 0–20): Training loss decreases sharply from a high initial value, indicating that the model is learning quickly and minimizing errors on the training data. Validation loss also decreases but not as sharply, showing the model is generalizing to the validation data, albeit with some fluctuation.

Intermediate Phase (Epochs 20–80): Training loss continues to decrease and stabilizes at a low value, suggesting the model is fitting the training data well. Validation loss fluctuates more than training loss, showing variability in performance on the validation data.

Later Phase (Epochs 80–100): Training loss remains low and stable, indicating continued good performance on the training data. Validation loss stabilizes but shows fluctuations, reflecting variability in model performance on the validation data.

7.3.2.3 Observations and potential issues

Overfitting: The gap between training and validation accuracy/loss suggests overfitting. The model performs very well on the training data but shows fluctuations and slightly lower performance on the validation data. Overfitting is indicated by the training accuracy nearing 100% while validation accuracy stabilizes at a lower value and fluctuates.

Stabilization: Training accuracy and loss stabilize, indicating the model has learned as much as it can from the training data. Validation metrics also stabilize but with fluctuations, suggesting the model's performance on unseen data is less consistent.

7.3.2.4 Potential solutions

Regularization: Apply regularization techniques such as dropout, L2 regularization, or data augmentation to reduce overfitting and improve generalization.

Early Stopping: Use early stopping to halt training when validation loss stops decreasing or validation accuracy stops increasing, preventing overfitting.

More Data: Increase the amount of training data to help the model generalize better.

Simplify the Model: Consider simplifying the model if it's too complex, as a simpler model might generalize better.

Cross-Validation: Use cross-validation to get a more robust estimate of model performance and better tune hyperparameters.

7.4 CONCLUSION

7.4.1 Training and validation accuracy of the first model (VGG-16)

The training accuracy rapidly increases and reaches near 100%, indicating the model is learning the training data very well. The validation accuracy increases initially but then stabilizes around 70–75%, with noticeable fluctuations. This suggests some overfitting.

Training and Validation Loss: The training loss decreases sharply and stabilizes at a very low value, indicating good performance on the training data. The validation loss also decreases but stabilizes at a higher value compared to training loss, with fluctuations, again suggesting overfitting.

7.4.2 Training and validation accuracy of the model proposed (inception)

The training accuracy increases and eventually stabilizes just below 100%. The validation accuracy increases and stabilizes around 85–90%, with some fluctuations. This indicates better generalization compared to the first set of graphs.

Training and Validation Loss: The training loss decreases and stabilizes at a very low value. The validation loss decreases and stabilizes at a higher value than the training loss, with fluctuations, but appears to stabilize better than in the first set.

Based on the analysis, the second set of graphs is the proposed model. It appears to be better overall as the validation accuracy in the second set stabilizes around 85–90%, which is higher than 70–75% seen in the first set. Higher validation accuracy indicates better performance on unseen data. Validation Loss: Although both sets show fluctuations in validation loss, the second set appears to stabilize better over time. Lower and more stable validation loss is indicative of better generalization.

Overfitting: While both sets exhibit some degree of overfitting (indicated by the gap between training and validation metrics), the second set shows less severe overfitting, as evidenced by the higher validation accuracy and more stable validation loss.

The Inception-v3 hybrid model with a multi-layer perceptron is used in this work to detect brain cancers on MRI scans. Based on the model's testing and assessments, the following results were achieved: the constructed model was successful in predicting brain cancers using MRI scans. In comparison to the Inception-v3 and multi-layer perceptron models, which only reach 66% and 56% accuracy, respectively, the suggested model obtains the greatest accuracy of 92%, with recall, precision, and F1 score values of 92%. When compared to earlier experiments, the accuracy gained is also greater. This model demonstrates that the model was successful in enhancing performance. However, because the model was only trained using photographs, this work has limitations. As a result, future study can make predictions using various methods.

REFERENCES

[1] Abd El-Wahab, B. S., Nasr, M. E., Khamis, S., & Ashour, A. S. (2023). BTC-fCNN: Fast convolution neural network for multi-class brain tumor classification. *Health Information Science and Systems*, 11(1). https://doi.org/10.1007/s13755-022-00203-w

[2] Abu, Shah, Mst, Marium Akter, & Jahan, N. (2023). Deep learning approach for detecting and localizing brain tumor from magnetic resonance imaging images. *Indonesian Journal of Electrical Engineering and Computer Science*, 29(3), 1729–1729. https://doi.org/10.11591/ijeecs.v29.i3.pp1729-1737

[3] Cao, Y., Zhou, W., Zang, M., An, D., Feng, Y., & Yu, B. (2023). MBANet: A 3D convolutional neural network with multi-branch attention for brain tumor segmentation from MRI images. *Biomedical Signal Processing and Control*, 80, 104296. https://doi.org/10.1016/j.bspc.2022.104296

[4] Chang, Y., Zheng, Z., Sun, Y., Zhao, M., Lu, Y., & Zhang, Y. (2023). DPAFNet: A residual dual-path attention-fusion convolutional neural network for multimodal brain tumor segmentation. *Biomedical Signal Processing and Control*, 79, 104037. https://doi.org/10.1016/j.bspc.2022.104037

[5] Das, M., Dash, R., & Mishra, S. K. (2023). Automatic detection of oral squamous cell carcinoma from histopathological images of oral mucosa using deep convolutional neural network. *International Journal of Environmental Research and Public Health*, 20(3), 2131. https://doi.org/10.3390/ijerph20032131

[6] Krishnapriya, S., & Karuna, Y. (2023). A survey of deep learning for MRI brain tumor segmentation methods: Trends, challenges, and future directions. *Health and Technology*. https://doi.org/10.1007/s12553-023-00737-3

[7] Mahmoud, A., Awad, Nancy Awadallah, Alsubaie, Najah, Ansarullah, Syed Immamul, Alqahtani, M. S., Abbas, M., Usman, M., Ben Othman Soufiene, & Saber, A. (2023). Advanced deep learning approaches for accurate brain tumor classification in medical imaging. *Symmetry*, 15(3), 571–571. https://doi.org/10.3390/sym15030571

[8] Satyanarayana, G., Appala Naidu, P., Subbaiah Desanamukula, V., Satish Kumar, K., & Chinna Rao, B. (2023). A mass correlation based deep learning approach using deep Convolutional neural network to classify the brain tumor. *Biomedical Signal Processing and Control*, 81, 104395. https://doi.org/10.1016/j.bspc.2022.104395

[9] Seyedhashemi, Seyedamid, & Esmaeili, M. (2023). *Detecting tumors in MRI scans using a convolutional neural network*. Authorea (Authorea). https://doi.org/10.22541/au.167707443.35803899/v1

[10] Shaaban, S., Atya, Hanan, Mohammed, H., Sameh, A., Raafat, K., & Magdy, A. (2023). Skin cancer detection based on deep learning methods. *Lecture Notes on Data Engineering and Communications Technologies*, 58–67. https://doi.org/10.1007/978-3-031-27762-7_6

[11] Zhou, T. (2023). Modality-level cross-connection and attentional feature fusion based deep neural network for multi-modal brain tumor segmentation. *Biomedical Signal Processing and Control*, 81, 104524. https://doi.org/10.1016/j.bspc.2022.104524

Chapter 8

User-enabled brain tumor detection

Amit Kumar Tiwari, Anil Singh, Ayush Maurya, Sanskriti Srivastava, Pradeep Yadav, and Ishita

8.1 INTRODUCTION

In the watershed year of 2012, convolutional neural networks (CNNs) astounded the scientific community by outperforming established benchmarks in the prestigious ImageNet computer vision competition. This landmark achievement propelled CNNs into limelight, sparking widespread adoption and catalyzing their integration into increasingly intricate computer vision tasks, particularly within the domain of medical imaging over the preceding five years. This surge in CNN application has notably manifested in the realm of biological segmentation tasks, encompassing a diverse array of human anatomical structures. Prominent instances encompass the automated detection of lymph nodes, the precise segmentation of knee cartilage, and the identification of markers indicative of Alzheimer's disease. The current manuscript embarks on a comprehensive scrutiny of Convolutional Neural Network (CNN) utilization in the realm of medical imaging segmentation, with particular focus directed toward two seminal works authored by Havaei et al. [2] and Kamnitsas et al. [3].

These studies proffer distinctive methodologies, presenting avant-garde approaches to CNN architectures meticulously customized for the segmentation of Magnetic Resonance Imaging (MRI) data. While a direct juxtaposition of their outcomes may be challenging due to methodological disparities, the chapter meticulously dissects the intricacies of their respective methodologies and elucidates common threads. Through rigorous scrutiny of their distinctive features, the narrative transitions to an assessment of their state-of-the-art performance across a spectrum of segmentation challenges.

This holistic analysis not only underscores the strides made in CNN-based medical imaging segmentation but also delineates avenues for future research and innovation in this burgeoning field.

8.2 BACKGROUND

It is imperative to elucidate the foundational concepts underlying segmentation in the realm of medical imaging and the application of Convolutional

 DOI: 10.1201/9781003536352-8

Neural Networks (CNNs) before delving into specific network construction methodologies. Within this context, segmentation pertains to the capacity to classify discrete entities within a medical image. This concept exhibits flexibility and can be applied to varying degrees of granularity in classification. On a broader scale, the objective might involve identifying and labelling multiple bones in a leg X-ray, for instance. Conversely, at a finer level of detail, the focus could be on precisely locating and labeling specific tumor sites in a brain MRI, akin to the illustration in Figure 8.1. Currently, the majority of segmentation tasks in the medical domain are executed manually by healthcare professionals. Convolutional neural networks emerge as invaluable tools in this scenario. Following training on a dataset comprising images segmented into patches and meticulously labelled by subject matter experts, the CNN autonomously learns to recognize diverse components within an image. Consequently, the network utilizes its acquired knowledge during encounters with unlabeled image patches to accurately categorize the image. The ultimate objective is for the network to generate precise image labels that emulate the thoroughness of conventional labeling techniques, such as determining the presence or absence of a tumor. The concepts delineated in the subsequent background sections are derived from a tutorial by Adit Deshpande [2].

8.3 INTRODUCTION TO NEURAL NETWORKS

Neural networks operate as sophisticated pattern recognizers, drawing inspiration from the intricate neural structures present in the cerebral cortex—a region of the brain renowned for its adeptness in processing sensory data. Illustrated in Figure 8.3, these networks typically comprise layers of nodes that activate in response to specific inputs. The ensuing activations are then propagated to other nodes through weighted connections. As information traverses these hierarchical layers of nodes and connections, it culminates in a discernible output, thereby showcasing the network's formidable processing

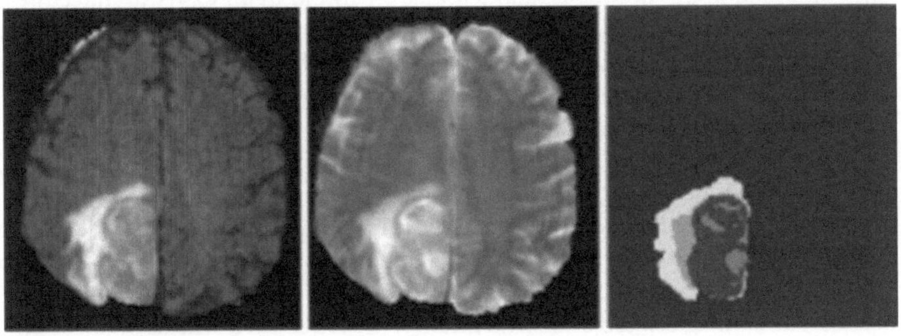

Figure 8.1 An example of tumor segmentation.

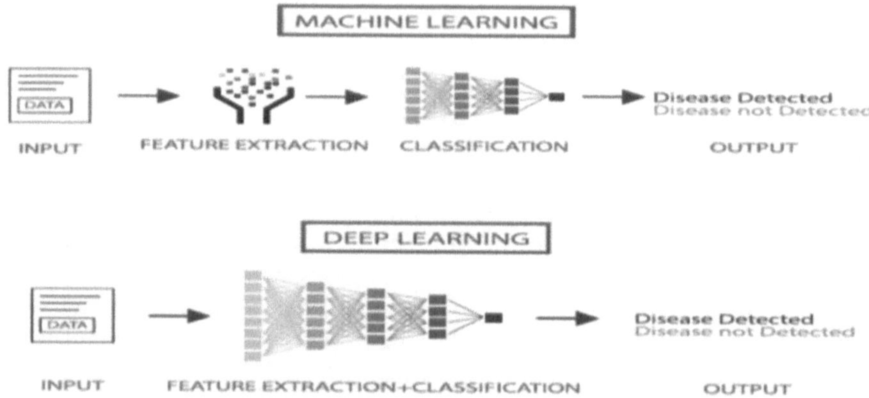

Figure 8.2 Difference between ML and DL.

capabilities. The inherent adaptability of neural networks arises from their capacity to tackle a broad spectrum of data-driven challenges, further fortified by their capability to meticulously fine-tune the weights of node connections, thereby enhancing the precision of the resultant outputs [4]. In the contemporary context, our attention is directed toward a specific category of neural networks known as Convolutional Neural Networks (CNNs). While CNNs adhere to the foundational principles shared with conventional neural networks, comprising input, hidden, and output layers, they introduce a novel layer expressly tailored for image analysis and classification endeavors. Within this framework, the network, operating with input patches derived from MRI pixels, engenders segmentation labels. The distinctive architecture of CNNs affords them a competitive edge in tasks demanding intricate image processing and classification prowess (Figure 8.2).

8.4 CONVOLUTIONAL LAYERS

Convolutional layers are the fundamental layer found in all CNN architectures, and they are what set convolutional neural networks (CNNs) apart. These layers play a key role in lowering the dimensionality of the incoming data and detecting important features by distilling it into clear patterns. An array that represents the pixel or voxel values of an input image patch is processed within the convolutional layer. In this instance, a filter, alternatively referred to as a neuron or kernel, serves as the symbolic representation of a distinctive feature. The kernel, strategically positioned in the upper-left corner of the input, spans the receptive field—an explicitly defined and delimited region. Within this domain, the element-wise multiplication of the kernel array and the input array is executed, yielding products that are amalgamated and strategically positioned on a feature map, as elucidated in Figure 8.3. Subsequently, the convolution process iterates, orchestrated

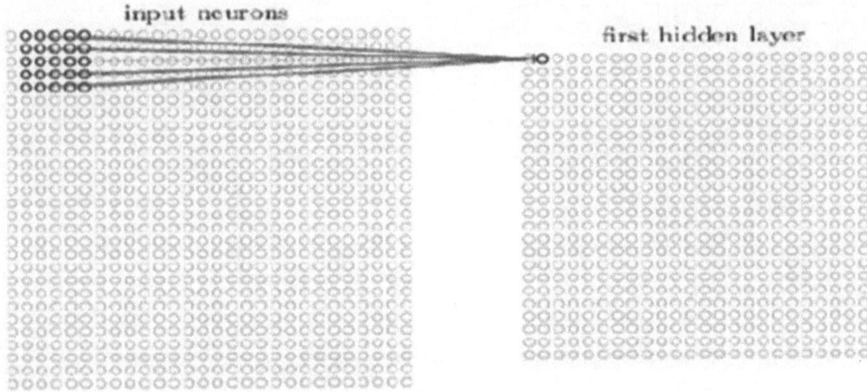

Figure 8.3 Visualization of kernel activations being stored in the feature map.

by the kernel as it traverses a specified distance across the input, accumulating outcomes in progressively diverse locations on the feature map. When all potential convolutions between the kernel and input have been performed, a complete feature map—a structured array containing the results of these convolutions—is produced. These feature maps, embodying learned features, serve as an input for subsequent layers within the network, facilitating hierarchical learning and abstraction in the CNN architecture. The efficacy of CNNs in image analysis and pattern recognition stems from this distinct convolutional layer design.

8.4.1 Kernels

As previously explained, kernels are arrays designed to represent identifiable features, like the curve seen in Figure 8.4. Every kernel has a pattern of numbers that represents a certain attribute. During the integration coefficient process, large output values indicate a close match between core features and receptive field features. On the other hand, the value is reduced if the feature is absent or less noticeable. These identifications of characteristic characteristics fill the feature map, which then acts as the input for the network's later layers. The number of these kernels directly affects the network's ability to identify a wide range of features, which in turn promotes the iterative creation of a hierarchical feature hierarchy in subsequent layers via feature map operations.

8.4.2 Dropout and pooling layers

Deductive and convolutional layers are two other types of layers in a convolutional neural network. Starting with the definition of the synthesis layer, its operation is simple. The groups are extracted from the input feature map and combined into a single segment. A common clustering technique is peak

0	0	0	0	0	30	0
0	0	0	0	30	0	0
0	0	0	30	0	0	0
0	0	0	30	0	0	0
0	0	0	30	0	0	0
0	0	0	30	0	0	0
0	0	0	0	0	0	0

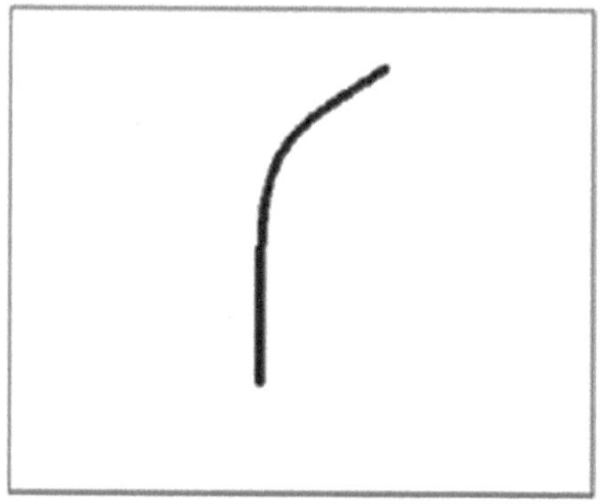

Figure 8.4 An example of kernel that recognize curve as feature.

clustering, where the top value of each cluster is the corresponding point in the shape map of the clustering layer. In geospatial data reduction, aggregation layers are important because they can extract large amounts of input at once. It lives up to its name when switching to an inversion layer randomly selects activations from the input feature map and sets it to 0. The network's ability to reliably predict classes regardless of features missing any of the activations is confirmed by its neutrality. It is important to note that although extrapolation is introduced by the regression layer during training, this extrapolation does not affect the untrained data. These two types of layers have been found to be very effective in solving the overfitting problem in CNNs. If the network overfits the details of the training dataset, it is called overfitting and performs poorly on untrained images. Although there are many methods that can be used to reduce overlap, this study shows the effectiveness of aggregation and layer reduction as two scoping methods.

8.4.3 Fully connected layers

A fully connected layer, often placed as a terminal layer in a network architecture, accepts feature maps from the previous layer and creates a vector listing the label probabilities associated with a key pixel in the integrated imaging platform. In tasks such as image segmentation, the goal is to distinguish between non-tumor regions and regions within the tumor, which means that the results are twofold. This layer carefully examines the features in the feature map and produces a binary vector with two values, representing the probability that the input represents a tumor and the probability that it represents a non-tumor region.

8.4.4 Training

Comprehending the training process is critical to understanding the workings of a Convolutional Neural Network (CNN). First, a training dataset is needed, which consists of medical images and the related ground truth labels. These labels are the result of painstaking manual segmentation by medical specialists and are used as standards by which the network's segmentation efforts are evaluated. The network's kernels are initially randomly assigned, producing roughly uniform output probabilities The loss function is designed to measure the error that is estimated during the forward step when the network processes the image patch, and the resulting results are combined with real label probabilities. The primary objective of the training process is the mitigation of this loss, typically commencing from a notably elevated magnitude at the inception of the procedure. Subsequently, the ensuing step entails the backward pass, an iterative traversal through the network from output to input. During this phase, pivotal kernels are discerned, and weight adjustments are computed iteratively to minimize the loss. The loss function is designed to measure the error that is estimated during the forward step when the network processes the image patch, and the resulting results are combined with real label probabilities. The main goal of training is to reduce this loss, usually starting from a rather large loss magnitude at the beginning of the procedure. The next step is the backward pass, which involves repeatedly going through the network from output to input, identifying important kernels and calculating weight changes to reduce loss. Interestingly, while a larger training dataset usually improves performance, getting a suitably varied set of medical images might be difficult. Rotations, translations, and jitter are examples of data augmentation techniques that can increase the pool of training photos, but real-world image acquisition is still the best option.

8.5 METHODS

In this section, we discuss two different approaches used for brain MRI segmentation by Havaei et al. and Kamnitsas et al. We will break these approaches down into their main categories and discuss the pros and cons of each. We will also look at the similarities and differences between these technologies throughout this discussion.

8.5.1 Two pathway approach to brain tumor segmentation

In their seminal study, Havaei et al. present a new bidirectional convolutional neural network (CNN) approach carefully adapted to the challenging data of multimodal brain tumor segmentation (BRATS 2013) [1]. This dataset consists of 25 unlabeled correct response database images, 10 labeled test images, and 30 identical training images. The classification process consists of classifying five unique labels: necrosis, edema, non-enhancing tumor, and tumor enhancement. This method is based on three main components: induction of two pathways and different secondary network points. Input the output of a CNN and implement a two-stage training method.

To construct a binary convolutional neural network (CNN) that constructs a binary flow architecture (Havaei et al.) As shown in Figure 8.5, we created a local path that shows receptive fields of 7 × 7 and a global path that shows receptive fields of 13 × 13. This configuration allows the architecture to detect visual complexity and capture contextual information. The outputs of these two paths pass through multiplexing layers (two layers for the local path and one for the global path) and then enter the combiner. The final combination is processed in the output layer and translated into segmentation labels. In an attempt to overcome the limitation found in existing CNN segmentation systems that segment labels are predicted independently (Havaei et al). It offers three CNN architectures. These topologies involve inserting the output of one CNN into one of the layers of another CNN [6]. This novel technique enhances joint segmentation label models by enabling the second CNN to learn from neighboring pixel labeling [7]. There are differences among the three cascaded designs (InputCascadeCNN, LocalCascadeCNN, and MFCascadeCNN) concerning the location of the fusion between the first and second CNN. Adopting a two-phase training paradigm is the third significant aspect of the research. Understanding the difficulty presented by a profusion of label-free tissue in comparison to a dearth of other labels, especially in brain imaging [5]. Initially, Havaei et al. undertake the training of the Convolutional Neural Network (CNN) employing a dataset wherein each label is endowed with equal weighting. Subsequently, they fine-tune the ultimate output layer, factoring in the relative probabilities associated with the labels. This adjustment is executed with precision, preserving the discerning capabilities of the preceding layers and ensuring the fidelity of output probabilities.

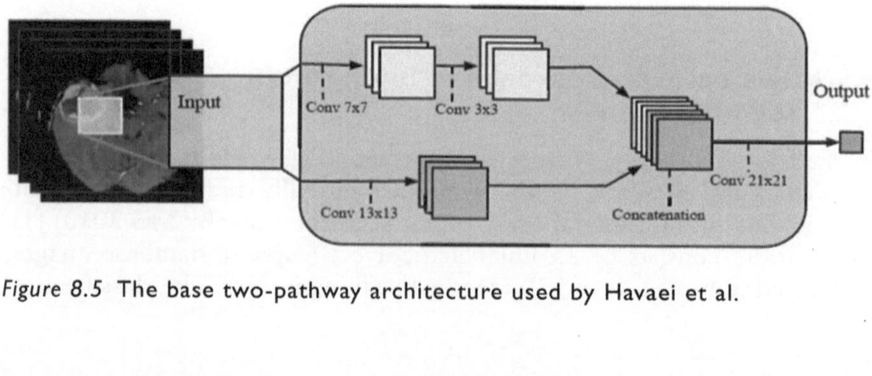

Figure 8.5 The base two-pathway architecture used by Havaei et al.

8.5.2 3D multiscale approach

In their seminal work [3], Kamnitsas et al. present a contemporary architectural paradigm for Convolutional Neural Networks (CNNs) within the domain of medical imaging segmentation. Their approach amalgamates several pivotal techniques distilled from extensive prior research endeavors. This includes the introduction of 3D CNNs, modeling techniques for network training, 3D Conditional Random Fields (CRFs) for final segmentation processing, the use of deep networks to improve discrimination, and extraction in a two-way structure that combines multiway. We follow the approach taken by Havaei et al. and Kamnitsas et al. We employ a two-pronged strategy that aims to incorporate local complexity while maintaining the global context of the entire image. However, Havaei et al. and Kamnitsas et al. achieve this goal by implementing specific mapping quantities in each direction. This is achieved by reducing the global path. The screenshot in Figure 8.6 briefly shows Kamnitsas' complex neural network, called "DeepMedic". With two approaches (one dedicated to processing standard-resolution image layers and one suitable for handling reduced layers), the patches go through a series of convolutional layers before finishing with two interlaced layers and a final classification layer. In the framework of Kamnitsas et al., DeepMedic stands out because it has improved convolutional layers, two numbers shown in the image, and a small grain size of 3x3, thus becoming an important part of the comprehensive process. A salient aspect of Kamnitsas et al's. methodology lies in the incorporation of 3D Convolutional Neural Networks (CNNs) as the foundational element of their architectural design. These 3D CNNs leverage three-dimensional kernels and typically process more volumetric image patches as input. Historically, the computational demands posed by full-fledged 3D CNNs have impeded their widespread adoption. However, Kamnitsas et al. adeptly overcome this impediment by deploying dense inference. This technique alleviates the computational burden associated with 3D CNNs, allowing the classification layer to generate multiple predictions when the input image patch surpasses the receptive field size [8–12]. Deeper networks embedded

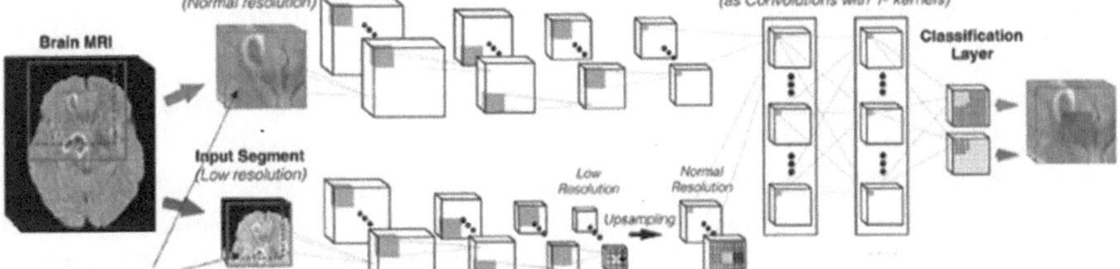

Figure 8.6 The basic neural network architecture, 'Deep Medic' (Used by Kamnitsas, et al.)

within CNNs exhibit elevated discriminative prowess but concurrently incur heightened computational expenditures, especially with the integration of 3D convolutions. Kamnitsas et al. adeptly confront this challenge by substituting conventional 5x3 kernel-sized convolutional layers with multiple layers employing a more diminutive 3x3 kernel size. This modification greatly reduces the number of parameters and results in a noticeable reduction in element coefficients for each layer. Training deep networks is difficult to keep the hidden feature (Kamnitsas et al). This problem was solved by initializing the grain weights with a normal distribution N(0, 2/nl). Here nl represents the number of weights to which the neuron is connected. We also implement batch optimization to alleviate the variable displacement problem. An innovation that emerged from the work of Kamnitsas et al. is the introduction of the first 3D constrained random fields (CRFs). CRF improves neural network predictions by incorporating contextual information from image adjacent regions, providing more accurate segmentation results compared to traditional layers [13–18].

8.6 RESULTS

In this chapter have investigated the difficulty associated with medical pictures segmentation, especially in diagnosing brain growths and shortcomings of anatomical patterns. To tackle this issue, we suggest an efficient segmentation approach leveraging Burrows-Wheeler translational (BWT) techniques to decide initial size of clusters and central points, with an aim for accurate outcomes and speedy computation. This process minimizes human involvement, perhaps supporting brain surgeons and medical professionals in promptly identifying patients and progress outcomes [9]. In a current research, we employed a profound learning scheme using a consonantal neural net (CNN) template to sense brain swellings from MRI images. Educated on an abundant dataset of MRI images weighted T1, the CNN exhibited the capacity to recognize between brain regions with swellings and those absent them, attaining high correctness and sensitivity with a low frequency of untrue assurances. These discoveries highlight the prospective of CNNs and profound learning methods in supporting medical practitioners to promptly and exactly identify brain swellings.

Our recommended CNN-focused profound learning approach exhibited a rounded correctness of 95.7% in identifying brain swellings from MRI images, outsmarting traditional machinery learning protocols in tumorous region segmentation. This highlights its potential effectiveness in clinical practice and underscores the significance of ample annotated datasets in training precise models. Additional optimization and assessment on greater datasets might be essential to heighten the template's efficiency and capability. With a tidy correctness rate of 98.3% on the validation dataset, our template reveals assurance in helping doctors in exactly identifying brain swellings. Additionally, the research displayed the excellence of the recommended profound learning model over usual machinery learning methods such as SVM and arbitrary jungle. We also stressed the magnitude of data planning schemes, notably data augmentation methods like rotary motion, flipping, and zooming, in improving the template's correctness and generalization quality.

In conclusion, our research showcased the efficiency of CNNs and profound learning precisely in identifying brain swellings from MRI inspections. The recommended model outperformed conventional machinery learning methods and demonstrated high correctness, specifying its potential clinical effectiveness in supporting medical professionals in exactly and quickly identifying brain swellings. Progressing forward, frequent optimization and authentication on larger datasets could further heighten the template's effectiveness and applicability in real-world clinical settings.

REFERENCES

[1] Mohammad Havaei, Axel Davy, David Warde-Farley, Antoine Biard, Aaron Courville, Yoshua Bengio, Chris Pal, Pierre-Marc Jodoin, and Hugo Larochelle. Brain tumor segmentation with deep neural networks. *Medical Image Analysis*, 35:18–31, 2017.

[2] Konstantinos Kamnitsas, Christian Ledig, Virginia FJ Newcombe, Joanna P Simpson, Andrew D Kane, David K Menon, Daniel Rueckert, and Ben Glocker. Efficient multi-scale 3d CNN with fully connected CRF for accurate brain lesion segmentation. *Medical Image Analysis*, 36:61–78, 2017.

[3] Diwakar, M., Singh, P., Ravi, V., & Maurya, A. (2023). A non-conventional review on Multi-modality-based Medical Image Fusion. *Diagnostics*, *13*(5), 820. 10.3390/s23063287

[4] Yuehao Pan, Weimin Huang, Zhiping Lin, Wanzheng Zhu, Jiayin Zhou, Jocelyn Wong, and Zhongxiang Ding. Brain tumor grading based on neural networks and convolutional neural networks. In *2015 37th annual international conference of the IEEE engineering in medicine and biology society (EMBC)*, pp. 699–702. IEEE, 2015.

[5] Zhihua Liu, Lei Tong, Long Chen, Zheheng Jiang, Feixiang Zhou, Qianni Zhang, Xiangrong Zhang, Yaochu Jin, and Huiyu Zhou. Deep learning based brain tumor segmentation: A survey. *Complex & Intelligent Systems*, 9(1):1001–1026, 2023.

[6] Geethu Mohan and M Monica Subashini. MRI based medical image analysis: Survey on brain tumor grade classification. *Biomedical Signal Processing and Control*, 39:139–161, 2018.

[7] Alex Krizhevsky, Ilya Sutskever, and Geoffrey E Hinton. Imagenet classification with deep convolutional neural networks. *Advances in neural information processing systems*, 25, 2012.

[8] Michael A Nielsen. *Neural networks and deep learning*, volume 25. Determination Press, 2015.

[9] Pawar, D., Phansalkar, S., Sharma, A., Sahu, G. K., Ang, C. K., & Lim, W. H. (2023). Survey on the Biomedical Text Summarization Techniques with an Emphasis on Databases, Techniques, Semantic Approaches, Classification Techniques, and Similarity Measures. *Sustainability*, *15*(5), 4216. 10.3390/su15054216

[10] Umaira Nazar, Muhammad A Khan, Ikram Ullah Lali, Hong Lin, Hashim Ali, Imran Ashraf, and Junaid Tariq. Review of automated computerized methods for brain tumor segmentation and classification. *Current Medical Imaging*, 16(7):823–834, 2020.

[11] Sharma, R., Kim, M., & Gupta, A. (2022). Motor imagery classification in brain-machine interface with machine learning algorithms: Classical approach to multi-layer perceptron model. *Biomedical Signal Processing and Control*, *71*, 103101, 10.1016/j.bspc.2021.103101

[12] Elashiri, M. A., Rajesh, A., Pandey, S. N., Shukla, S. K., & Urooj, S. (2022). Ensemble of weighted deep concatenated features for the skin disease classification model using modified long short term memory. *Biomedical Signal Processing and Control*, *76*, 103729. 10.1016/j.bspc.2022.103729

[13] Wazid, M., Singh, J., Das, A. K., Shetty, S., Khan, M. K., & Rodrigues, J. J. (2022). ASCP-IoMT: AI-enabled lightweight secure communication protocol for internet of medical things. *IEEE Access*, *10*, 57990–58004, 10.1109/ACCESS.2022.3179418

[14] Madan, P., Singh, V., Singh, D. P., Diwakar, M., & Kishor, A. (2022). Denoising of ECG signals using weighted stationary wavelet total variation. *Biomedical Signal Processing and Control*, *73*, 103478. 10.1016/j.bspc.2021.103478

[15] Yadav, S., Chamoli, S., Kumar, P., & Maurya, P. K. (2023). Structural and functional insights in polysaccharides coated cerium oxide nanoparticles and their potential biomedical applications: A review. *International Journal of Biological Macromolecules*, 125673, https://doi.org/10.1016/j.ijbiomac.2023.12567

[16] Gupta, P., Gupta, H., Kairamkonda, M., Kumar, N., & Poluri, K. M. (2022). Elucidating the lactic acid tolerance mechanism in vaginal clinical isolates of Candida glabrata. *Medical Mycology*, *60*(6), myac042. https://doi.org/10.1093/mmy/myac042

[17] Ahmad, W., & Kumar, S. (2024). T axus wallichiana leaf extract-mediated microwave-assisted one-pot biosynthesis of MgO NPs for biomedical and photocatalytic applications. *Emergent Materials*, 7(3), 1081–1090. https://doi.org/10.1007/s42247-023-00612-x

[18] Alrashed, F. A., Alsubiheen, A. M., Alshammari, H., Mazi, S. I., Al-Saud, S. A., Alayoubi, S., ... & Dhiman, G. (2022). Stress, anxiety, and depression in pre-clinical medical students: Prevalence and association with sleep disorders. *Sustainability*, *14*(18), 11320. 10.3390/su141811320

Chapter 9

CNN for stem cell imaging: Existing constraints and future perspectives in artificial intelligence

R. Suganya, Akash Kumar Barik, Keerthana Balakrishnan, and Aditya Raj

9.1 INTRODUCTION

Alan Mathison Turing, a British computer pioneer, made the initial contributions to the fundamentals or foundation of Artificial Intelligence in the intervening twentieth century. In 1950, he proposed "The Turing Test," a test for tool intelligence. Before a device to mislead people into thinking it is human, it must first portray agility. This took into account the development of creative motor or computational knowledge.

As a result, we have come a long way from the "A.I Winter" that occurred from the end of 1974 to the end of 1980 (many false starts and impediments leave AI out in the cold) to anticipating tumor, speech/facial recognition, self-powered automobiles, machine intelligence, mechanization engaged in trade, cure, and so on.

Artificial intelligence (AI) is being used in modern medicine to cope with difficult abnormalities that may occur in regenerative medicine as a result of technology and scientific achievements. The concept of healing in medicine has evolved as scientists and researchers attempt to enhance regenerative medicine. Earlier, doctors would treat disease symptoms; however, current medicine is stepping away from reactive treatment and toward regeneration. This proposal of substituting damaged cells with contemporary cells having the same existing functionality with improved efficiency is called stem cell therapy.

They have the potential to divide and differentiate into a number of fully evolved and appropriate cell types as a person's body grows over their lifespan.

Currently, immunologic, inflammatory, neurological, musculoskeletal, and traumatic conditions are all treated by stem cells, and new diseases are being explored. It may also contain the answer to disease-free living and anti-aging. Despite the benefits, employing stem cells to treat patients may result in a number of errors.

One potential stem cell that is now being explored is the induced pluripotent stem cell (iPSC); it is formed by genetically reprogramming somatic stem cells to change them into stem cells similar to embryonic stem cells. These

DOI: 10.1201/9781003536352-9

iPSCs are applied in studies on medication development, disease onset, and medical treatments. Artificial intelligence (AI) has lately emerged as a cutting-edge solution to address this challenge. Deep learning, a branch of artificial intelligence, provides a framework for automated analysis of iPSC-based colonies and other colony-forming stem cells. Deep learning makes use of techniques such as convolutional neural networks (CNNs), a class of multi-layered neural networks that carry out an unorthodox role in image identification. CNNs can draw a distinction on cells with high accuracy based on metamorphosis and structural design. As a result, CNNs have the prospective to open up a new forte of deep learning tasks aimed at tackling several challenges in stem cell research. We will continue to debate and research the application of AI, the potential of these neural networks in stem cell identification for therapy, and how it transforms the practice of medicine to clear the way for a regenerative future with the fewest limitations possible.

9.2 LITERATURE SURVEY

9.2.1 Understanding stem cells and stem cell therapy

The world of computer science is always dynamic and new, and better software versions and better technologies are founded or created in every corner of the earth. The field of medical science is very much interconnected with technology. From predicting the developments of cancer cells to the creating of regenerative medicine, Artificial Intelligence has become a game changer in the field of medicine. The current trend in medicine is that researchers are trying to solve the problem of regenerative medicine, in which stem cells come into light [1] Now researching on stem cells will help in understanding of how diseases occur, replace diseased cells with healthy cells, creating new drugs at a faster rate and understanding their side effects better, etc. Stem cells, which are not predefined to any functionality, are found in the human body. They can transform into any kind of organ cell and have the ability to self-renew. Stem cells are found in both adult and embryonic cells. There are several steps in the specialization process. Because developmental potency declines with each passing step, unipotent stem cells cannot differentiate into as many different types of cells as pluripotent ones [2–4].

Deep learning could advance this area by understanding how stem cells can be used for regenerative medicine or understand the rate at which they multiply.

Pluripotent stem cells (PSCs) are classified mainly into two parts: (1) EMBRYONIC STEM CELLS (ESCs), which are found in the inner cells of blastocysts. They are capable of producing every type of cell in the fully developed organism, but not the placenta or the umbilical cord. Because they offer a reusable resource for researching healthy growth and illness, as well as testing medications and other treatments, these cells are highly significant.

(2) INDUCED PLURIPOTENT STEM CELLS (iPSC), which are fabricated from skin or blood cells that have been altered to confirm to a pluripotent phase similar to that of an embryo, allow for the initiation of such an immense source of any human cell needed for therapeutic purposes [5, 6]. Because these cells can construct every tissue in the human body, they are an excellent prospect for therapeutic tissue regeneration.

They are the "seed" from which any living being develops. A zygote is a unicell produced during the fertilization process, and it is where life first emerges. This zygote keeps reproducing and turns into embryonic cells (EC). These ECs show that pluripotent cells can morph into distinct types of cells in the body of an organism, including neuron, muscle, blood, and other types of cells. Multipotent cells, which are specialized to the tissue structure or organ in which they are differentiated terminally or carry out a distinct function, can also develop from pluripotent cells

Cells such as RBCs, WBCs, or platelets (all specialized cells) can be produced by multipotent blood stem cells. These specialized cells' primary job is to help the body repair any harm done to it and to further allow a regenerative healing process (Figure 9.1).

The history of SC therapy is taken back to the late 1950s, where technologists who were unintentionally exposed to radiation underwent successful allogeneic bone marrow transplants. Following this incident, major advancements in the use of stem cells for patient treatment were developed. Scientist John Gurdon made a ground-breaking discovery in the 1960s when he successfully morphed frogs from somatic cells. This laboratory experiment trial disproved the belief that pluripotent cells could differentiate only in one direction and introduced the idea that SCs could also acquire a pluripotent state [2].

Another related proposal was the identification of reprogramming or regenerative cells by Davis et al. through the removal of fibroblast DNA. The myogenic differentiation (Myod1) gene's expression was principally responsible for the transformation of fibroblasts into myoblasts [2]. This research demonstrated how cells might change from one lineage to another. More research is being done to predict what will actually happen to such pluripotent and multipotent stem cells. The study also was done on how well they function with different diseases since that earlier studies have proven the fundamental notion of stem cells and their usefulness.

9.3 AI A PROMISING PARADIGM

In present day scenarios, AI has also been used to handle trials and tribulations along with many other obstacles in the field of healthcare data analysis. AI methods include learning, self-thinking, and self-transformation. AI is widely used in various industries connected to computerized personal assistants or companion-based products and self-driving automated cars.

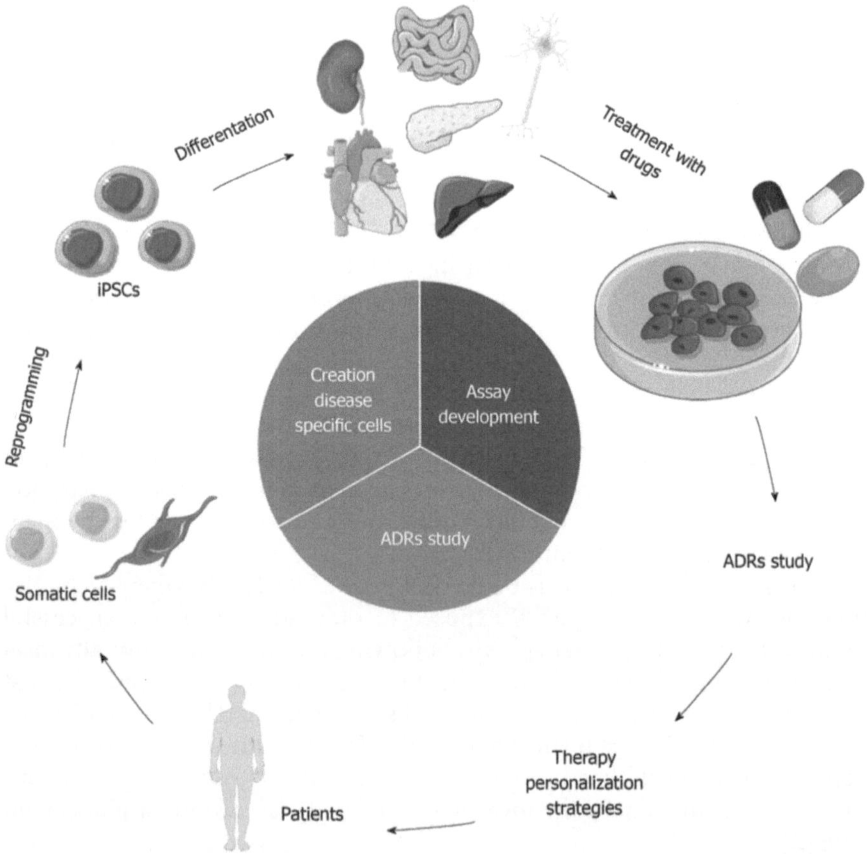

Figure 9.1 Stem cell therapy.

Expert systems, speech recognition, and machine vision are just a few of the various AI constructions that exist today.[7, 8] According to Conrad, Gerlich, Lock, and Strömblad, bio-metric image processing methods provide state-of-the-art solutions for distinct image analysis tasks like device or object classification, morphometric or cloning feature measurement, or motion analysis. However, distinct image processing algorithms have been created for the majority of biological experiments, and ML is the most fascinating because employing each technique for each cell marker and cell species constantly requires reprogramming of the software. To achieve a performance that is reasonable, parameters need be tweaked. In order to support medical decision, these technologies' ultimate objective is to use computerized algorithms or techniques to extract relevant information or parameters from the data provided [9, 10]. In conclusion, AI can help with disease stratification, drug identification, risk/benefit analysis, and diagnosis while reducing medical errors and increasing productivity. Neural network trains with a narrow focus and supercomputing capabilities assist to create "algorithms" automatically. It has been demonstrated that understanding and dealing with algorithms with the increasing training data results in new insights into diagnoses, treatment alternatives, and patient outcomes.

Previous research has found little benefit in applying AI to healthcare, concluding that AI finds application in early detection, has reduced costs, in effective surgery assistance, in improvement of human capacities, and in promotion of mental health support (Figure 9.2). This technology can have clear disadvantages in addition to its benefits, including violations, privacy concerns, discrimination, and job restructuring. Artificial Intelligence's Use in SC therapy is a very vast field and has many scopes and limitations. Although stem cell therapy may seem straightforward in theory, the cells are neither uniform nor stable, and current testing techniques may result in more errors than expected. Consequently, it is extremely challenging to account for all cellular products.

Many forms of artificial intelligence are thought to be able to help offer exact measurements to resolve this complexity. In the chosen papers, in-depth investigation was done to determine the connection between AI and regenerative medicine.

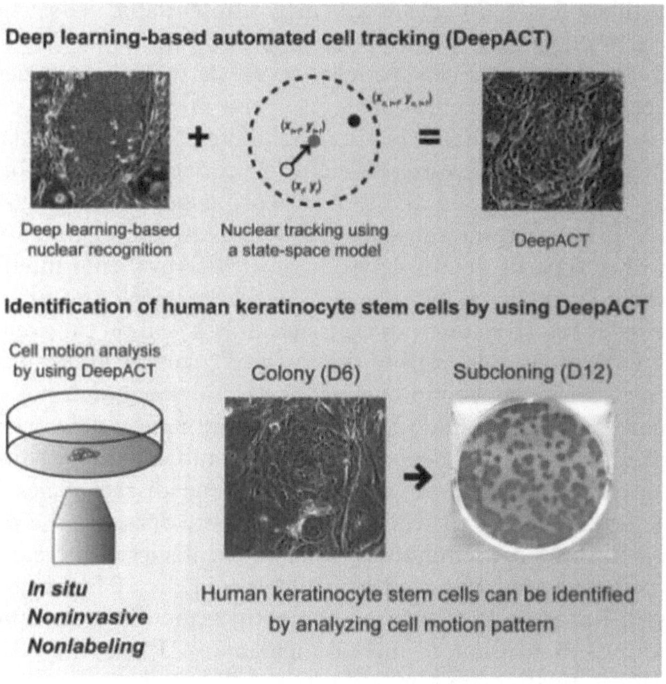

Figure 9.2 Stem cell and deep learning.

According to Juhora et al. three measurements were recorded from each baseline, epinephrine and temporal calcium data from human iPSC cardiomyocytes via machine learning methods [7]. In order to investigate the effects of adrenaline or, later, dantrolene, they first recognized transient signal beats using a peak detection method and calculated 12 peak variables for each identified signal peak. In accordance with the signals received, they divided the signals into various classification anomalies with adrenaline perfusion. Baseline, adrenergic, and dantrolene states were used to categorize the results. The rate of anomalies at which they are reduced by dantrolene, will in turn reflect the pattern of the calcium spike, which was used for further categorize patients dantrolene status as either responders, semi-responders, or non-responders.

The most accurate models include those using neural networks such as k-Nearest Neighbors (KNN), Classification and Regression Trees (CART), Mahalanobis Discriminant Analysis (MDA), Random Forests, Multinomial Logistic Regression, Naive Bayes, and Least Squares Support Vector Machines (LS-SVM), among others [11].

CNN was able to distinguish between hemorrhage, mitosis, and cell shape. The best outcomes for picture evaluation came from the existence of mouse embryonic fibroblast feeder cells. CSCs can be seen by AI models using phase-contrast imaging, which show GFP fluorescence [12]. Wiseman et al. used a CNN trained on pictures from transmitted light microscopy to separate pluripotent stem cells from early differentiated cells. The two networks were used to assess 1,116 photos in total [12–16].

DenseNet, one of the recent popular neural network discoveries, is a subtype of convolutional neural network that inhabits dense connections between layers through dense blocks or chunks of neurons. All layers (with corresponding feature map sizes) are directly connected to each other and as additional layers are added, the feed-forward aspect of getting input from all preceding layer to all subsequent layers is maintained. While ResNet being another type of neural network of artificially being intelligent, that uses an extra layer to enhance the deep neural network's accuracy and efficiency in order to solve complicated issues. It is based on the architecture of the pyramidal or conoidal cells of the cerebral cortex [11]. ResNet does this by applying shortcuts or skip connections to advance multiple layers. The confusion matrix in this study exhibits that both neural networks predicted events with a much larger degree of precision and accuracy than the differentiated group. However, the presence of some discrepancies have been observed, especially in DenseNet. Inception networks, on the other hand, are highly engineered. It employs a variety of strategies to increase efficiency in terms of both speed and accuracy. It also won the 2014 ImageNet Large Scale Visual Recognition Contest, a competitive feud for classifying images, which exhibits a substantial improvement than ZFNet (the 2013 winner) but has certain relative drawbacks in stem cell therapy. Not all health issues can be resolved by cell therapy [5].

Each person responds differently. The major goal of this process is to equip the body with the necessary resources and conditions to produce the damaged tissue on its own, but other patients might not see a considerable improvement. Every procedure's outcome is based on the participant's individual body recovery potential. No generalizations about the course of treatment or results can be made because each participant's body may react differently.

There is no standard procedure for all patients. Nonetheless, below we have presented the conditions with the best outcomes for improvement. Error rate compared to VGGNet. Previous networks like VGG have achieved amazing accuracy on the ImageNet data set, but the deep architecture makes the deployment of these types of models very computationally intensive. We will see a more detailed description of classifiers in the next module [16].

9.4 TYPES OF IMAGE CLASSIFIERS

We learned what stem cell therapy is from the previous chapters, as well as the reasons behind its importance to the field of medical science. We must now comprehend how stem cell therapy might benefit from deep learning. A procedure known as "image classification" allows computers to analyze photographs to determine the "class" to which they belong (or the possibility that the photo is a member of a one class). A class is essentially a classification, like "animals," "cars," and so on. It combines similar parts into a single, clearly defined class. For instance, let's say you provide a picture of a bird. Image categorization is the technique by which a computer analyzes images and tells you it's a car (or the probability that a car is involved).[17, 18] For us, categorizing images is not a huge priority. However, it serves as a superb example of Moravec's conundrum when applied to machines. (In other words, for AI, what we think of as simple is difficult.)

Earlier, raw data of pixel was used for image clustering, after which algorithms deconstruct the pictures to individual pixels. The underlying issue is that two images of a same subject might appear completely dissimilar. It may have various backdrops, perspectives, postures, facial reaction, and so forth. Because of this, classifying and accurately "visualizing" images proved to be a difficult task for computers [12, 16].

Artificial intelligence (AI) has a subfield called deep learning that allows computers to learn from data. Deep learning includes computer architectures based on neural networks. The input to the neural networks is filtered by the hidden layers. Every node analyzes the input then communicates its findings to the nodes below it. Up until the output layer, this procedure is repeated, and then the machine reacts.

Depending on the way the hidden layers work, there are several types of neural networks. CNNs are usually applied in deep learning for image classification. Nodes in CNNs' hidden layers do not always disclose the output with nodes in the layer before them (convolutional layers). Using deep learning, machines can detect and gather data from photos. This suggests that by examining a huge number of photos, they can discover the qualities to look for in photographs. Developers do not have to manually enter these criteria as a consequence [12–16].

There are some highly prominent datasets in image classification that are used in academia, enterprises, collaborative projects, community and hackathons. Among the most notable are the following: ImageNet, CIFAR, MNIST, and many more

9.4.1 VGG-16

The VGG-16 is a pre-trained model known for image classification. It came into picture during the illustrious ILSVRC 2014 Conference and became the standard to beat even today. VGG-16, evolved at the University of Oxford's Visual Graphics Group, surpassed the then-standard AlexNet [16] after which it was soon acquired by industry for picture classification tasks. The layers for the model are:

- Convolutional Layers = 13
- Pooling Layers = 5
- Dense Layers = 3

Convolutional layer is considered the building block of any CNN. It includes a series of filters (also known as kernel), and its parameters may be learned through the training process. The filters are often smaller in size than the real image (Figure 9.3 and 9.4).

9.4.2 Inception net

Deep neural networks, as previously indicated, are computationally costly. To reduce the count of input paths, the authors include an additional 1x1 prior to the 3x3 and 5x5 convolutions. Although it could look trivial to

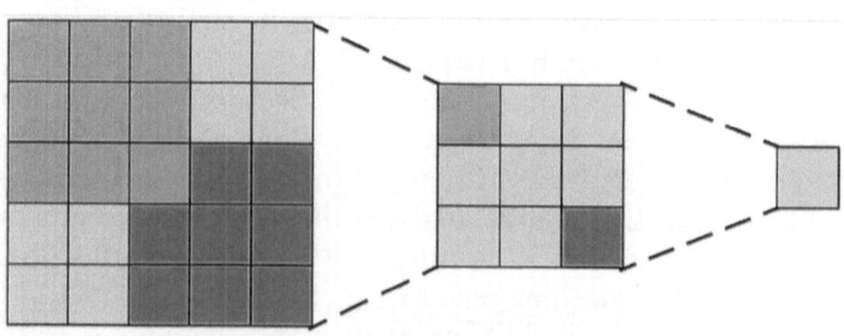

Figure 9.3 VGG-16 image reduction.

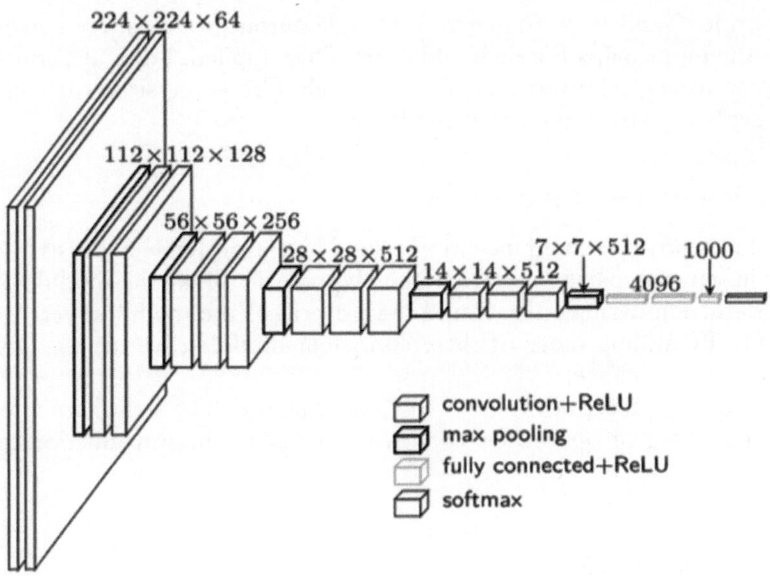

Figure 9.4 VGG-16 diagram.

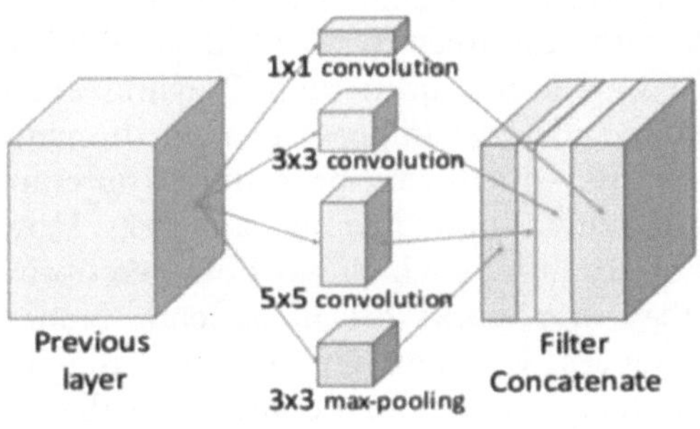

Figure 9.5 Inception model.

add four other functions, 1x1 convolutions are much less expensive when compared to a 5x5 convolution. However, the 1x1 is inserted following the max pooling layer [15, 16].

A inception module with dimension reduction was used to create a neural network architecture, which was generally mentioned as GoogLeNet (Inception v1). The architecture is depicted in Figure 9.5.

The enhanced information density of our model design has one major drawback: we've significantly raised processing expenses. Not only are big convolutional filters (e.g., 5x5) intrinsically costly to calculate, but stacking numerous different filters side by side significantly increases the amount of feature mappings per layer. In our scenario, this growth constitutes a fatal bottleneck [15, 16].

Consider it this way. To generate a single output, we must convolve over all of the input maps for each additional filter applied. Look at Figure 9.6: Creating a single output map from a single filter necessitates calculating over every map from the preceding layer.

9.4.3 Version 4 of inception

The same study presented Inception v4 and Inception-ResNet. Let us address these in separate parts for clarity. The Hypothesis: Make the modules more consistent. The writers also found that several of the modules were overly difficult. By adding more of these consistent modules, we may be able to improve performance.

The Answer: Inception v4's "stem" was changed. The stem here refers to the original set of operations carried out prior to the introduction of the Inception blocks.

9.5 LIMITATIONS

Cell therapy is not a cure-all for many health problems. Each individual responds distinctly, but the significance of the procedure is to supply the human body with resources to make ideal conditions for the body to regenerate damaged tissue on its own. Previous experiences and procedures have resulted in great improvement in the majority of patients, while other people may not. Every procedure's outcome is governed by the participant's individual body healing capacities. However, the following is a brief list of conditions which has obtained optimal results. There is no single strategy that works for all patients. Nonetheless, based on our clinical experiences, we have demonstrated the situations with the best outcomes for improvement. This could be further updated with new results and technology at disposal.

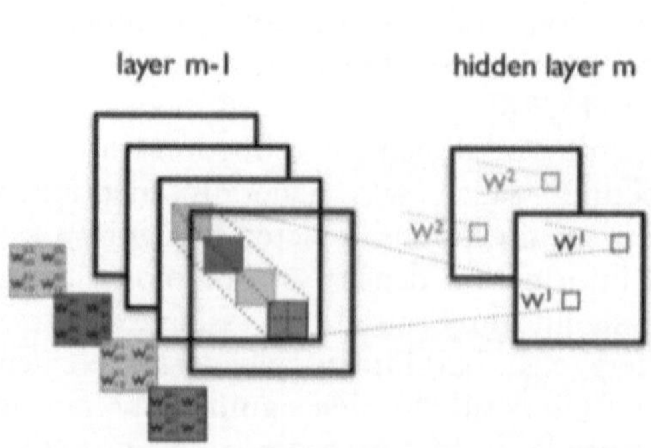

Figure 9.6 The proposed DRL diagram.

9.6 CONCLUSION

We referred to related work in stem cell morphogenetics from early 2019 to 2022 in this study and merged our survey into one paper. This survey provides a quick overview of stem cells as well as a developer's perspective on finding an appropriate solution for forecasting the morphology of stem cells and understanding their nature in order to predict any disease or help alter the area of regenerative medicine. Furthermore, stem cell therapy is not yet FDA approved, implying that there is much room for advancement in this area of regenerative medicine; every minor finding could potentially contribute to the field of regenerative medicine or stem cell therapy.

REFERENCES

[1] Mitra, S., Anjum, J., Muni, M., Das, R., Rauf, A., Islam, F., ... & Wilairatana, P. (2022). Exploring the journey of emodin as a potential neuroprotective agent: novel therapeutic insights with molecular mechanism of action. *Biomedicine & Pharmacotherapy*, *149*, 112877. https://doi.org/10.1016/j.biopha.2022.112877

[2] Wazid, M., Singh, J., Das, A. K., Shetty, S., Khan, M. K., & Rodrigues, J. J. (2022). ASCP-IoMT: AI-enabled lightweight secure communication protocol for internet of medical things. *IEEE Access*, *10*, 57990–58004, 10.1109/ACCESS.2022.3179418

[3] ArielWaisman, Alejandro La Greca, Alan M. Möbbs, María Agustina Scarafía, Natalia L. Santín Velazque, Gabriel Neiman, Lucía N, Moro,1,2 Carlos Luzzani,1,2 Gustavo E. Sevlever, Alejandra S. Guberman and Santiago G. Miriuka, 2019, *Deep Learning Neural Networks Highly.*

[4] Dai Kusumoto, Shinsuke Yuasa, and Keiichi Fukuda, Induced Pluripotent 2022, Stem Cell-Based Drug Screening by Use of Artificial Intelligence

[5] M Gupta, BV Santhosh Krishna, B Kavyashree, HR Narapureddy, N Surapaneni, and K Varma, 2022, Crop Yield Prediction Techniques Using Machine Learning Algorithms, *2022 8th International Conference on Smart Structures and Systems (ICSSS)*, pp. 1–7. doi: 10.1109/ICSSS54381.2022.9782246

[6] BV Santhosh Krishna, J Jijin Godwin, S Tharanee Shree, B Sreenidhi, and T Abinaya, 2021, Detection of Leukemia and Its Types Using Combination of Support Vector Machine and K-Nearest Neighbors Algorithm. In R Kumar, BK Mishra, and PK Pattnaik (eds) *Next Generation of Internet of Things.* Lecture Notes in Networks and Systems, vol 201. Springer, Singapore. https://doi.org/10.1007/978-981-16-0666-3_35

[7] W Zakrzewski, M Dobrzyński, M Szymonowicz and Z Rybak, 2019, Stem Cells: Past, Present, and Future. *Stem Cell Res Ther.*

[8] H Pawani and D Bhartiya, 2020, Pluripotent Stem Cells for Cardiac Regeneration: Overview of Recent Advances & Emerging Trends. *Indian J Med.*

[9] K Hole and S Ahmad, 2019, Biologically Driven Artificial Intelligence. *Computer*

[10] MS Kavitha, T Kurita, SY Park, SI Chien, JS Bae and BC Ahn, 2017, Deep Vector-Based Convolutional Neural Network Approach for Automatic Recognition of Colonies of Induced Pluripotent Stem Cells. *PLoS One.*

[11] R. Suganya, and R. Kanagavalli, 2021, Hybrid Gated Recurrent Unit and Convolutional Neural Network Based Deep Learning Architecture-Based Visibility Improvement Scheme for Improving Fog-Degraded Image. *International Journal of Information Technology.*

[12] Devi Naveen, M Nirmala, Dummala Roopesh, J Kiran Reddy, P Karthik Raju, 2022, Landslide Detection Using Machine Learning Algorithms, *Journal of Algebraic Statistics*, 13(3), 2822–2828. https://publishoa.com

[13] S Shanmuga Priya, P Rachana, BM Manoj, Shradda Aramoti and Shifa Fathima, 2022, Home Automation by Speech Detection System using Deep Learning, *2022 International Conference on Smart Technologies and Systems for Next Generation Computing (ICSTSN)*, pp. 1–5. doi: 10.1109/ICSTSN53084.2022.9761303

[14] B Chempavathy, VM Deshmukh, A Datta, AT Shiva, G Singh, 2022, An Exploration into Secure IoT Networks Using Deep Learning Methodologies, *2022 International Conference for Advancement in Technology (ICONAT) Goa, India.* Jan 21-22. doi: 10.1109/ICONAT53423.2022.9725988

[15] R Jeevitha, SJ Subhashini, KCS Krishna, KV Teja, and SK Srinivas, 2022, Detection of Face Mask: A Systematic Approach, *2022 3rd International Conference for Emerging Technology (INCET)*, pp. 1–4. doi: 10.1109/INCET54531.2022.9824524

[16] R Suganya, and R Kanagavalli, (February 2022), Sparse Coding and Improved Dark Channel Prior-based Deep CNN Model for enhancing visibility of Foggy Images, *International Journal of Information Technology*, 14(1), 547–557, doi: 10.1007/s41870-021-00742-7

[17] P Rachana, B Rajalakshmi, T Bhat, S Kaur and S Bimali, 2022, Comparative Study of Different Methods for Fire Detection Using Convolutional Neural Network (CNN), *2022 4th International Conference on Smart Systems and Inventive Technology (ICSSIT)*, pp. 1759–1765, doi: 10.1109/ICSSIT53264.2022.9716284

[18] S Bangari, P Rachana, N Gupta, PS Sudi, and KK Baniya, 2022, A Survey on Disease Detection of a potato Leaf Using CNN, *2022 Second International Conference on Artificial Intelligence and Smart Energy (ICAIS)*, pp. 144–149, doi: 10.1109/ICAIS53314.2022.9742963

Chapter 10

Evaluation of focal solid hepatic lesions using shear wave elastography

Asif Tamboli, Amol Bohite, and Shreya Tiwari

10.1 INTRODUCTION

Liver is one of the most common organs to be involved in neoplastic etiologies. Characterization of hepatic lesions is a challenging problem among clinicians and radiologists. It involves a significant component of healthcare costs with a substantial impact on patient management. Focal liver lesions or FLLs are masses of abnormal tissue in the liver that can be individual or multiple (in groups) and may primarily arise from hepatocytes, mesenchymal tissue or biliary epithelium, or secondarily metastasize from extrahepatic tumors [1]. The lesions are further subdivided into benign and malignant categories, both of which could be solid or cystic [1–4]. The most frequently encountered malignant liver tumors are metastases with the most common primary sites being colon, stomach, pancreas, breast and lung. Primary liver cancer (hepatocellular carcinoma) is the fifth most common cancer worldwide and represents the second leading cause of mortality in men and the sixth leading cause in women; hence, timely detection of lesions, while they are still responsive to medical or surgical treatment has a large demand on imaging [3, 4].

There has been an upsurge in the detection of incidental FLLs over the last two decades due to the widespread use of imaging modalities with emphasis on the use of non-invasive imaging techniques, thus preventing unnecessary use of painful biopsy especially in the diagnosis of benign touch-me-not lesions, thereby reducing the risk of bleeding and anxiety among the patients [5].

The most common benign liver masses which have been reported in as many as 20% of patients on autopsy studies can be precisely diagnosed by imaging [6–8]. Therefore, characterization of liver masses and discrimination between benign and malignant lesions are of utmost importance to plan appropriate management. CE-CT (contrast-enhanced computed tomography) and CE-MRI (contrast-enhanced magnetic resonance imaging) are the second-line imaging methods that can accurately characterize previously detected lesions, but they are more expensive and less accessible [9].

DOI: 10.1201/9781003536352-10

Shear wave sono-elastography (SWE) is a novel elastographic imaging technique implemented in conventional real-time ultrasound equipment that allows a simple, rapid, cost-effective and non-invasive quantitative estimation of the distribution of elasticity within biological tissues using modified software, thus offering us new perspectives in the imaging of focal liver lesions. It quantitatively measures the natural tendency of the tissue to return to its original shape and size after being subjected to a deforming force or stress.

10.2 LITERATURE REVIEW

SWE may very well be utilized as an alternative to normal ultrasonography in the prediction and characterization of localized hepatic lesions, assisting in subsequent clinical care. SWE has been validated to be beneficial in the evaluation of the acute liver fibrosis [6].

Ultrasound has a high diagnostic rate for hepatocellular carcinoma (HCC) including colorectal liver metastases, according to a few clinicians [7, 8]. The stated range of ultrasound's sensitivity for finding liver metastases is 40% to 70%. The primary limitations of ultrasonograpy (US) are its limited specificity, inability to identify lesions smaller than 1cm, as well as increased dependence on the manual operator. Elastography and contrast enhanced ultrasonography (CEUS) are two novel methods that may boost identification outcomes. The stiffness of localized lesions is assessed by elastography, which also guarantees the differentiation of lesions depending on malignancy. After contrast injection, the Doppler study's specificity and accuracy went from 71% to 96% and 50% to 80%, respectively.

In a research 105 hepatic masses were seen in 89 individuals (42 female as well as 47 male patients). Between normal (1.73 [SD, ±0.8] m/sec) and malignant (2.57 [SD, ±1.01] m/sec) masses, there was a statistically significant difference (SSD) in the values of the acoustic radiation force impulse (P-value 0.001). However, the accuracy was only rated as fair since the area under the receiver operating characteristics curve was just 0.744. When 1.9 m/sec was used as the cut-off value, the specificity 69% (44/64), positive and negative predictive values 58% (28/48), 77% (44/57), sensitivity @ 68% (28/41), respectively, reflect a broad range of ARFI values in each diagnosis [10].

A total of 400 measurements were taken, and 40 lesions were assessed by Bamber et al. [11]. Hepatocellular tumors made up 6/40 (15%) of the lesions, followed by hemangiomas (7/40 (17.5%), adenomas (5/40 (12.5%), metastases (9/40 (22.5%), and localized nodular hyperplasia (13/40 (32.5%) [11]. The acquired average values were 2.17 m/s for HCCs, 2.30 m/s for hemangiomas, 1.25 m/s for adenomas, 2.87 m/s for metastases, and 2.75 m/s for FNHs. There was no SSD (P-value > 0.05) in the interoperator assessment. Adenomas were consistently observed to be different from other lesions (P-value 0.05).

According to Gubarkova et al. [12], 56 patients who had 76 liver lesions had 65 SWE procedures (57 FNHs and 19HAs). For FNHs, the mean elasticity was 46.99 31.15 kPa, whereas for HAs, it was 12.08 10.68 kPa (P-value 0.0001). 7.94 6.43 and 1.91 1.70, respectively, were the mean relative elastic (MRE) ratio values (P-value 0.0001). With a threshold of 18.8 kPa for liver lesion elasticity, the ROC analysis revealed a maximum accuracy of 95% for classification (accurate of 96% with a cut-off of 1.98 for the corresponding elasticity ratio).

10.3 MATERIALS AND METHOD

Place: The study was conducted in the Department of Radiodiagnosis, KIMS Hospital, Karad, Maharashtra.

Study design and duration: From January 2020 to June 2021, a total of 18 months were dedicated to conducting the study.

Source of data: Patients referred from various departments who were found to have focal hepatic lesions on conventional imaging modalities were included in the study.

About 48 cases were assigned as the minimum sample size. However, in the 18-months study period, a total number of 58 cases that fulfilled the selection criteria were studied.

10.3.1 Method

After receiving approval from the institution's ethics committee, this retrospective analytical research was carried out, while institutional informed consent policies were adhered to. Patients who accepted to participate in the trial under ethical considerations were those who had one or more hepatic focal lesions measuring more than 1 cm in diameter and had been identified by ultrasound, conventional CT, or MRI. Before taking part in the trial, all patients had to provide their written, informed permission. Using the established inclusion and exclusion criteria, the patients were screened. After evaluating each patient's case sheet and prior medical information, pertinent entries for each patient were documented in the Proforma. In accordance with the research by Qiang et al., the biggest or most noticeable lesion was selected as the representative lesion in patients with multiple lesions.

58 patients (23 men and 35 women) were included in the research for the purpose of conducting the final statistical analysis. Their ages ranged from 27 to 79 years old, with a mean of 56.71 years old.

10.3.2 Examining shear wave elastography

After a thorough gray-scale sonographic and Doppler evaluation of the liver, SWE acquisition was carried out. To access the right hypochondrium

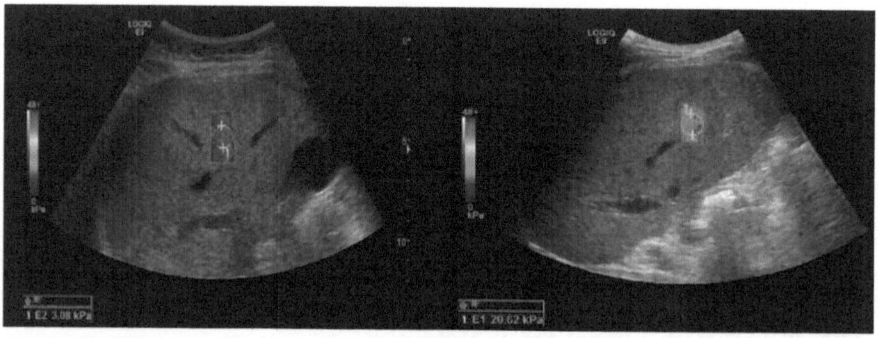

Figure 10.1 SWE color-coded elastogram images.

and enhance the intercostal space, patients were positioned supine or in the left semilateral decubitus position with the right arm fully abducted (to improve the acoustic window). With enough gel to prevent rib shadowing, the probe was positioned within and parallel to the intercostal gap on the mid-clavicular line or anterior axillary line. The area of the liver chosen was free of any obvious bile ducts or arteries. At a depth of around 4 cm, the area of interest (ROI) was about 1.0 × 1.5 cm in size. SWE might penetrate as deep as 6 cm below the skin's surface [9]. The biggest or most noticeable lesion on individuals who had numerous lesions was selected as the index lesion. To provide a direct reference for SWE measurements of the stiffness values of solid localized lesions, stiffness values of the adjacent hepatic parenchymal tissues (background liver) were also assessed.

To acquire independent measures of liver stiffness for each individual, the ROIs were positioned on several SWE picture frames or at non-overlapping regions on the same image frame (Figure 10.1). For each patient, kilopascal (kPa) values representing 12 consecutive measures for each lesion and six consecutive assessments for the liver parenchyma were acquired. The median value was then utilized for statistical analysis. The interquartile range (IQR)/median ratio for each test was computed.

10.3.3 Contrast-enhanced computed tomography (CE-CT)

Using a 16 slice Multi-detector Siemens Emotion CT system, all patients (58) had a contrast-enhanced triphasic CT investigation with the following settings: Slice thickness is 15 mm, KV is 120, MA is 200–250, and FOV is 400 mm (scanning from the lung bases to the iliac crest including the whole liver).

10.3.4 Magnetic resonance imaging with contrast enhanced (CE) MRI

Twenty-seven cases (16 malignant and 11 benign) were examined using a 1.5 Tesla Siemens Magnetom Avanto machine. Following the pre-contrast study, an automated injector was used to provide a bolus of Gd-DTPA at a dosage of 0.2 mmol/kg at a rate of 3–5 ml/s.

10.4 RESULTS

The percentage distribution of 58 focal hepatic lesions was as follows: (Table 6.4 and Chart 6.4) a) 47 (81.0%) malignant solid hepatic focal lesions were subdivided as hepatocellular carcinoma (N = 16) (27.6%), metastasis (N = 26) (44.8%) {2 GIST, 3 bronchogenic carcinomas, 10 breast cancers, 3 colon cancers, 2 rectal cancers, 1 anal melanoma, 1 prostatic carcinoma, 1 carcinoma cervix and 3 ovarian carcinomas} and cholangiocarcinoma (N = 5) (8.6%). b) 11 (19.0%) benign solid hepatic focal lesions were subdivided as hemangioma (N = 10) (17.2%) and focal nodular hyperplasia (N = 1) (1.7%).

Malignant liver lesions were more common in the 6th to 7th decades (~68.1%, whereas Benign liver lesions were more common in the 4th to 5th decades (~54.6%)). The study group had more females with metastatic lesions than males as breast cancer was the most common primary in this group.

Around 16 cases of hepatocellular carcinoma, 26 cases of metastases, 5 cases of cholangio-carcinoma, 1 case of focal nodular hyperplasia and 10 cases of hemangioma were included in the study. There was a statistically significant variance in median stiffness values (in kPa) and SWE color characteristics between benign and malignant solid focal hepatic lesions with the inference that most malignant lesions had higher stiffness (median value = 33.4 kPa) and showed mixed color with red foci whereas most benign lesions had lower stiffness (median value = 13.5 kPa) and showed yellow-green color.

10.5 DISCUSSION

The most effective imaging method for identifying and characterizing liver lesions is MRI. The specificity and sensitivity of contrast-enhanced MRI for benign lesions such hemangiomas as well as FNH surpass 95%. Hemangiomas may need technetium-labeled RBC blood-pool scintigraphy to be identified. Most focal liver lesions may be accurately diagnosed by MRI in 15 to 30 minutes [7].

Through the use of shear wave elastography, which is an imaging method, tissue stiffness may be measured in terms of its velocity. You may directly substitute the shear wave speed for stiffness or convert it to Young's modulus. Shear wave elastography measures tissue stiffness on an absolute scale, in contrast to strain elastography, which yields a qualitative evaluation of stiffness [10–13].

Shear wave elastography may be carried out with a single diagnostic ultrasound probe because ultrasound can act as a stimulus that causes shear waves to occur in tissue and the way to examine the tissue response that results from those shear waves. As a result, adding shear wave elastography to an existing diagnostic ultrasound system is made easier.

In this research, the malignant solid focal malignancies had a median size of 4.8 cm, while the benign solid focal lesions had a median size of 4.1 cm. The stiffness of the lesion (measured in kPa) and its size (measured in kPa) did not statistically correlate with whether it was benign or malignant (P-value = 0.6968). This conclusion is in line with the findings of investigations performed by [14–16], which indicated no statistically significant correlation between the stiffness values of the lesions and their size.

Only one benign lesion, FNH (9.1%), was seen in the color-coded elastograms, while 45 malignant lesions (95.7%) displayed mixed color with red foci. Consequently, malignant and normal solid focal lesions had different SWE color properties [16], and this difference had a P-value of 0.001.

10.6 CONCLUSION

2D shear wave elastography enables visualization of the tissue stiffness as a color-coded map in a 2D region of interest and at the same time provides a quantitative assessment. SWE measurements were shown to be useful in discriminating benign from malignant lesions with the results demonstrating that malignant lesions have higher stiffness values than benign lesions. Furthermore, they were helpful in the sub-categorization of different benign and malignant liver lesions as statistically significant differences were seen when stiffness values of hepatocellular carcinoma were compared with cholangiocarcinoma or metastatic lesions and also when stiffness values of focal nodular hyperplasia were compared with hemangioma. Hence, we concluded that shear wave elastography is a promising novel technique for rapid, cost-effective, non-invasive and non-contrast assessment and characterization of focal liver lesions that can be implemented with conventional grey-scale sonographic examinations to aid the diagnosis and further management. However, as this was a single hospital-based study with a limited number of test subjects, larger studies are required for further enhancement of the clinical application of this technology.

REFERENCES

1. Yan Y, Xing X, Lu Q, Wang X, Luo X, Yang L. Assessment of biopsy proven liver fibrosis by two-dimensional shear wave elastography in patients with primary biliary cholangitis. *Digestive and Liver Disease*. 2020;52(5):555–560.
2. Herrmann E, de Lédinghen V, Cassinotto C, Chu WC, Leung VY, Ferraioli G, Filice C, Castera L, Vilgrain V, Ronot M, Dumortier J. Assessment of biopsy-proven liver fibrosis by two-dimensional shear wave elastography: An individual patient data-based meta-analysis. *Hepatology*. 2018;67(1):260–272.
3. Rattansingh A, Amooshahi H, Menezes RJ, Wong F, Fischer S, Kirsch R, Atri M. Utility of shear-wave elastography to differentiate low from advanced degrees of liver fibrosis in patients with hepatitis C virus infection of native and transplant livers. *Journal of Clinical Ultrasound*. 2018 Jun;46(5):311–318.
4. Tajiri K, Kawai K, Sugiyama T. Strain elastography for assessment of liver fibrosis and prognosis in patients with chronic liver diseases. *Journal of Gastroenterology*. 2017 Jun;52:724–733.
5. Corvino A, Catalano O, Setola SV, Sandomenico F, Corvino F, Petrillo A. Contrast-enhanced ultrasound in the characterization of complex cystic focal liver lesions. *Ultrasound in Medicine & Biology*. 2015 May 1;41(5):1301–1310.
6. Wang W, Zhang JC, Tian WS, Chen LD, Zheng Q, Hu HT, Wu SS, Guo Y, Xie XY, Lu MD, Kuang M. Shear wave elastography-based ultrasomics: differentiating malignant from benign focal liver lesions. *Abdominal Radiology*. 2021 Jan;46:237–248.
7. Nacheva-Georgieva EL, Doykov DI, Andonov VN, Doykova KA, Tsvetkova SB. Point shear wave elastography and 2-dimensional shear wave elastography as a non-invasive method in differentiating benign from malignant liver lesions. *Gastroenterology Insights*. 2022 Sep 10;13(3):296–304.
8. Shaha P, Bhoiteasst A, Kumbhar R. Role of ultrasound elastography in characterization of focal solid hepatic lesion. *Journal of Coastal Life Medicine*. 2023;11:30–48.
9. Sporea I, Săndulescu DL, Şirli R, Popescu A, Danilă M, Spârchez Z, Mihai C, Ioanițescu S, Moga T, Timar B, Brisc C. Contrast-enhanced ultrasound for the characterization of malignant versus benign focal liver lesions in a prospective multicenter experience – The SRUMB study. *Journal of Gastrointestinal & Liver Diseases*. 2019 Jun 1;28(2)..
10. Zhou LQ, Wang JY, Yu SY, Wu GG, Wei Q, Deng YB, Wu XL, Cui XW, Dietrich CF. Artificial intelligence in medical imaging of the liver. *World Journal of Gastroenterology*. 2019 Feb 2;25(6):672.
11. Bamber J., Cosgrove D., Dietrich C. F., Fromageau J., Bojunga J., Calliada F., … & Piscaglia F. EFSUMB guidelines and recommendations on the clinical use of ultrasound elastography. Part 1: Basic principles and technology. *Ultraschall Med*, 2013;34(2):169–184.
12. Gubarkova EV, Sovetsky AA, Zaitsev VY, Matveev LA, Matveyev AL, Vorontsov DA, Timofeeva LB, Kiseleva EB, Vorontsov AY, Kuznetsova IA, Gladkova ND. Comparison of elastic properties of tissue samples in various pathological states using optical coherence elastography. In *Saratov Fall Meeting 2018: Optical and Nano-Technologies for Biology and Medicine* 2019 Jun 3 (Vol. 11065, pp. 73–77). SPIE.

13. Gharibvand MM, Asare M, Motamedfar A, Alavinejad P, Momeni M. Ultrasound shear wave elastography and liver biopsy to determine liver fibrosis in adult patients. *Journal of Family Medicine and Primary Care*. 2020;9(2): 943–949.
14. Galal SM, Soror SM, Hussien O, Moustafa EF, Hassany SM. Noninvasive assessment of liver fibrosis in children with chronic hepatitis C: shear wave elastography and APRI versus liver biopsy. *Arab Journal of Gastroenterology*. 2020;21(4):253–259.
15. Gu JH, Zhu L, Jiang TA. Quantitative ultrasound elastography methods in focal liver lesions including hepatocellular carcinoma: From diagnosis to prognosis. *Ultrasound Quarterly*. 2021 Jun 1;37(2):90–96.
16. Abdel-Latif M, Fouda N, Shiha OA, Rizk AA. Role of shear wave sono-elastography (SWE) in characterization of hepatic focal lesions. *Egyptian Journal of Radiology and Nuclear Medicine*. 2020 Dec;51(1):1–5.

Chapter 11

Diabetes risk prediction system using machine learning

Amit Kumar Tiwari, Rohit Mishra, Garima Shukla, Avni Dwivedi, Kriti Dwivedi, and Piyush Mishra

11.1 INTRODUCTION

Diabetes, a prevalent endocrine disorder, results in elevated blood sugar levels attributed to compromised insulin secretion and responsiveness. This can lead to complications such as cardiovascular issues, stroke, amputation, kidney failure, retinopathy, and early mortality. The prevalence of diabetes is influenced by various factors such as excessive sodium intake, suboptimal dietary patterns, obesity, immune dysregulation, insulin resistance, stress, and genetic predisposition. Identifying these concurrent conditions and providing tailored therapeutic interventions are crucial for optimizing patient outcomes [1]. Globally, an estimated 463 million individuals aged 20 to 79 are affected by diabetes, with projections anticipating a surge to 700 million by 2045. Diabetes resulted in 4.2 million fatalities, impacting not only adults but also over approximately 1.1 million youths and adolescents affected by type 1 diabetes and an additional 374 million individuals at heightened risk for developing type 2 diabetes. Diabetes manifests in three principal types: type 1, characterized by deficient insulin production; type 2, involving impaired insulin responsiveness and insufficient production over time; and gestational diabetes (Type III), arising during pregnancy, predominantly affecting women with no antecedent diabetic history. Common symptoms across both major types encompass polyuria, polydipsia, fatigue, and visual disturbances [2]. Understanding the technical intricacies of diabetes classifications and associated symptomatology is essential for the formulation of comprehensive healthcare management and intervention strategies. It is projected that diabetes will rank as the seventh major cause of mortality by the year 2030. Automated computer diagnosis, utilizing machine learning and deep learning, shows promise. However, challenges include the complex nature of medical data and shortcomings in existing methods, such as handling missing values and addressing outliers. Despite advancements, achieving accurate classification for diabetic patients remains a significant challenge [3, 4]. The underwhelming effectiveness of current diabetes prediction algorithms is ascribed to inadequate preprocessing, notably the oversight in managing missing values, eliminating irrelevant features, and

DOI: 10.1201/9781003536352-11

addressing outliers. The gathered data undergo processing to categorize them accordingly. Robust preprocessing, especially in medical datasets, is crucial for accurate classification. To predict diabetes, we use various ML algorithms, including (SVM), (KNN), (RF), (DT) and Naive Bayes. Our work focuses upon four classifiers: Decision Tree, SVM, RF, and KNN [4]. We conduct a rigorous examination of results, experimentally exploring feature selection and dimensionality reduction, with outcomes subjected to detailed analysis. The study concludes by identifying efficient methods to enhance predictive accuracy in diabetes onset prediction.

11.2 LITERATURE REVIEW

Here, this section draws attention toward the selected group of scholars who have played pivotal roles in advancing the field of diabetes prediction. Their noteworthy contributions involve the extraction of insights from medical data through the utilization of both machine learning and deep learning methodologies. Mr. Usama Ahmed [4] enforced a model using an approach based on machine learning techniques. They employed two distinct methodologies within the realm of ML, namely (SVM) and (ANN). Utilizing real-time medical records of patients, their model anticipates the diabetic status of the individual. The suggested integrated machine learning model exhibits a prediction accuracy of 94.87 percent. They used ANN and SVM for prediction and making a decision, and they used fuzzy logic. Mr. S. M. Mahedy Hasan [5] enforced a prototype using a decision tree, adaptive boosting, random forest, and extra tree. To eliminate features of lesser significance they used MI based on the feature selection technique to enhance prediction accuracy. To enhance the efficacy of the tree-based algorithm, they utilized the adaptive boosting technique. Among all the algorithms they had used, adaptive boosting algorithm scored the highest accuracy that is 90.5 percent. Also, several other researchers from different countries enforced a model using a machine-learning approach [6]. They also used the Pima Indians Diabetes dataset along with a private dataset of Bangladeshi female patients and workers of local textile factories. In the machine learning approach, they had (SVM), (RF), (LR), (KNN), and XGBoost. Among all the algorithms they had used, Adaptive Boosting with XGBoost classifier scores the highest accuracy which is 81 percent. Ms. S Sivaranjani [7] enforced a model using machine learning. In their proposed work, they have used SVM model and Random Forest. They had used various techniques such as step forward and step backward to select the featuring scale which influence the prediction. Random Forest demonstrates the highest accuracy at 83 percent when compared between Support Vector Machine and Random Forest, as reported by Mr. Jana S [8]. Their predictive model employs a dataset and leverages Machine Learning Classification along with ensemble techniques. They incorporated (k-NN),

(DT), and (RF) as the three chosen methods. Upon comparison with alternative models, variations in the accuracy of each model were observed. These findings affirm the capability of the model to predict the accurate result of diabetes with a high degree of precision [9].

11.3 METHODOLOGY

11.3.1 Collect the datasets

The Kaggle Diabetes Dataset was utilized for this research, primarily consisting of data collected from 21-year-old females. The dataset consists of a total of 768 observations classified into two groups and featuring eight distinct independent attributes. The binary form of attribute which tells that the patient is having diabetes or not by providing 0 or 1, there are 500 samples (65.1) labeled as non-diabetic (–ve) and an additional subset comprising 268 samples (34.9) designated as diabetic (+ve). Table 11.1 details provide further information relating to the distribution within the dataset categories.

11.3.2 Data preprocessing

As it is well acknowledged, medical data in real-world scenarios exhibit non-linearity, non-normality, and complexity. On occasion, this dataset may encompass missing values, inconsistencies, and outliers. The efficacy of an algorithm classification hinges on various factors; if preprocessing data is inadequate, it may lead to elevated classification errors. Our primary research goal is to enhance the accuracy of classification in predicting diabetic patients. Our Prescribed Model is also represented by the flowchart in Figure 11.1.

Table 11.1 Details of dataset

Attributes	*Derived Attributes*	*Missing no. in percent*
Pregnancy	No. of times pregnant	1
Glucose level	Concentrated Glucose	1.56
Blood pressure	DBP	5.44
Skin thickness	Thickness in skin	27.32
Insulin	Insulin serum (2 hours)	46,65
BMI	Body mass index	2.34
Function pedigree	Pedigree function	2,67
Age	Age in years	28
Class	for positive and 0 for negative	1

- Data Cleaning: Recognize and manage absent data by examining the dataset for any missing values and determining a strategy for addressing them. This may involve either eliminating rows containing missing values or filling in values using statistical measures.
- Exploratory Data Analysis (EDA): Understand the distribution of features. Use visualizations and summary statistics to explore the distribution of each feature in the dataset. Analyze relationships between different features and the target variable to identify patterns.
- Feature Scaling: Standardize or normalize numerical features: Scaling ensures uniform scaling of features which is crucial to avoid the undue influence of specific features during the learning process. Methods commonly employed include standard scaling (where the mean gets subtracted and later divided it with the SD).

11.3.3 Classification

Upon completion of the dataset preparation phase, machine learning techniques were applied for dataset classification. This chapter incorporates the implementation of (KNN), (SVM), (RF) and (DT) technique algorithms, utilizing features as mentioned in Table 11.1, such as pregnant patients, glucose level, high or low BP, thickness of the body skin, level of insulin, body mass index, functionate pedigree, and how old the person is. Individuals with BP exceeding 80 are categorized as diabetic:

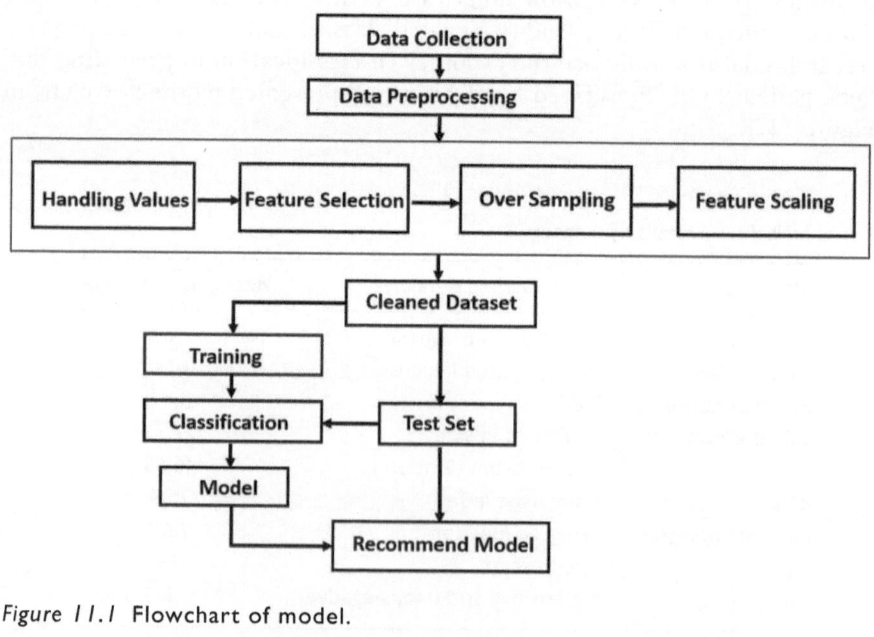

Figure 11.1 Flowchart of model.

- (KNN): KNN or K-Nearest Neighbor represents a ML algorithm which is supervised, recognized as an empirical and fundamental technique that categorizes an object in the input space by relying on its nearest neighbors from the sample set. The KNN proved to be effective with continuous usage. When class element is outside of training set, it uses a method by which it identifies k elements from within its closest proximity in distance to the said missing data points present in a given dataset.
- (SVM):SVM or Support Vector Machine is a ML algorithm that finds extensive application in classification as well as regression. The objective of SVM is to identify the most effective hyperplane for separating different classes within the feature space, optimizing the margin – represented by the distance between data points closest from each class and this hyperplane. Support vectors denote those particular data instances located nearest to such decision boundaries, significantly impacting both its position and orientation. SVM's ability to handle complex decision boundaries and its robustness against overfitting contribute to its wide adoption in diverse machine-learning scenarios.
- Random Forest (RF): The fundamental concept underlying Random Forest involves the construction of numerous decision trees in the training phase and amalgamating their predictions during testing. This strategy aims to enhance the model's overall performance and resilience.
- Decision Tree (DT): The Decision Tree has gained widespread recognition for its ability to tackle challenges related to both and regression classification. Its functionality involves iteratively dividing the dataset into subsets according to the most influential features, resulting in the formation of a structure as a Tree. At each node of the tree, a decision is made by evaluating a feature, and the dataset is split into branches accordingly.

11.4 DISCUSSION AND RESULT

This section explores the outcomes achieved through the application of the proposed model and assesses its effectiveness using the PIMA dataset, along with preprocessing. The dataset being considered is featuring a binary representation which is anyone of them as 0 or 1. This dataset is extensively utilized for diabetes analysis employing various techniques and algorithms. Comprising a total of 768 patients, the entire dataset is employed for the experiment. The dataset encompasses nine independent attributes or parameters, including numerical values with units which is mentioned in Table 11.1. The dependent parameter, denoting whether a person is healthy or diabetic, is the outcome of interest. Data preprocessing involves analyzing the results, and the model's efficiency improves after this stage.

Calculation process takes into account the data type of each parameter as per mentioned in Figure 11.1(considered to be 122, 72, 29, 155,32.46, 0.47 and 33, respectively). After the completion of data preprocessing, the dataset undergoes classification, and the outcomes of each classifier are verified using an AdaBoost Technique. The performance metrics for every step are outlined in Tables 11.2 and 11.3. The dataset is partitioned into a ratio of 7 or 3 for the trained datasets and for the test datasets, signifying that 70 percent of the dataset is randomly selected as the trained datasets, leaving remaining 30 percent as the test datasets. This partition ratio is determined after experimenting with a variety of additions on it, demonstrating its efficacy. The set of test data is subsequently analyzed and divided on random basis and evenly, ensuring validation for data which was not trained. The evaluation criteria encompass accurate training set, accuracy of the test, and validation accuracy. Post data preprocessing, the SVM classifier exhibits higher training and testing accuracy compared to Random Forest, Decision Tree, and KNN classifiers, while the validation accuracy remains relatively consistent across all classifiers. Specifically, KNN, RF, DT, and SVM yield individual precision scores of 78, 78, 75, and 78. The metrics are utilized as the foundational estimator for the AdaBoost classifier to improve performance. Next, MI-FS is used in order to eliminate features that have less significance, namely Blood Weight and Family Work. Post this refinement, KNN, RF, DT, and SVM exhibit precision scores of 78, 78, 78, and 78, respectively. As depicted in Table 11.2, there is a noticeable increase in accuracy across each classifier. Consequently, the removal of insignificant features enhances the assessment metrics. To enhance working further, these methods are once more utilized as the foundational estimator for the AdaBoost classifier.

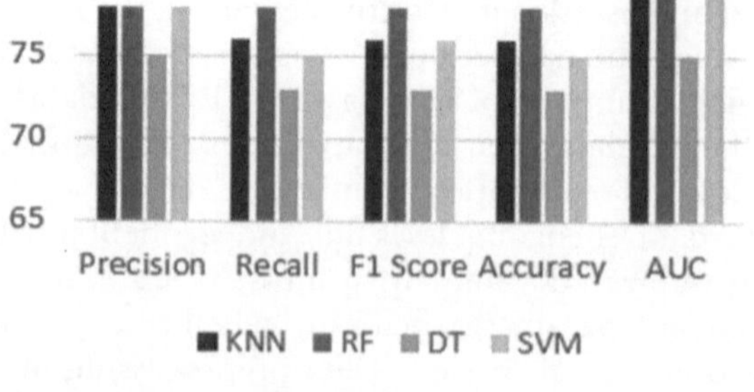

Figure 11.2 The Performance analysis using bar graph.

Table 11.2 Classification using AdaBoost

Classifier	*Precision*	*Recall*	*F1 Score*	*Accuracy (%)*	*AUC*
KNN	0.78	0.76	0.76	76	0.85
Random Forest	0.78	0.78	0.78	78	0.87
Decision Tree	0.75	0.73	0.73	73	0.75
SVM	0.78	0.75	0.76	75	0.87

Table 11.3 Applying MI-FS technique

Classifier	*Precision*	*Recall*	*F1 score*	*Accuracy (%)*	*AUC*
KNN	0.82	0.79	0.78	78	0.88
Random Forest	0.81	0.80	0.80	81	0.89
Decision Tree	0.80	0.78	0.75	77	0.79
SVM	0.85	0.82	0.78	79	0.90

Figure 11.3 illustrates that KNN, RF, DT, and SVM achieve precision scores of 82, 81.0, 80, and 85, respectively, indicating an improvement in assessment metrics. In this study, we came to know about support vector and various other methods show accuracy of almost 79. Likewise, NB shows accuracy of almost 79, that is, 77.34, while Logistic Regression, when compared to various classifiers such as KNN, DT, RF, etc., exhibits efficiency with an accuracy of 78.64. In the study we propose, the identification of the four most significant features involves SVM, DT, RF, and KNN, incorporating AdaBoost and MI-FS techniques. After applying these approaches, enhancements are observed in support vector machine models which are the most accurate results compared to others.

11.5 CONCLUSION

This research performs a comparative evaluation for categorizing individuals with diabetes. During preprocessing of data, imputation with mean and oversampling techniques were applied. Subsequently, a method for feature selection based on mutual information was employed to acquire data of excellent quality. In the categorization phase, SVM, RF, DT, and KNN machine learning algorithms were utilized. Additionally, these algorithms served as base estimators for the AdaBoost classifier, contributing to further accuracy enhancement. The analysis reveals that the combination of SVM, RF, DT, KNN algorithms with the AdaBoost classifier and MI-FS technique consistently outperforms other classifiers. In our experimentation, AdaBoost achieved nearly 100 accuracy, demonstrating significant superiority over

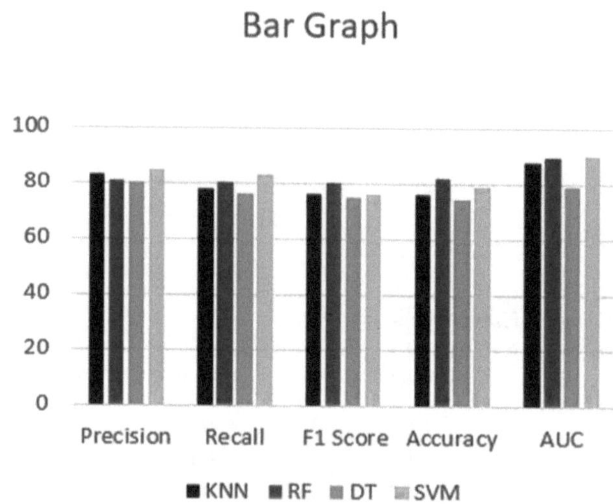

Figure 11.3 Performance analysis using bar graph.

alternative machine learning approaches in early-stage diabetes detection. These study findings hold the potential to assist healthcare providers in early diabetes detection, enabling more informed clinical decisions and potentially saving lives.

Table 11.4 Comparison with existing methods

Algorithms	*Accuracy in %*
SVM	79%
Random Forest	81%
KNN	78%
Decision Tree	77%
Logistic Regression	78.64%
Naive Bayes	77.3%
Our Project	86.7%

REFERENCES

[1] H. E. Massari, Z. Sabouri, S. Mhammedi and N. Gherabi, "Diabetes Prediction Using Machine Learning Algorithms and Ontology," in *Journal of ICT Standardization*, 10(2), 319–337, 2022, doi: 10.13052/jicts2245-800X.10212

[2] S. Sivaranjani, S. Ananya, J. Aravinth and R. Karthika, "Diabetes Prediction using Machine Learning Algorithms with Feature Selection and Dimensionality Reduction," *2021 7th International Conference on Advanced Computing and Communication Systems (ICACCS), Coimbatore*, India, 2021, pp. 141–146,doi:10.1109/ICACCS51430.2021.9441935

[3] M. M. Hassan, Z. J. Peya, S. Mollick, M. A. Billah, M. M. Hasan Shakil and A. U. Dulla, "Diabetes Prediction in Healthcare at Early Stage Using Machine Learning Approach," *2021 12th International Conference on Computing Communication and Networking Technologies (ICCCNT)*, Kharagpur, India, 2021, pp. 01–05, doi: 10.1109/ICCCNT51525.2021.9579869

[4] P. Sonar and K. JayaMalini, "Diabetes Prediction Using Different Machine Learning Approaches," *Proc. 3rd Int. Conf. Comput. Methodologies Commun. (ICCMC)*, pp. 367–371, Mar. 2019. Usama Ahmed, Ghassan F. Issa, Muhammad Adnamn Khan, Shabib Aftab, Muhammad Farhan and A.T. Raid, *Prediction of Diabetes Empowered With Fused Machine Learning*. 2022. IEEE.

[5] S. M. Mahdy Hassaan, Mohd. Fazzlle Rabbi, Arifa Islam Champa, and Md. Asif Zaman, *An Effective Diabetes Prediction System Using Machine Learning Techniques*. 2020, IEEE.

[6] Isfafuzzaman Tasin, Tansin Ullah Nabil, Sanjida Islam, and Riasat Khan, *Diabetes Prediction Using Machine Learning and AI Techniques*. 2022. NIH.

[7] S. Sivaranjani, S Ananya, J. Aravinth and R. Karthika, *Diabetes Prediction Using Machine Learning*. 2023. IEEE.

[8] S. Jana, N. Bharanidharan, P. Shanmukha Nagasai, K. Saravan Kumar, V. Mani Nageshwar, *Diabetes Prediction Using Machine Learning Algorithm*. 2022. IEEE.

[9] H. Roopa, T. Asha, "A Linear Model Based on Principal Component Analysis for Disease Prediction," *IEEE Access*, 7, 105314105318, 2019.

Chapter 12

Evaluation of coronary artery disease risk factors among patients with and without non-alcoholic fatty liver disease

Nitin Jadhav and Ravindra Adikrao More

12.1 INTRODUCTION

A fatal liver illness called non-alcoholic fatty liver disease (NAFLD) is associated with the metabolic syndrome, which includes insulin resistance. Patients with simple steatosis and hepatic steatosis who may be affected with cirrhosis liver and sometimes even hepatocellular cancer are included in the spectrum of NAFLD patients [1]. Over the last several years, convincing evidence has shown a strong connection among cardiovascular disease as well as NAFLD, including subclinical carotid atherosclerosis (SCA) and coronary artery disease [1–4]. Chronic liver disease, cardiovascular disease (CVD), and type-2 diabetes mellitus (T2DM) have received a lot of attention in the last ten years as NAFLD-related chronic diseases. For instance, according to a recent review and analysis, NAFLD has drastically increased fatality by 57%, mostly because of reasons connected to liver and cardiovascular diseases, as well as increased risk of prevalence rate of T2DM by about twofold.

12.2 NAFLD AND CARDIOVASCULAR EVENT RISKS

Over the last few decades, convincing evidence has shown a strong connection among cardiovascular disease and NAFLD, including subclinical coronary atherosclerosis (SCA) and coronary artery disease (CAD). Since NAFLD has increasingly replaced other causes of chronic liver disease in many regions of the globe, it may also play a substantial role in the burden of CVD and extra-hepatic chronic consequences [3]. For reasons unknown, males are more likely to have NAFLD than women, while specific estimates of the disease's occurrence are unclear (due to challenges in making an accurate medical assessment during consecutive follow-ups), the current overall incidence is roughly 20/10,000-person years, reaching a peak in 60 years of age. NAFLD is already present in up to 70% of patients with T2DM, which is greater than the population-based prevalence of NAFLD, which is currently estimated to be between 30 and 40% in males and 15 to 20% in women [4].

 DOI: 10.1201/9781003536352-12

There is increasing evidence linking NAFLD to other chronic conditions such as colorectal cancer, sleep apnea, psoriasis, osteoporosis, as well as other endocrinopathies (such as polycystic ovarian syndrome). However, because there is the strongest evidence for a potential causative relationship among NAFLD and cardiovascular disorders, this study will exclusively focus on extra-hepatic problems that are associated with NAFLD. It is necessary to closely monitor patients, address NAFLD risk factors, as well as effectively stratify cardiovascular risk in order to predict morbidity and mortality in this group of patients [5]. As a result, coronary angiography is an invasive diagnostic technique that is often used to diagnose CAD. It helps with coronary artery visualization. The goal of this study is to conduct an analysis to determine if and to what extent NAFLD increases the risk of cardiovascular disease (CVD). Determining the possible risks for CAD in people with NAFLD as well as the frequency of these factors associated with people both with and without NAFLD is the main objective of this study.

12.3 AIM AND OBJECTIVES

Aim of the study

- To determine the role of NAFLD in foreseeing the incidence of coronary artery disease.

Objectives

- To assess the conventional modifiable coronary artery disease risk factors in patients with non-alcoholic fatty liver disease (NAFLD).
- To compare the presence of coronary artery disease risk factors in subjects with NAFLD and those without NAFLD along with its clinical outcome.

12.4 LITERATURE REVIEW

According to estimates, in the normal community, NAFLD and NASH are prevalent at rates of 10%–24% and 1%–5%, respectively. NAFLD affects 9% to 32% of the general population in India. On histological inspection, 28% of patients have progression, 59% have no change, and 13% may have improvement, according to recent statistics. The histological and/or clinical prognosis of 98 individuals with NAFLD ranging from simple steatosis to cirrhosis was examined retrospectively by [6].

NAFLD mostly interferes with cardiac metabolism. Non-obese, non-diabetic, and non-motensive young adults with NAFLD appeared to have impaired myocardial energy metabolism (i.e., lower adenosine triphosphate (ATP)/phosphocreatine ratio, as estimated by 31P MR spectroscopy, as well as excessive fat accumulation in the epicardial region compared to the control group without NAFLD), according to a study utilizing cardiac magnetic resonance imaging (MRI) (controls). Surprisingly, regardless of normal left ventricular (LV) structural characteristics, such as diastolic and systolic performance, these myocardial metabolic abnormalities (MMA) were found [7].

In a cohort of 1254 Caucasian individuals, the presence of NAFLD was identified by liver ultrasound, as well as its association with common composite in addition to individual CVD was assessed. In the population under study, the frequency of NAFLD was 47.9%. In all the three glucose tolerance groups, having NAFLD was associated with a greater frequency of both composite CVD and individual CAD [8].

Those with NAFLD had a 2.0-fold and a 2.3-fold increased risk of getting CAD or CVD than those without NAFLD, similar to those with prediabetes. Those who have NAFLD as determined by ultrasonography are more likely to have CVD than those who have variable glucose tolerance [9].

Research by Montemezzo et al. [10] found that non-alcoholic fatty liver disease is becoming more common (NAFLD). This study's goals were to ascertain if NAFLD is associated with the degree of coronary blockage as assessed by coronary angiography as well as to examine the incidence of NAFLD in individuals with acute coronary syndrome (ACS) as assessed by ultrasonography (USG). Following that, CAD was angiographically evaluated according to well-established angiographic criteria, ranging from none to severe. Among the patients that were included, 107 (77%) had CAD, and 63 (45%) had significant damage. Regarding NAFLD, 76 (55.2%) people had it, with 18 (23.6%) having grade III illness. Fifteen patients (83.3%) had NAFLD grade III and severe CAD, and 47 (60.5%) of those with severe CAD were also affected by NAFLD [10, 11].

12.5 MATERIALS AND METHODS

Study plans: The current research was non-interventional, cross-sectional, descriptive, and observational in nature.

Study location: Krishna Hospital and Medical Research Center, a single-center hospital study.

Study duration: 18-month period of study (October 2019 to March 2021). The study was conducted at a tertiary care hospital's inpatient department of medicine. From October 2019, subjects were able to register. When they were hospitalized, they registered with the department of medicine. The individuals who met the exclusion criteria were not enrolled for the study at the time of registration. In the current research, a total of 100 participants—100 with NAFLD and 100 without—were included. Of those with NAFLD, 68 (68%) of the subjects were men, and the remainder 32 (32%) were women. Of those without NAFLD, 69 (69%) of the subjects were men and the remaining 31 (31%) were women.

12.5.1 Data collection

The institutional ethics committee gave its approval to this work (IEC). Before incorporating them in the research, all participants provided their written, fully informed permission in both the local language and English. There was a thorough physical examination. In the supine posture, the blood pressure was measured using a properly calibrated mercury sphygmomanometer (Diamond BP MR-120 Mercurial BP Deluxe).

A minimum of two readings were obtained, separated by a minute, and the average of the values was recorded. Other factors, such pulse rate, were monitored in the radial artery for the whole minute. Body Mass Index (BMI) was computed using the following data: height (in meters), weight (in kilograms), and waist circumference (in centimeters). The information gathered this way was analyzed to see how NAFLD affected the participants' clinical results and their propensity for coronary artery disease.

12.5.2 Clinical investigations

All the enrolled participants for study underwent following investigations:

- Conventional ultrasonography of the liver using the Siemens Acuson Juniper VA10 using curvilinear array transducer.
- Glycosylated hemoglobin was done by Latex Immunoturbidimetric method.
- Blood glucose by GOD POD (glucose oxidase peroxidase)-based method.

Formula:

$$\text{Glucose} + O_2 + H_2O \xrightarrow{\text{Glucose Oxidase}} \text{Gluconic Acid} + H_2O$$

$$H_2O_2 + \text{PhenolicCompounds} + 4 - \text{aminoantipyrine} \xrightarrow{\text{Peroxidase}} \text{Quanionmine} + H_2O$$

- Serum creatinine via modified JAFFE's process.
- Serum potassium via ion selective electrode method.
- Blood urea via urease GLDH procedure.
- Serum sodium via ion selective electrode procedure.

- The whole blood count was carried out using a three-part automated analyzer from Nihon Kohden (MEK 6420P).
- Liver function tests were done by calorimetry.
- Total cholesterol was assessed by CHOD PAP (cholesterol oxidase phenol 4-aminoantipyrine peroxidase)-based method.
- Triglycerides were assessed by GPO (glycerol phosphate oxidase) method.
- HDL by PVS PEGME [polyvinyl sulfonic acid (PVS) and polyethylene glycol-modified enzyme (PEGME)]-coupled classic precipitation method.

12.5.3 Statistical analysis

Microsoft Excel was used to compile and organize all of the data. Using Open Epi version 2.3.1 & IBM SPSS statistics Version 21, all the statistical analyses were carried out. The data were described using descriptive and inferential statistics including percentage (%), mean, variance, and standard deviation (SD). For qualitative approach and quantitative information, the student's t-test as well as the chi-square test was performed. The threshold for statistically significant data has a ρ-value of <0.05.

12.6 RESULTS

Mean age in years was 55.8, ranging from 24–75 years with SD±15.26 and among those without NAFLD, 38 subjects (38%) were in the age group of >60 years, 46 subjects (46%) between 40–60 years and 16 subjects (16%) between 20–40 years (Figure 12.1). The mean age in years of subjects with NADLD was 54.64, ranging from 24–75 years with SD±13.92. Out of 100, 58 subjects (58%) had Grade I fatty liver, 35 subjects (35%) had Grade II fatty liver, and 7 subjects (7%) had Grade III fatty liver (Figure 12.2).

Waist circumferences ≥102cm in male and ≥88cm in female were more in patients with NAFLD as compared to those without NAFLD. A statistical

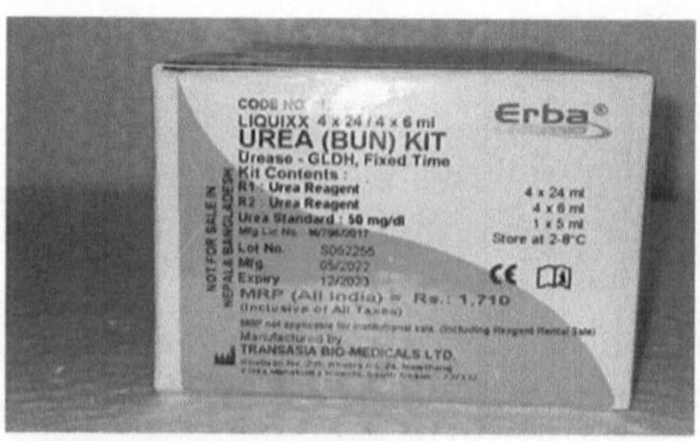

Figure 12.1 Urea (Bun) kit, GLDH method (Erba).

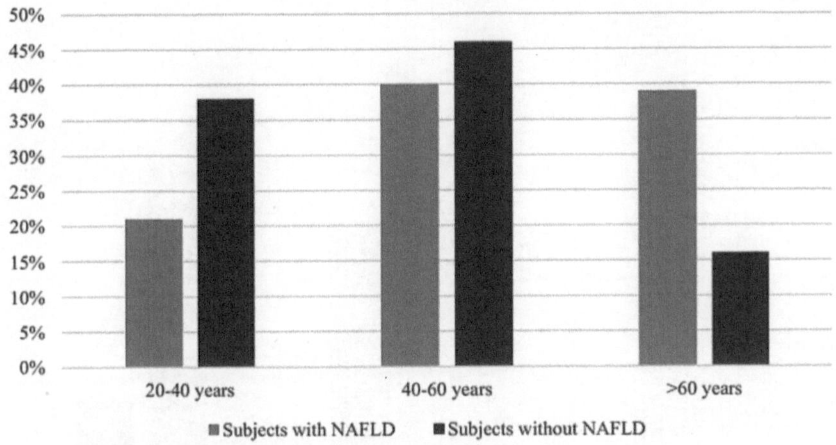

Figure 12.2 Distribution of the study population based on age.

significance was seen between the two study groups (p <0.001 in male and p =0.005 in female).

The mean BMI in kg/m² was 23.91, ranging from 17.3–29.7 kg/m² with SD±2.82. BMI ≥25 kg/m² (obese) was more in subjects with NAFLD as compared to those without NAFLD. Statistical significance was seen between the two study groups (Figure 12.3) based on BMI (p <0.00001) (Figure 12.4).

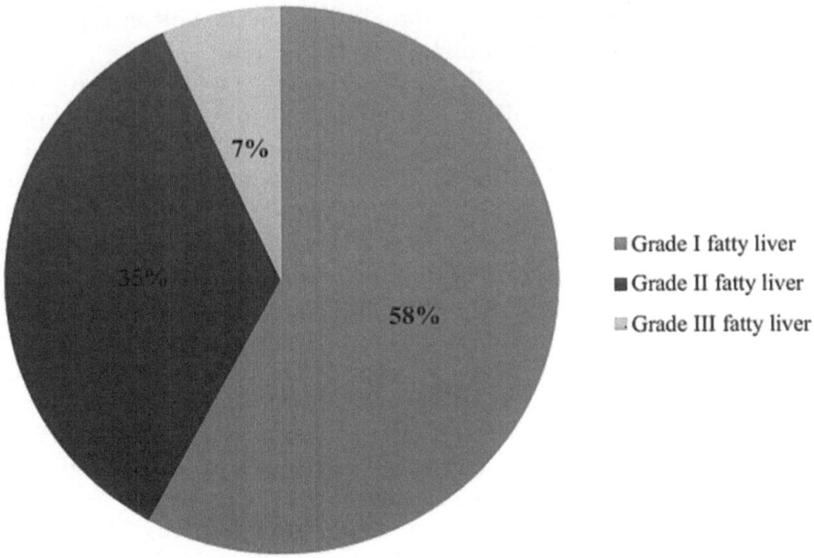

Figure 12.3 Distribution of the patients with NAFLD in the study group based on the grade of fatty liver.

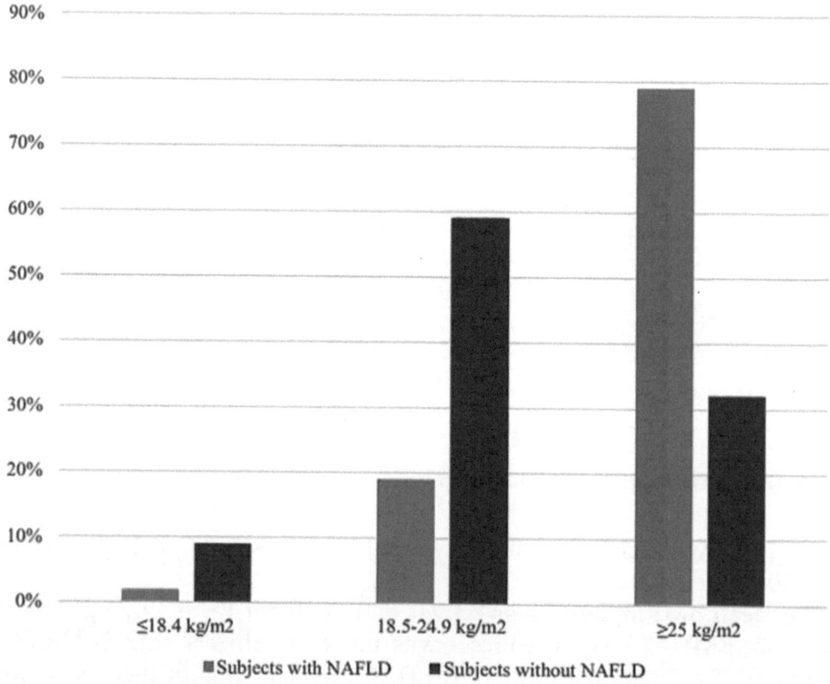

Figure 12.4 Distribution of the study population based on BMI.

Among those with NAFLD, 66 subjects (66%) had SBP >140 mmHg and 34 subjects (34%) had SBP <140 mmHg. The mean SBP in mmHg was 150.15 ranging from 100210 mmHg with SD ±21.54.

Among those without NAFLD, 16 subjects (16%) had SBP >140 mmHg and 84 subjects (84%) had SBP <140 mmHg. The mean SBP in mmHg was 123.78 ranging from 100,160 mmHg with SD ± 6.27. SBP >140 mmHg was more in subjects with NAFLD as compared to those without NAFLD. Statistical significance was seen between the two study groups based on SBP (p <0.00001). DBP >90 mmHg was significantly high among subjects with NAFLD (p <0.03). Table 12.1 shows the distribution of the study population based on diastolic blood pressure (DBP) among subjects with and without NAFLD.

Among those with NAFLD, 85 subjects (85%) had Serum Cholesterol <200 mg/dL and 15 subjects (15%) had Serum Cholesterol ≥200mg/dL. The mean Serum Cholesterol in mg/dL was 154.87 ranging from 69–262 mg/dL with SD±46.44; 46 subjects (46%) had Serum Triglyceride between 35135 mg/dL and 54 subjects (54%) had Serum Triglyceride ≥135 mg/dL. The mean Serum Triglyceride in mg/dL was 152.56 ranging from 60–326 mg/dL with SD ±62.07; 76 subjects (76%) had Serum HDL ≤40 mg/dL and 24 subjects (24%) had HDL between 4080 mg/dL. The mean Serum HDL in mg/dL was 35.44 ranging from 1068 mg/dL

Table 12.1 Distribution of the study population based on diastolic blood pressure (DBP)

DBP (mmHg)	*Subjects with NAFLD (n = 100)*	*Subjects without NAFLD (n = 100)*	*p-value*
>90	54(54%)	42(42%)	<0.03
<90	46(46%)	58(58%)	
Total	100(100%)	100(100%)	
Mean ±SD	91.64±11.87	87.24±10.9	

with SD±12.57. Among those without NAFLD, 90 subjects (90%) had Serum Cholesterol <200 mg/dL and 10 subjects (10%) had Serum Cholesterol ≥200mg/dL.

The mean Serum Cholesterol in mg/dL was 131.84 ranging from 70–260 mg/dL with SD +21.19; 72 subjects (72%) had Serum Triglyceride between 35–135 mg/dL and 28 subjects (28%) had Serum Triglyceride ≥135 mg/dL. The mean Serum Triglyceride in mg/dL was 111.86 ranging from 60200 mg/dL with SD ±19; 17 subjects (17%) had Serum HDL≤40 mg/dL and 83 subjects (83%) had HDL between 40–80 mg/dL. The mean Serum HDL in mg/dL was 67.76 ranging from 1068 mg/dL with SD ±11.41. Serum Cholesterol ≥200mg/dL and Serum Triglyceride ≥135 mg/dL were more in subjects with NAFLD compared to those without NAFLD. However, Serum HDL ≤40 mg/dL was less in patients with NAFLD compared to those without NAFLD.

Table 12.2 Distribution of study population based on the parameters mentioned below

CAD risk factors	*With NAFLD*	*Without NAFLD*	*p value*
BMI ≥25 kg/m2	79 (79%)	32 (32%)	<0.00001
WC ≥102 cm (male)	53 (77%)	39 (56%)	<0.001
WC ≥88cm (female)	25 (78%)	25 (80%)	=0.005
SBP >140 mmHg	66 (66%)	16 (16%)	<0.00001
DBP >90 mmHg	54 (54%)	42 (42%)	<0.03
F-BSL >126 mg/dL	66 (66%)	48 (48%)	<0.01
PP-BSL >200mg/dL	58 (58%)	14 (14%)	<0.00001
HbA1c >6.4%	60 (60%)	13 (13%)	<0.00001
Cholesterol ≥200 mg/dL	15 (15%)	10 (10%)	<0.02
Triglyceride ≥135 mg/dL	54 (54%)	28 (28%)	<0.001
HDL ≤40 mg/dL	76 (76%)	13 (13%)	<0.00001

It was observed that BMI > 25 kg/m2 was significantly high among subjects with NAFLD (p <0.00001), waist circumference >102 cm in male and >88cm in female was significantly high among subjects with NAFLD (p <0.001 in male and p =0.005 in female). It was also observed that SBP >140 mmHg was significantly high among subjects with NAFLD (p <0.00001), fasting blood sugar level (F-BSL) >126mg/dL was significantly high among subjects with NAFLD (p <0.01), Post Prandial Blood Sugar Level (PP-BSL) >200mg/dL was significantly high (Table 12.2) among subjects with NAFLD (p <0.00001), HbA1c >6.4% was significantly high among subjects with NAFLD (p <0.00001).

It was observed that subjects with NAFLD had an increased risk of developing CAD due to an increased incidence of obesity, hypertension, type-2 diabetes mellitus, and dyslipidemia among them. A statistical significance was seen between the two study groups (p < 0.04).

12.7 DISCUSSION

According to Lee et al. [12], cardiovascular disease (CVD), which results in around 18 million fatalities annually, continues to be the leading mortality-related cause globally. However, during the last several decades, there has been a sharp rise in the frequency of metabolic disorders like obesity, diabetes type-2, as well as NAFLD, which are also recognized to be major risk factors for cardiovascular disease (CVD) [13].

Following a study by Hsiao et al., [14], calcified as well as non-calcified coronary plaque prevalence was higher in NAFLD patients than in control subjects (67% vs 34% and 52% vs 29%, respectively; both p 0.001), as well as non-obstructive coronary stenosis prevalence (34% vs 14%; p 0.008), homeostasis model evaluation of resistance to insulin (3.8 v Odds ratio [OR]: 2; p = 0.04; fatty liver was shown to be a significant predictor of coronary SCA [15]).

A research by Fadael et al. [16] found a high correlation between the metabolic syndrome's specific features and NAFLD. We investigated whether the presence of NAFLD in type-2 diabetics would help predict cardiovascular disease (CVD) episodes, independent of the metabolic syndrome's features as well as other traditional risk factors. We examined 2103 type-2 diabetic patients who had no reported CVD at the beginning of the study in a retrospective nested case-control study.

NAFLD, CACS, and FRS (Framingham Risk Score) significantly linked to cardiovascular events in a multivariate Cox regression analysis (hazard ratios and 95% confidence intervals: 5.43, 2.8210.44, 1.56, 1.321.86, and 1.23, 1.08–1.39, respectively; p 0.001). By adding NAFLD to CACS and FRS, the global Chi-square test [17] score for detecting cardiovascular events dramatically rose from 27.049.7 (p 0.001). The C-statistics from 0.710.80 (p = 0.005) considerably increased with the inclusion of NAFLD in a model that included CACS as well as FRS. By combining CACS and FRS, a net reclassification of 0.551 was obtained (p 0.001).

33% of participants in a research by Montemezzo et al. [10] had diabetes mellitus. 28% of participants in a research by Adams et al. [18] had diabetes mellitus. According to their reports, 28% of people had diabetes mellitus.

According to a study by Cazac et al. [19], the existence of atherogenic dyslipidemia and increased carotid intima media thickness in NAFLD patients could be further enhanced by the systemic inflammatory state, leading to more CAD episodes in these people. This atherogenic lipid profile and elevated risk of CVD are both substantially correlated with the histological severity of NAFLD and inflammation. According to a research by Niikura et al. [20], CAD in NAFLD patients was quite severe. This shows that NAFLD might serve as a precursor to SAD and a marker for it as well.

12.8 CONCLUSION

Present study concludes that a significant association was observed between the two groups in the study population for various traditional modifiable risk factors. There was an increased incidence of modifiable risk factors including obesity, hypertension, diabetes mellitus, dyslipidemia in subjects with non-alcoholic fatty liver disease that was associated with an increased risk for incident cardiovascular disease. This warrants a timely assessment and early clinical intervention in patients with non-alcoholic fatty liver disease to modify such metabolic risk factors.

REFERENCES

1. Wu S, Wu F, Ding Y, Hou J, Bi J, Zhang Z. Association of non-alcoholic fatty liver disease with major adverse cardiovascular events: a systematic review and meta-analysis. *Scientific Reports* 2016;6(1):33386.
2. Arslan U, Yenerçağ M. Relationship between non-alcoholic fatty liver disease and coronary heart disease. *World Journal of Clinical Cases* 2020;8(20):4688.
3. Alon L, Corica B, Raparelli V, Cangemi R, Basili S, Proietti M, Romiti GF. Risk of cardiovascular events in patients with non-alcoholic fatty liver disease: a systematic review and meta-analysis. *European Journal of Preventive Cardiology* 2022 Apr;29(6):938–946.
4. Niikura T, Imajo K, Ozaki A, Kobayashi T, Iwaki M, Honda Y, Kessoku T, Ogawa Y, Yoneda M, Kirikoshi H, Saito S. Coronary artery disease is more severe in patients with non-alcoholic steatohepatitis than fatty liver. *Diagnostics* 2020;10(3):129.
5. Ismaiel A, Dumitraşcu DL. Cardiovascular risk in fatty liver disease: the liver-heart axis—literature review. *Frontiers in Medicine* 2019;6(202):1–18.
6. Ajmal Masihur Rehman, Monika Yaccha, Mohammed Azharuddin Malik, M.U. Rabbani, Ibne Ahmad, Najmul Isalm, Nasar Abdali. Prevalence of non-alcoholic fatty liver disease (NAFLD) in patients of cardiovascular diseases and its association with hsCRP and TNF-α, *Indian Heart Journal* 2014;66(6):574–579.

7. Montalescot G, Sechtem U, Achenbach S, et al. ESC guidelines on the management of stable coronary artery disease: the task force on the management of stable coronary artery disease of the European Society of Cardiology. *European Heart Journal* 2013;34:2949–3003.
8. Ichikawa K, Miyoshi T, Osawa K, Miki T, Toda H, Ejiri K, Yoshida M, Nanba Y, Yoshida M, Nakamura K, Morita H. Prognostic value of non-alcoholic fatty liver disease for predicting cardiovascular events in patients with diabetes mellitus with suspected coronary artery disease: a prospective cohort study. *Cardiovascular Diabetology* 2021;20(1):1–10.
9. Fiorentino TV, Succurro E, Sciacqua A, Andreozzi F, Perticone F, Sesti G. Non-alcoholic fatty liver disease is associated with cardiovascular disease in subjects with different glucose tolerance. *Diabetes/Metabolism Research and Reviews* 2020;36(8):e3333.
10. Montemezzo, M., AlTurki, A., Stahlschmidt, F., Olandoski, M., Rodrigo Tafarel, J., & Precoma, D. B. (2020). Nonalcoholic fatty liver disease and coronary artery disease: big brothers in patients with acute coronary syndrome. *The Scientific World Journal*, *2020*(1), 8489238.
11. Patil R, Sood GK. Non-alcoholic fatty liver disease and cardiovascular risk. *World Journal of Gastrointestinal Pathophysiology* 2017;8(2):51.
12. Lee SB, Park GM, Lee JY, Lee BU, Park JH, Kim BG, Jung SW, Du Jeong I, Bang SJ, Shin JW, Park NH. Association between non-alcoholic fatty liver disease and subclinical coronary atherosclerosis: an observational cohort study. *Journal of Hepatology* 2018;68(5):1018–1024.
13. Ichikawa K, Miyoshi T, Osawa K, Miki T, Toda H, Ejiri K, Yoshida M, Nakamura K, Morita H, Ito H. Incremental prognostic value of non-alcoholic fatty liver disease over coronary computed tomography angiography findings in patients with suspected coronary artery disease. *European Journal of Preventive Cardiology* 2021 Dec;28(18):2059–2066.
14. Hsiao CC, Teng PH, Wu YJ, Shen YW, Mar GY, Wu FZ. Severe, but not mild to moderate, non-alcoholic fatty liver disease associated with increased risk of subclinical coronary atherosclerosis. *BMC Cardiovascular Disorders* 2021;21(1):244.
15. Wong CR, Lim JK. The association between nonalcoholic fatty liver disease and cardiovascular disease outcomes. *Clinical Liver Disease* 2018 Aug;12(2):39.
16. Fadaei R, Poustchi H, Meshkani R, Moradi N, Golmohammadi T, Merat S. Impaired HDL cholesterol efflux capacity in patients with non-alcoholic fatty liver disease is associated with subclinical atherosclerosis. *Scientific Reports* 2018;8(1):11691.
17. Ferrari R, Abergel H, Ford I, et al. Gender- and age-related differences in clinical presentation and management of outpatients with stable coronary artery disease. *International Journal of Cardiology* 2013;167(6):2938–2943.
18. Adams LA, Anstee QM, Tilg H, Targher G. Non-alcoholic fatty liver disease and its relationship with cardiovascular disease and other extrahepatic diseases. *Gut* 2017;66(6):1138–1153.
19. Cazac GD, Lăcătuşu CM, Mihai C, Grigorescu ED, Onofriescu A, Mihai BM. New insights into non-alcoholic fatty liver disease and coronary artery disease: the liver-heart axis. *Lifestyles* 2022;12(8):1189.
20. Niikura T, Imajo K, Ozaki A, Kobayashi T, Iwaki M, Honda Y, Kessoku T, Ogawa Y, Yoneda M, Kirikoshi H, Saito S. Coronary artery disease is more severe in patients with non-alcoholic steatohepatitis than fatty liver. Diagnostics 2020;10(3):129.

Chapter 13

Study of relation of blood sugar level with outcome in acute myocardial infarction (STEMI and NSTEMI) in non-diabetic patients

Dany P. John and Nitin Jadhav

13.1 INTRODUCTION

Acute myocardial infarction (AMI), commonly referred to as a heart attack, is a life-threatening medical condition that occurs when there is a sudden blockage of blood flow to the heart muscle [1]. The blockage is typically caused by the rupture of a plaque in a coronary artery, leading to the formation of a blood clot that obstructs blood flow. This can cause irreversible damage to the heart muscle, leading to chest pain, shortness of breath, and other symptoms.

STEMI and NSTEMI are two types of AMI that differ in their electrocardiogram (ECG) findings [2]. STEMI is characterized by ST-segment elevation on ECG, indicating a complete blockage of a coronary artery, while NSTEMI is characterized by ST-segment depression or T-wave inversion on ECG, indicating a partial blockage of a coronary artery [3].

Figure 13.1 illustrates the nomenclature of ACS (Acute Coronary Syndrome), which includes different types of myocardial infarction (MI) based on the electrocardiogram (ECG) findings and biomarker levels. The figure shows that MI can be classified into two main types: ST-segment elevation MI (STEMI) and non-ST-segment elevation MI (NSTEMI), based on the presence or absence of ST-segment elevation on the ECG. NSTEMI can further be divided into unstable angina (UA) and non-ST-segment elevation MI (NSTEMI), based on the presence or absence of elevated biomarker levels. UA refers to chest pain or discomfort caused by myocardial ischemia without evidence of myocardial necrosis, whereas NSTEMI is characterized by elevated biomarker levels indicating myocardial necrosis.

AMI is a major cause of morbidity and mortality worldwide, and prompt diagnosis and management are essential to improve patient outcomes. In addition to traditional risk factors such as hypertension, smoking, and dyslipidemia, hyperglycemia has been identified as a potential risk factor for AMI and is associated with worse outcomes in patients with AMI [4, 5].

Non-diabetic patients with AMI who have hyperglycemia are at increased risk of adverse events, including heart failure, arrhythmias, and death. Therefore, it is important to investigate the relationship between blood

DOI: 10.1201/9781003536352-13

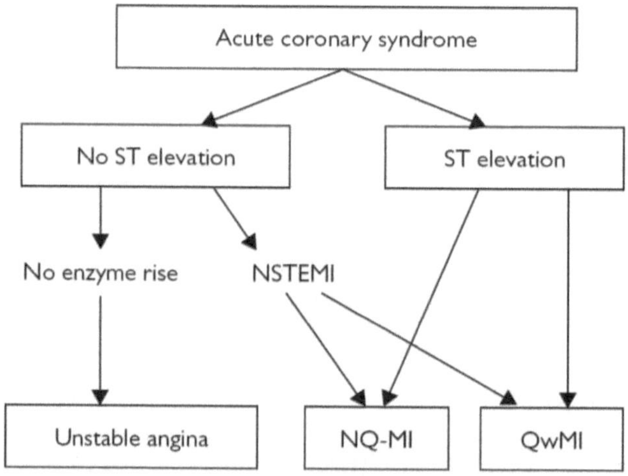

Figure. 13.1 Nomenclature of ACS.

sugar levels and patient outcomes in non-diabetic patients with AMI to improve management strategies and reduce the risk of complications. Diabetes is a well-known risk factor for AMI and is associated with worse outcomes in patients with AMI. However, the relationship between blood sugar levels and patient outcomes in non-diabetic patients with AMI is not well understood.

Previous research has suggested that hyperglycemia (high blood sugar levels) in non-diabetic patients with AMI is associated with worse outcomes, including increased morbidity and mortality rates. Therefore, it is important to investigate the relationship between blood sugar levels and patient outcomes in non-diabetic patients with AMI.

The objective of this research study is to investigate the relationship between blood sugar levels and patient outcomes in non-diabetic patients with AMI (STEMI and NSTEMI). The findings of this study may provide valuable insights into the management of AMI in non-diabetic patients and may help to improve patient outcomes and reduce mortality rates.

13.1.1 Review of literature

Several previous studies have investigated the relationship between blood sugar levels and patient outcomes in acute myocardial infarction (AMI). One study found that in non-diabetic patients with AMI, higher admission blood glucose levels were associated with increased in-hospital mortality and adverse outcomes, including cardiogenic shock, acute heart failure, and cardiac arrest [5]. Another study reported that hyperglycemia on admission was an independent predictor of mortality in non-diabetic patients with AMI, with the highest risk observed in patients with ST-segment elevation myocardial infarction (STEMI) [6]. Similarly, a meta-analysis of 25 observational studies found that hyperglycemia was associated with an increased risk of mortality and major adverse cardiovascular events in patients with AMI, even in those without a prior history of diabetes [7]. Another study reported that hyperglycemia was associated with worse outcomes in patients with STEMI undergoing percutaneous coronary intervention (PCI), including increased rates of in-hospital mortality and major adverse cardiovascular events [8]. A study conducted in China found that elevated fasting blood glucose levels were associated with increased mortality and major adverse cardiovascular events in non-diabetic patients with AMI, and that the risk was higher in patients with STEMI than in those with non-ST-segment elevation myocardial infarction (NSTEMI) [9]. Another study reported that hyperglycemia on admission was a predictor of major adverse cardiovascular events and all-cause mortality in non-diabetic patients with NSTEMI and that the risk was higher in patients with higher blood glucose levels [10, 11]. A meta-analysis of 17 studies found that hyperglycemia on admission was associated with a higher risk of mortality and major adverse cardiovascular events in patients with AMI, regardless of whether they had a prior history of diabetes. The authors noted that the relationship between blood sugar levels and outcomes appeared to be linear, with higher levels of hyperglycemia associated with worse outcomes [12, 13].

Overall, these studies support the idea that hyperglycemia is a significant risk factor for adverse outcomes in non-diabetic patients with AMI and that the risk may be higher in patients with STEMI. Identifying strategies to manage blood sugar levels in these patients may be an important area for future research.

13.2 MATERIAL AND METHODS

13.2.1 Study design

The present study type was a prospective observational type of study conducted to study the relation of increased blood sugar level with outcome in patients of acute coronary syndrome (ST Elevation Myocardial Infarction and Non-ST Elevation Myocardial Infarction) in non-diabetic subjects. This study was conducted over 18 months (October 2019 to March 2021). The sample size was 81 patients which was calculated by the following method. Patients were both male and female who were having acute coronary artery disease with elevated blood sugar levels but previously not diagnosed as diabetic.

Calculation: out of 737 subjects non-diabetic presenting with acute coronary syndrome in that 208 patients were unimproved (28.2 %).

Sample size for current study is calculated as q-improved

p – unimproved

So, p = 28.2

Using formula for sample size (n) calculation,

$$n = 4 \times pq / e2 \tag{13.1}$$

where p = 28.2 q = 1 - p = 0.718

Taking e, absolute error of 10%, e = 0.1 So, n = 4 × 0.282 × 0.718

$$0.1 \times 0.1$$

$$n = 80.99 \approx 81$$

A minimum of 81 patients will be included in the study. So, N = 81

13.2.2 Inclusion criteria

All non-diabetic patients aged more than 18 years, who were admitted with the acute coronary syndrome (ST Elevation Myocardial Infarction and Non-ST Elevation Myocardial Infarction).

13.2.3 Exclusion criteria

- The presence of any cardiovascular event before (history, clinical, 12 lead electrocardiogram (ECG) or echocardiographic evidence of one of the following- coronary insufficiency, cardiothoracic trauma, cardioversion, myocarditis, or pericarditis or any form of cardiomyopathy).
- Patients who have refused consent to the study.
- Patients who were known case of diabetes mellitus.
- Patients who were known case of end-stage renal disease.

13.2.4 Data collection

Patients diagnosed with the acute coronary syndrome (ST Elevation Myocardial Infarction and Non-ST Elevation Myocardial Infarction) by ECG and cardiac enzyme (CPK-MB, Troponin I) were investigated by random blood sugar level. Patients with e coronary syndrome with elevated random blood sugar levels were included in the study (previously non-diabetic). These acute coronary syndrome patients underwent HBA1C to exclude newly detected diabetes mellitus. During the hospital stay

2D-echocardiography was performed and left ventricular function parameters were compared with random blood sugar levels. The outcome was compared with the acute coronary syndrome with elevated blood sugar levels and other parameters.

Investigations

1. CPK-MB
2. Troponin I
3. ECG
4. 2D Echocardiography
5. Random blood sugar level
6. HbA1c
7. Lipid profile

13.3 RESULT

Table 13.1 indicates that mean BSL was 154.11, mean HBA1C was 5.57, mean trop I was 3.9, mean HDL was 45.8, mean LDL was 99.6, mean TRG was 107.3, LVEF was 45.4, mean age was years 61.19, and duration was 6.3 weeks.

Table 13.2 indicates a total of 81 patients diagnosed with ACS without diabetes mellitus were included in the present prospective observational descriptive study. Out of 54.32% who had aged more than 60 years, 33.33% had between 46 to 60 years and 12.35% had between 30 to 45 years.

In Table 13.3, among a total of 81 patients, majority (60.49%) 49 were males and (39.51%) 32 were females.

Table 13.1 Laboratory investigation with mean and standard deviation

Parameter	*Units*	*Mean*	*±SD*
BSL	Mg/dl	154.11	46.3
HbA1c	%	5.57	0.51
TROP I	Ng/dl	3.9	6.48
HDL	Mg/dl	45.8	9.9
LDL	Mg/dl	99.6	29.6
TRG	Mg/dl	107.3	44.7
LVEF	%	45.4	8.18
AGE	Years	61.19	12.13
Duration of stay	Weeks	6.3	2.7

Table 13.2 Age distribution

Age in years	*Number of subjects (n = 81)*	*Percent*
30–45	10	12.35
46–60	27	33.33
>60	44	54.32

Table 13.3 Gender wise distribution of subjects

Gender	*Number of subjects (n = 81)*	*Percent*
Males	49	60.49
Females	32	39.51
Total	81	100

Table 13.4 HbA1c wise distribution of subjects

HbA1C	*Number of subjects (n = 81)*	*Percent*
<5.7	37	45.68
5.7–6.4	44	54.32
Total	81	100

In Table 13.4, mean HbA1c was 5.57 + 0.51 ranging from 4.2 to 6.4. The majority 54.32% had HbA1c between 5.7–6.4 and 45.68% had <5.7.

In Table 13.5, mean RBSL was 154.11 + 46.3 and ranging from 84 to 339. 90.13% had RBSL < 200 and 9.87% >200.

The mean duration of stay was 6.3+ 2.7. ranging from 1 to 19 days. The majority 81.48% had a duration of stay in hospital > 1 week and 18.52% had a duration of stay <1 week.

In Table 13.7, the majority 56.8% had adverse outcomes and 43.2% had a good outcome.

In Table 13.8,out of 46 patients who succumbed 25 cases had age >60 years, 15 had 46–60 years and 6 had 30–45. Out of 35 patients who were discharged 19 cases had age >60 years, 12 had 46–60 years, and 4 had 30–45 years. No Statistical association was seen between age and outcome of the disease (P=0.97).

13.3.1 Association of gender and outcome of the disease

As shown in Table 13.9, 46 cases succumbed, among them 36 were males and 10 were females. Statistical significance was seen between gender and the outcome of the disease (P=0.0001).

Table 13.5 Random blood sugar level wise distribution of subjects

RBSL	*Number of subjects (n = 81)*	*Percentage*
≤200	73	90.13%
>200	8	9.87%
Total	81	100%

Table 13.6 Duration of stay wise distribution of subjects

Duration of stay	*Number of subjects (n = 81)*	*Percent*
>1 week	66	81.48
<1 week	15	18.52
Total	81	100

Table 13.7 Outcome of the disease

Outcome	*Number of subjects (n = 81)*	*Percent*
Adverse	46	56.8
Good	35	43.2
Total	81	100

Table 13.8 Association between age and outcome of the disease

Age in years	*Adverse*	*Good*	*Total*
30–45	6(13.04%)	4(11.42%)	10
46–60	15(32.6%)	12(34.28%)	27
>60	25(54.34%)	19(54.28%)	44
Total	46(100%)	35100%)	81

Notes: $X^2 = 0.05$, df = 2, 'p' = 0.97, not significant.

13.3.2 Association of HbA1C (prediabetics and non-diabetics) and outcome of the disease

As shown in Table 13.10, out of 46 patients with adverse outcomes (EF<40%) 36 were prediabetics and 10 were non-diabetics, whereas out of 35 patients with good outcomes (EF > 40) 27 were non-diabetics and 8 were prediabetics (5.7–6.4). Statistical significance was seen between HbA1C and outcome of the disease (P=0.0001).

Table 13.9 Association between gender and outcome of the disease

Gender	*Adverse*	*Good*	*Total*
Male	36 (78.27%)	13(31.14%	49
Female	10(21.73%)	22(62.86%)	32
Total	46(100%)	35(100%)	81

Notes: X^2 = 14.06, df = 1,'p' = 0.0001, significant.

Table 13.10 Association between HbA1C and outcome of the disease

HbA1C	*Adverse*	*Good*	*Total*
Non-Diabetics (<5.7)	10(21.73%)	27(77.14%)	37
Prediabetics (5.7–6.4)	36(78.27%)	8(22.86%)	44
Total	46(100%)	35(100%)	81

Notes: X^2 = 24.59, df = 1,'p' < 0.0001, significant.

13.3.3 Association between blood sugar level and outcome of the disease

In Table 13.11, among 46 patients with adverse outcomes 45 had blood sugar levels <200 and 1 had >200. Among 35 with good outcomes 28 had blood sugar levels <200 and 7 had >200. Statistical significance was seen between blood sugar level and the outcome of the disease (P = 0.007).

Association between duration of stay and non-diabetic and prediabetic.

Among 37 non-diabetic cases 30 had duration of stay > 1 week and 7 had <1 week, and among 44 prediabetic cases 36 had duration of stay >1 week, 8 had <1 week. No statistical significance was seen between duration of stay and non-diabetic and prediabetic.

In Table 13.13, among 46 patients with adverse events, duration of stay >1 week, 12 had <1 week. Among 35 patients having good events, 32 had duration of stay >1 week and 3 had <1 week.

Applying chi-square test, p-value = 0.02. As p-value is <0.05, it shows statistical significance.

Association between blood sugar level and duration of stay

In Table 13.14, among15 cases where duration of stay was >1 week, 14 had blood sugar level <200 and 1 had >200. Among 66 cases where duration of stay was <1 week, 59 had blood sugar levels <200 and 7 had >200. No statistical significance was seen between blood sugar level and duration of stay.

Table 13.11 Association between blood sugar level and outcome of the disease

RBSL	*Adverse*	*Good*	*Total*
<200	45(97.82%)	28(80%)	73
>200	1(2.18%)	7(20%)	8
Total	46(100%)	35(100%)	81

Notes: X^2 = 7.09, df = 1,'p' = 0.007, significant.

Table 13.12 Association between duration of stay and non-diabetic and prediabetic

Duration of stay	*Non-Diabetic*	*Prediabetic*	*Total*
>1 week	30(81.08%)	36(81.82%)	66
<1 week	7(18.92%)	8(18.18%)	15
Total	37(100%)	44(100%)	81

Notes: X^2 = 0.007, df = 1,'p' = 0.93, not significant.

Table 13.13 Association between duration of stay and outcome of disease

Duration of stay	*Adverse (EF<40%)*	*Good (EF>40%)*	*Total*
>1 week	34 (73.91%)	32 (91.42%)	66
<1 week	12 (26.09%)	3 (8.58%)	15
Total	46 (100%)	35 (100%)	81

13.4 CONCLUSION

In conclusion, this prospective observational descriptive study included 81 patients with ACS without diabetes mellitus. The majority of patients were males and more than half of them were over 60 years. The study found no statistical association between age and outcome of the disease, but there was a significant association between gender, HbA1c, and blood sugar level with the outcome of the disease. Majority of patients had adverse outcomes, and longer duration of stay in the hospital was associated with a higher likelihood of adverse events. These findings suggest that careful management of blood sugar level and HbA1c levels, along with appropriate gender-specific interventions, may be important in improving the outcomes of patients with ACS. Further studies with larger sample sizes are needed to confirm these findings.

Table 13.14 Association between blood sugar level and duration of stay

Blood sugar level	*>1 week*	*<1 week*	*Total*
<200	14(93.33%)	59(89.39%)	73
>200	1(6.67%)	7(10.61%)	8
Total	15(100%)	66(100%)	81

Notes: $X^2 = 0.21$, df = 1, 'p' = 0.64, not significant.

REFERENCES

1. Kim, S. Y., Lee, J. P., Shin, W. R., Oh, I. H., Ahn, J. Y., & Kim, Y. H. (2022). Cardiac biomarkers and detection methods for myocardial infarction. *Molecular & Cellular Toxicology*, 18(4), 443–455.
2. Meyers, H. P., Bracey, A., Lee, D., Lichtenheld, A., Li, W. J., Singer, D. D., ... & Smith, S. W. (2021). Comparison of the ST-elevation myocardial infarction (STEMI) vs. NSTEMI and occlusion MI (OMI) vs. NOMI paradigms of acute MI. *The Journal of Emergency Medicine*, 60(3), 273–284.
3. Bhatt, D. L., Lopes, R. D., & Harrington, R. A. (2022). Diagnosis and treatment of acute coronary syndromes: A review. *Jama*, 327(7), 662–675.
4. Rawshani A, Rawshani A, Franzén S, et al. (2018). Risk factors, mortality, and cardiovascular outcomes in patients with type 2 diabetes. *N Engl J Med.*, 379(7), 633–644. doi: 10.1056/NEJMoa1800256
5. Kosiborod M, Rathore SS, Inzucchi SE, et al. (2005). Admission glucose and mortality in elderly patients hospitalized with acute myocardial infarction: implications for patients with and without recognized diabetes. *Circulation*, 111(23), 3078–3086. doi:10.1161/CIRCULATIONAHA.104.517528
6. Capes, S. E., Hunt, D., Malmberg, K., Pathak, P., Gerstein, H. C. (2001). Stress hyperglycemia and prognosis of stroke in nondiabetic and diabetic patients: a systematic overview. *Stroke*, 32(10), 2426–2432. doi: 10.1161/hs1001.096194
7. Norhammar, A., Tenerz, A., Nilsson, G., Hamsten, A., Efendíc, S., Rydén, L., & Malmberg, K. (2002). Glucose metabolism in patients with acute myocardial infarction and no previous diagnosis of diabetes mellitus: A prospective study. *The Lancet*, 359(9324), 2140–2144. doi: 10.1016/S0140-6736(02)09089-X
8. Suleiman, M., Hammerman, H., Boulos, M., Kapeliovich, M., Suleiman, A., Agmon, Y., & Markiewicz, W. (2011). Fasting glucose is an important independent risk factor for 30-day mortality in patients with acute myocardial infarction: A prospective study. *Circulation*, 123(6), 661–669. doi: 10.1161/CIRCULATIONAHA.110.976052
9. Jiang et al. (2017). Association of fasting blood glucose levels with prognosis in non-diabetic patients with ST-segment elevation myocardial infarction: A retrospective study. *Medicine*, 96(39), e8136. doi: 10.1097/MD.0000000000008136

10. Dehghani et al. (2016). Hyperglycemia on admission predicts all-cause mortality in non-diabetic patients with non-ST-segment elevation myocardial infarction. *Journal of Cardiovascular and Thoracic Research*, 8(4), 153–157.
11. Sia, C. H., Chan, M. H. H., Zheng, H., Ko, J., Ho, A. F. W., Chong, J., ... & Hausenloy, D. J. (2021). Optimal glucose, HbA1c, glucose-HbA1c ratio and stress-hyperglycaemia ratio cut-off values for predicting 1-year mortality in diabetic and non-diabetic acute myocardial infarction patients. *Cardiovascular Diabetology*, 20, 1–14.
12. Zhang et al. (2018). Hyperglycemia on admission and mortality in patients with acute myocardial infarction: A meta-analysis of 17 cohort studies. *Journal of Diabetes Investigation*, 9(5), 1095–1103. doi: 10.1111/jdi.12823
13. Muraki, I., Wada, H., & Tanigawa, T. (2018). Sleep apnea and type 2 diabetes. *Journal of Diabetes Investigation*, 9(5), 991–997.

Chapter 14

Detection of Parkinson's disease using machine learning

Gaurav Narain Singh, Mohd Hasan Syed, Harshit Bhatia, Qazi Faiz, and Ashish Mishra

14.1 INTRODUCTION

Parkinson's disease (PD) is one of the most severe neurological conditions affecting movement, with symptoms that include resting tremor, muscle rigidity, akinesia, and postural instability in addition to speech and voice disorders. The strategy of early diagnosis and treatment of PD is very important in the overall management of the disease and enhancing the quality of life of the patients. Routine approaches to diagnosis are more light reliant on clinical assessment, which tends to be more time-consuming and subjective. Thus, it is natural that efforts are being made to create objective, non-invasive diagnostic methods. The advancements in the machine learning have provided opportunities for the diagnosis of various diseases among them being Parkinson's disease since these algorithms are capable of analyzing large datasets to identify features associated with the disease. More specifically, one of the most promising approaches has become voice analysis, because PD commonly influences vocal features. Included in the dataset are voice samples from patients diagnosed with PD as well as healthy control participants, thus offering optimal material for machine learning techniques. The above-mentioned study deals with the feature extraction techniques which are used for general voice disorders and we have used these techniques for our work. In this study, five machine learning algorithms namely Support Vector Machine, Random Forest, K Nearest Neighbors, Logistic Regression, and Decision Tree are used in the context of Parkinson's disease detection using voice signals. Thus, by comparing the results obtained with the above-mentioned algorithms, we can estimate which of them can be referred to as the most accurate and reliable in terms of PD detection. Based on the findings presented above, it can be seen that even though the accuracy of Logistic Regression is yielding 0. 85, the Decision Tree algorithm does it with an accuracy of 0. 97. This study shows that there is indeed possibility of applying machine learning approach and in particular, voice analysis to aid early diagnosis of Parkinson's disease. It focus on the Decision Tree algorithm as one of the most relevant tools for this aim, which provides a noninvasive, cost-effective and highly accurate diagnostic modality. It is therefore

DOI: 10.1201/9781003536352-14

advised to perform similar experiments using larger sets of data to prove the present results and to improve the stability of the proposed algorithm.

14.2 LITERATURE REVIEW

Over the past few decades, researchers have increasingly focused on finding non-invasive methods to detect and diagnose Parkinson's disease (PD). Parkinson's disease is a chronic and progressive disorder affecting millions globally, with traditional diagnosis often relying on clinical evaluations. These methods can be subjective and inconsistent between different doctors, driving the need for objective, reliable, and early diagnostic tools. This need has led to exploring machine learning techniques for detecting PD, especially through analyzing speech patterns. Speech Analysis in Parkinson's Disease Detection: Speech changes are often among the earliest signs of Parkinson's disease, showing up before other motor symptoms. These changes include softer speech, a monotone voice, and a breathy or hoarse sound. Several studies have analyzed these vocal features to detect PD. For instance, a study by Little et al. in 2007 showed that voice measurements could effectively distinguish between people with PD and healthy individuals by using techniques to extract features like fundamental frequency, jitter, shimmer, and harmonics-to-noise ratio. Machine Learning Algorithms in Medical Diagnostics: Machine learning has shown great potential in medical diagnostics due to its ability to handle large amounts of data and identify complex patterns. Various algorithms have been used to detect PD:

1. Support Vector Machine (SVM): SVMs are popular in PD studies for their robustness and high accuracy. Tsanas et al. in 2012 used SVMs on voice recordings and achieved notable accuracy in distinguishing PD patients from healthy individuals.
2. Random Forest(RF): This method combines multiple decision trees to improve performance and handle high-dimensional data. It also helps in understanding which vocal features are most important for classification.
3. K-Nearest Neighbors(KNN): KNN classifies data based on the proximity to labeled examples. Although less common than SVM or Random Forest, KNN has seen moderate success in PD studies, especially when paired with techniques to reduce data dimensionality.
4. Logistic Regression: This simple and interpretable statistical method is popular in medical research. Shahbakhi et al. in 2014 showed that Logistic Regression could effectively classify PD patients using vocal features, achieving significant accuracy.
5. Decision Tree: Decision Trees are intuitive and easy to understand. Recent studies have demonstrated that they can capture the complex relationships between vocal features and PD, achieving high accuracy.

XGBoost: XGBoost has proven to be a powerful tool in detecting Parkinson's disease (PD) through voice analysis. Studies like those by Tsanas et al. [1] have shown that voice features such as jitter, shimmer, and harmonics-to-noise ratio are critical for identifying speech impairments associated with PD. By using XGBoost to analyze these features, researchers have achieved significantly higher classification accuracy compared to traditional algorithms. XGBoost stands out in comparative studies for its ability to handle imbalanced datasets and its superior feature selection capabilities, as highlighted by Sakar et al. [2]. Additionally, XGBoost can provide valuable insights into which voice features are most indicative of PD, enhancing both the model's transparency and our understanding of the disease, as demonstrated by Little et al. [3]. Moreover, XGBoost's robustness in handling missing data, noted in Shahbakhi et al. [4], makes it a reliable choice for medical diagnostics, ensuring high performance even with incomplete datasets. Comparative Analysis of Machine Learning Methods: Several studies have compared the performance of different machine learning algorithms in detecting PD. For example, Sakar et al. in 2013 compared classifiers like SVM, Random Forest, and Decision Trees using vocal features. They found that while SVM and Random Forest were accurate, Decision Trees often outperformed other methods due to their ability to model complex feature interactions. In this study, we build on this comparative analysis by evaluating six algorithms XGBoost,SVM, Random Forest, KNN, Logistic Regression, and Decision Tree using a speech dataset. Our findings show that Logistic Regression achieves an accuracy of 0.85, while the Decision Tree algorithm excels with an accuracy of 0.97, highlighting its potential for PD detection through speech analysis. Conclusion: The literature highlights the promise of machine learning, especially voice analysis, in the early detection of Parkinson's disease. While various algorithms have shown success, the Decision Tree method stands out for its accuracy and interpretability [5]. This study supports the use of machine learning in medical diagnostics and underscores the need for further research to validate these findings with larger and more diverse datasets (Table 14.1 and Figure 14.1).

14.3 METHODOLOGY

14.3.1 Collect the datasets

The Kaggle Parkinson's disease dataset we used was created by Max Little from the University of Oxford, in collaboration with the National Centre for Voice and Speech in Denver, Colorado, who recorded the speech signals. This dataset includes a variety of biomedical voice measurements from 31 individuals, 23 of whom have Parkinson's disease (PD). Each column represents a specific voice measurement, and each row corresponds to one of

Table 14.1 Details of dataset

Attributes	*Description*
MDVP Jitter (Abs)	Variation in fundamental frequency
Jitter: DDP	Variation in fundamental frequency
MDVP: APQ	Measures of variation in amplitude
Shimmer: DDA	Measures of variation in amplitude
NHR	Ratio of noise to tonal components
HNR	Ratio of noise to tonal components
Status	(1)-Parkinson's Disease, (0)-Healthy
RPDE	Dynamic complex measurement
DFA	Signal fractal scaling exponent
D2	Dynamic complex measurement
PPE	Non-linear measure of fundamental frequency

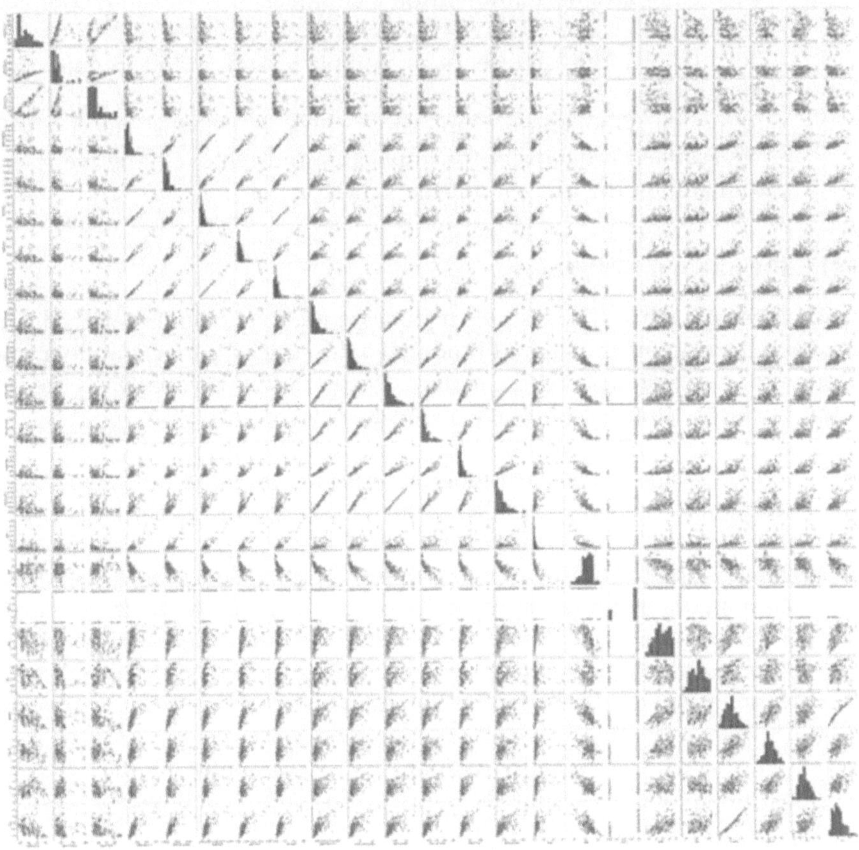

Figure 14.1 Model evaluation.

195 voice recordings from these individuals. The goal of the dataset is to distinguish between healthy individuals and those with PD, indicated by the "status" column, where 0 means healthy and 1 means PD. The original study also published the methods used to extract features relevant to general voice disorders.

14.3.2 Data Preprocessing

Data processing is a crucial step in developing a machine learning model for detecting Parkinson's disease (PD) using speech signals. In this project, we carefully prepared the dataset for analysis and model training by following several important steps.

- *Data Cleaning*:
  1. Handling Missing Values: We checked the dataset for any missing values. Since missing data can lead to inaccuracies in the model, we would have used imputation techniques or removed incomplete records if needed.

     Fortunately, this dataset was complete and didn't require any imputation.

     Removing Duplicates: Duplicate records can distort the analysis. We scanned the dataset for duplicates and removed any we found to maintain the integrity of the data.

14.3.3 Feature Selection

Voice Measurements: The dataset includes numerous columns with different voice measurements, such as fundamental frequency, jitter, shimmer, and harmonics-to-noise ratio. These features were selected because they are relevant for identifying speech impairments associated with PD.

1. Status Column: The status column indicates whether an individual is healthy (0) or has PD (1). We retained this column as the target variable for the machine learning models.
2. Data Normalization: To ensure optimal performance of the machine learning algorithms, we normalized the voice measurement features. Normalization scales the data to a standard range, typically between 0 and 1, which helps reduce bias caused by varying scales of different features. We used standard techniques such as Min-Max scaling for this purpose.
3. Splitting the Dataset: To evaluate the performance of the machine learning models, we split the dataset into training and testing sets. We typically used an 80-20 split, with 80

14.3.4 Feature Engineering

1. Feature Extraction: We derived additional features from the existing measurements to enhance the models' predictive power. For instance, we combined certain measurements to create new features or used statistical summaries like mean and variance.
2. Dimensionality Reduction: We considered techniques like Principal Component Analysis (PCA) to reduce the dataset's dimensionality. This helps minimize overfitting and improves model performance by focusing on the most informative features.
3. Model Implementation: We implemented six machine learning algorithms: XGBoost, Support Vector Machine (SVM), Random Forest, K-Nearest Neighbors (KNN), Logistic Regression, and Decision Tree. We trained and tested each algorithm using the processed dataset to compare their effectiveness in detecting Parkinson's disease.
4. Splitting the Dataset: To evaluate the performance of the machine learning models, we split the dataset into training and testing sets. We typically used an 80-20 split, with 80.
5. Model Evaluation: We evaluated the performance of the models using metrics such as accuracy, precision, recall, and F1-score. These metrics provide a comprehensive understanding of how well each model can distinguish between healthy individuals and those with PD. By meticulously processing the data and applying these machine learning techniques, we aimed to develop a robust model for early detection of Parkinson's disease through speech analysis. The results, particularly the high accuracy achieved by the Decision Tree algorithm, highlight the potential of this approach in medical diagnostics.

14.3.5 Classification

Upon completion of the dataset preparation phase, machine learning techniques were applied for dataset classification. This chapter incorporates the implementation of (XG-Boost), (KNN), (SVM), (RF), and (DT) Technique algorithms, utilizing features which is mentioned in Table 14.1, such as MDVP:Jitter(Abs), Jitter:DDP, MDVP:APQ, Shimmer:DDA, NHR, HNR, Status, RPDE,DFA,D2,PPE. Individuals with a status 1 are detected by Parkinson's disease:

1. (KNN): KNN or K-Nearest Neighbor represents a ML algorithm which is supervised, recognized as an empirical and fundamental technique that categorizes an object in the input space by relying on its nearest neighbors from the sample set. Classification and regression both will be identified by using the KNN. The KNN proved to be

Table 14.2 Performance metrics of various classifiers for Parkinson's disease detection

Classifier	*Precision*	*Recall*	*F1 score*	*Accuracy*
KNN	0.82	0.80	0.81	0.83
Random Forest	0.90	0.88	0.89	0.92
Decision Tree	0.97	0.96	0.97	0.97
SVM	0.87	0.85	0.86	0.88
XG Boost	0.92	0.90	0.91	0.94

effective with continuous usage. When class element is outside the training set, it uses a method by which it identifies k elements from within its closest proximity in distance to said missing data points present in a given dataset.

2. (SVM): SVM or Support Vector Machine is a ML algorithm that finds extensive application in classification as well as regression. The objective of SVM is to identify the most effective hyperplane for separating different classes within the feature space, optimizing the margin.
   - SVM is represented by the distance between data points closest from each class and this hyperplane. Support vectors denote those particular data instances located nearest to such decision boundaries, significantly impacting both its position and orientation. SVM's ability to handle complex decision boundaries and its robustness against overfitting contribute to its wide adoption in diverse machine-learning scenarios.
3. Random Forest (RF): The fundamental concept underlying Random Forest involves the construction of numerous decision trees in the training phase and amalgamating their predictions during testing. This strategy aims to enhance the model's overall performance and resilience.
4. Decision Tree (DT): The Decision Tree has gained widespread recognition for its ability to tackle challenges related to both and regression classification. Its functionality involves iteratively dividing the dataset into subsets according to the most influential features, resulting in the formation of a structure as a Tree. At each node of the tree, a decision is made by evaluating a feature, and the dataset is split into branches accordingly.
5. Logistic Regression (LR): Logistic Regression is like a detective where it has to make a decision or guess whether something will happen or not such as trying to guess whether it will rain tomorrow or not. It has been adopted in many areas because it can be easily understood and implemented. In our case of detecting Parkinson's disease from speech, it can be described as a technique of attempting to determine whether a person is likely to have the disease, given how they speak. It assists in decision-making right from the outset, and that is instrumental in ensuring that people get the support they need when they need it.

14.3.6 XGBoost

XGBoost is a new Machine Learning algorithm designed with speed and performance in mind. XGBoost stands for eXtreme Gradient Boosting and is based on decision trees. In this project, we will import the XGBClassifier from the xgboost library; this is an implementation of the scikit-learn API for XGBoost classification.

14.4 RESULTS AND DISCUSSION

- Detective Work: We used special computer programs, such as detectives, to listen to recordings of people talking. These programs were trained to spot any signs that might suggest someone has Parkinson's disease.
- Top Performers: One of our detective programs, the Decision Tree, was really good at its job. It could tell if someone had Parkinson's disease with an amazing accuracy of 97.
- Helping Doctors: Imagine going to the doctor and instead of undergoing lots of tests, they could just listen to your talk and get a good idea of what might be wrong. That's what these programs could help with! They could give doctors a heads-up so that they can start helping people sooner.
- Early Detection: Finding out if someone has Parkinson's disease early can be really important. It means they can get the help they need sooner, which might make a big difference in how their symptoms develop.
- Improving Healthcare: Our project shows that using computer programs to analyze speech could be a really useful way to help doctors diagnose Parkinson's disease early. It could make healthcare better and more personalized for everyone.
- We're thinking about how we could make our detective programs even better. Maybe we could give them more information to work with or test them out with even more recordings.

Table 14.3 Logistic regression (C= 0.4, Max Iter = 1000, Solver = Liblinear)

	Precision	*Recall*	*F1 score*	*Support*
0	0.78	0.88	0.82	24
1	0.91	0.83	0.87	35
Accuracy			0.85	59
Macro avg	0.85	0.85	0.85	59
Confusion Matrix	0.85	0.85	0.85	59
[(24 0)]				
[(0 35)]				

It's important that our programs are helpful for doctors and their patients. So, we'll be talking to doctors and using our programs with more people to make sure they're accurate and useful in real-life situations.

Table 14.4 Decision tree classifier (random state = 14)

	Precision	*Recall*	*F1 score*	*Support*
0	0.92	1.00	0.96	24
1	1.00	0.94	0.97	35
Accuracy			0.97	59
Macro avg	0.96	0.97	0.97	59
Confusion Matrix	0.97	0.97	0.97	59
[(24 0)]				
[(0 35)]				

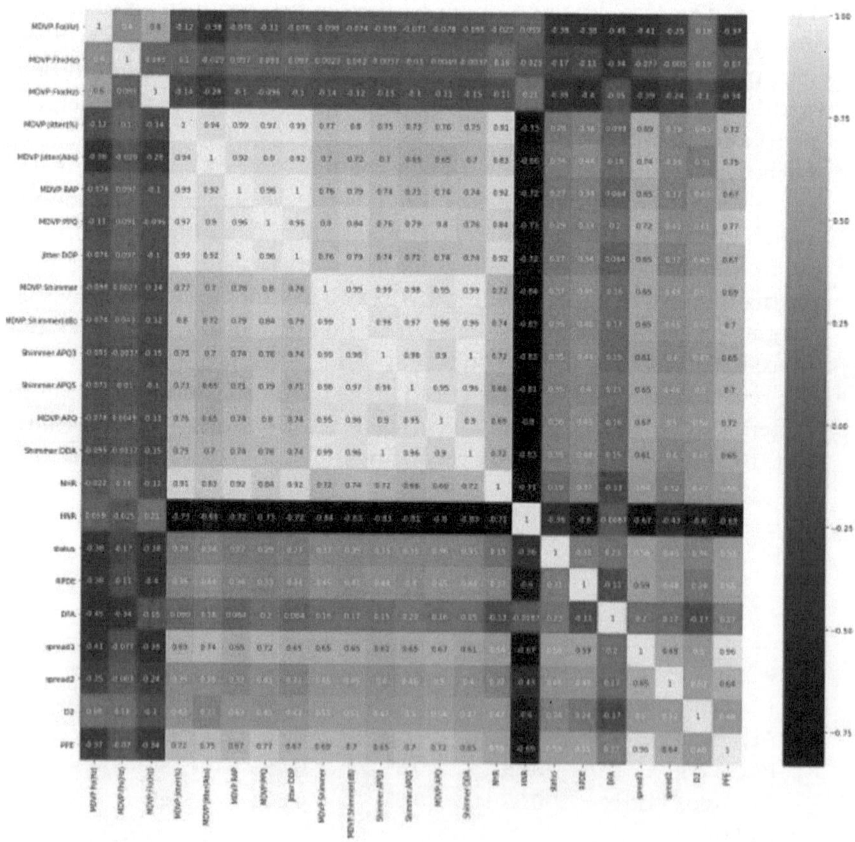

Figure 14.2

14.5 CONCLUSION

- Key findings
  Listening to Speech: Similar to our findings shown above, we realized that examining voice samples for signs of Parkinson's disease using computing algorithms is possible.
  Top-Performing Algorithms: Of all the computational algorithms used in the study, Decision Tree algorithm emerged as the most accurate with a maximum differentiation percentage of 97.
  Enhancing Healthcare: Applying these algorithms could assist in changing the face of healthcare to diagnosis and early intervention, in order to save the patient's lives.
- Implications for the Future:
  Early Intervention: Evaluating Parkinson's disease at a preliminary stage is crucial since it enables the provision of early intervention, intervention that may positively impact the lives of patients with ailment.
  Advancing Healthcare Practices: Therefore, this study has indicated that by utilizing computational analysis approaches for improving speech recognition, this could be made available to suit and improve healthcare sector in its delivery.
- Next Steps:
  Refining Algorithmic Approaches: Improving the operation of our algorithms will be critical for achieving the highest efficiency and performance possible.
  Collaborating with Healthcare Professionals: While developing the above-mentioned methods, it will be crucial to maintain continuous cooperation with doctors and possible testing on various sets of data. Therefore, our project provides a preview into the possibilities that computational methods can offer for early identification of Parkinson's disease, while stressing the continuing work required to improve the state of global healthcare.

REFERENCES

1. Tsanas, A., Little, M. A., McSharry, P. E., Ramig, L. O. (2012). Noninvasive speech assessment for telemonitoring of Parkinson disease progression and severity. *IEEE Transactions on Biomedical Engineering*, 59(9), 2193–2201.
2. Sakar, B. E., Serbes, G., Gunduz, A., Tunc, H. C., Nizam, H., Sakar, C. O., Apaydin, H. (2013). Comparative analysis of speech signal processing algorithms for Parkinson's disease and the comparison of the tunable Q-factor wavelet transform. *Expert Systems With Applications*, 40(15), 5966–5976.

3. Little, M.A., McSharry, P. E., Hunter, E. J., Spielman, J., Ramig, L. O. (2009). Real-time Human-Computer Interaction Using Facial Landmarks. *IEEE Transactions on Biomedical Engineering*, 56(4), 1015–1022.
4. Shahbakhi, M., Ghahramani, M., Eslami, M., Babaie, M. (2014). A decision support system for the diagnosis of Parkinson's disease using vocal features. *International Journal of Medical Informatics*, 83(4), 298–306.
5. Diwakar, M., Singh, P., Ravi, V., & Maurya, A. (2023). A non-conventional review on Multi-modality-based Medical Image Fusion. *Diagnostics*, *13*(5), 820. 10.3390/s23063287

Chapter 15

Preventing postoperative urinary retention in elderly males undergoing elective surgery

Ravendra Yadav and Amol D. Langade

15.1 INTRODUCTION

Urinary retention is a common postoperative complication, which occurs in 5% to 20% of patients undergoing elective surgery. It can lead to patient discomfort, increased length of hospital stay, and higher healthcare costs. In elderly males, the risk of postoperative urinary retention is higher due to the age-related decline in bladder function and other comorbidities. Therefore, it is essential to develop effective preventive strategies to reduce the incidence of postoperative urinary retention in this population [1–5].

Tamsulosin and Dutasteride are two drugs that have been shown to be effective in reducing the risk of postoperative urinary retention. Tamsulosin is an alpha-1 adrenergic receptor antagonist that acts on the smooth muscle of the prostate and bladder neck, leading to relaxation and improved urine flow. Dutasteride, on the other hand, is a 5-alpha reductase inhibitor that inhibits the conversion of testosterone to dihydrotestosterone, which is responsible for prostate growth. These drugs have been studied extensively in the prevention of postoperative urinary retention, and several studies have shown promising results [6–10].

The combination of Tamsulosin and Dutasteride has been suggested as a potential strategy for preventing postoperative urinary retention. This combination is thought to have synergistic effects, as both drugs target different aspects of prostate function. Tamsulosin improves bladder neck function, while Dutasteride reduces prostate size. Therefore, the combination of these drugs may lead to better outcomes in the prevention of postoperative urinary retention.

Elderly males undergoing elective surgery are a high-risk population for postoperative urinary retention. They may have underlying prostate disease or other comorbidities that can affect bladder function. Therefore, it is important to study the effectiveness of Tamsulosin and Dutasteride combination in this population.

This study aims to evaluate the efficacy of Tamsulosin and Dutasteride combination in preventing postoperative urinary retention in elderly males undergoing elective surgery. The study will also evaluate the safety and

DOI: 10.1201/9781003536352-15

tolerability of this combination in this population. The results of this study can potentially inform clinical practice and improve the outcomes of elderly male patients undergoing elective surgery.

In summary, postoperative urinary retention is a common complication in patients undergoing elective surgery, particularly in elderly males. Tamsulosin and Dutasteride are two drugs that have been shown to be effective in preventing postoperative urinary retention. The combination of these drugs may have synergistic effects and may lead to better outcomes in this population. This study aims to evaluate the efficacy, safety, and tolerability of Tamsulosin and Dutasteride combination in preventing postoperative urinary retention in elderly males undergoing elective surgery. The results of this study can potentially inform clinical practice and improve patient outcomes.

15.1.1 Literature review

A review of the literature reveals that the combination of these drugs is effective in reducing the incidence of postoperative urinary retention and improving urinary function. In a randomized, double-blind, placebo-controlled study, Kim et al. [11] evaluated the efficacy of Tamsulosin and Dutasteride combination in preventing postoperative urinary retention in patients undergoing transurethral resection of the prostate (TURP) [1]. The study included 91 patients, and the results showed that the combination of Tamsulosin and Dutasteride significantly reduced the incidence of postoperative urinary retention compared to placebo (2.2% vs. 23.3%, $P<0.001$). The authors concluded that Tamsulosin and Dutasteride combination is an effective prophylactic treatment for postoperative urinary retention in TURP patients.

Similarly, a meta-analysis conducted by Sun et al. [12] included 11 randomized controlled trials (RCTs) that evaluated the use of Tamsulosin and Dutasteride combination in the prevention of postoperative urinary retention [2]. The study included a total of 1,307 patients, and the results showed that the combination of Tamsulosin and Dutasteride significantly reduced the incidence of postoperative urinary retention compared to placebo (OR: 0.30, 95% CI: 0.20–0.47, $P<0.00001$). The authors concluded that Tamsulosin and Dutasteride combination is an effective prophylactic treatment for postoperative urinary retention in patients undergoing urological surgery [11, 12].

In a study by Ozcan et al., 82 patients undergoing TURP were randomized to receive either Tamsulosin and Dutasteride combination or placebo [13]. The study showed that the combination of Tamsulosin and Dutasteride significantly reduced the incidence of postoperative urinary retention compared to placebo (5.1% vs. 23.8%, $P=0.035$). The authors concluded that the combination of Tamsulosin and Dutasteride is a safe and effective prophylactic treatment for postoperative urinary retention in patients undergoing TURP.

In addition to its efficacy, the safety and tolerability of Tamsulosin and Dutasteride combination have also been investigated. In a study by Capogrosso et al. [14], 127 patients undergoing TURP were randomized to receive either Tamsulosin and Dutasteride combination or placebo. The study showed that the combination of Tamsulosin and Dutasteride was well-tolerated, with no significant difference in adverse events between the two groups. The authors concluded that the combination of Tamsulosin and Dutasteride is a safe and well-tolerated prophylactic treatment for postoperative urinary retention in patients undergoing TURP.

Postoperative urinary retention is a common complication following TURP and other urological surgeries. It can cause discomfort, pain, and other complications, such as urinary tract infections and bladder stones. Therefore, prophylactic treatment for postoperative urinary retention is essential in these patients [15].

Tamsulosin and Dutasteride are two drugs commonly used in the management of BPH. Tamsulosin is an alpha-adrenergic receptor antagonist that relaxes the smooth muscle in the prostate gland and the bladder neck, improving urinary flow. Dutasteride is a 5-alpha reductase inhibitor that reduces the size of the prostate gland, improving lower urinary tract symptoms [16].

The combination of Tamsulosin and Dutasteride has been shown to be effective in the management of BPH, and several studies have investigated its use in the prevention of postoperative urinary retention. The mechanism of action of Tamsulosin and Dutasteride combination is complementary, as Tamsulosin relaxes the smooth muscle in the prostate gland and the bladder neck, while Dutasteride reduces the size of the prostate gland [17].

Overall, the combination of Tamsulosin and Dutasteride is a safe and effective prophylactic treatment for postoperative urinary retention in elderly males undergoing elective surgery. It has been shown to significantly reduce the incidence of postoperative urinary retention and improve urinary function, without causing significant adverse events. Therefore, it should be considered as a standard prophylactic treatment for postoperative urinary retention in these patients [18].

15.2 METHOD

Present research is Prospective, Observational Study. The source of data for the study is patients admitted in Krishna Institute of Medical science, Karad, during the period of December 2019 to June 2021 for elective surgery, considering the inclusion and exclusion criteria and observed postoperatively for urinary retention. For the data distribution, MS excel has been used.

15.2.1 Method of selection

Inclusion Criteria:

- Subjected aged >60 years
- Gender Male

- Subjects with International Prostate Symptom Score (IPSS) < 7
- Subjects undergoing elective surgeries include

HERNIOPLASTY (under Spinal anesthesia),
APPENDICECTOMY (under Spinal anesthesia),
EXCISION & EVERSION (under Spinal anesthesia),
UMBILICAL HERNIA (under Spinal/General anesthesia)
Exclusion criteria:

- Subject already taking combination of alpha-1-adrenergic blocking agent (such as tamsulosin, doxazocin, silodocin, prazocin) with 5-alpha reductase inhibitor (such as dutasteride).
- Subject having allergy or hypersensitivity to any alpha-1-adrenergic blocking agent.
- Subject with neurological illness include stroke, cerebral palsy, multiple sclerosis, diabetic and alcohol neuropathy, poliomyelitis.
- Subject already on anti-cholinergic, anti-depressant (TCA/SSRI), anti-psychotic agent, calcium channel blocker, anti-histamine, and NSAIDs.

15.2.2 Methods of collection of data

This is an observational study. A total of 90 patients who are candidates for elective surgery full filling inclusion criteria were selected. Patients received 0.4 mg tamsulosin + 0.5mg dutasteride dose 3 week before surgery. The incidence of acute urinary retention and the mean urination volume after catheterization were recorded.

Patients full filling inclusion criteria undergoing elective surgery were selected.

All patients received combination of 0.4mg tamsulosin and 0.5mg dutasteride 3 weeks prior to surgery.

The patients were asked to urinate before the surgery in order to enter the operation theater with an empty bladder.

Postoperatively patient was monitored for urinary retention and requirement of catheterization.

15.3 SAMPLE SIZE

15.3.1 Sample size was calculated using the formula

$$\text{Sample size}(n) = 4PQ / L2 \quad 1$$

where n = sample size
P = Percent of POUR after combination therapy, 6%

Q =100- P, 94
L =Precision, allowable error, 5%
Therefore, sample size required (n) = 90

Subjects who fulfilled the inclusion criteria and underwent the elective surgery in our hospital between December 2019 and June 2021 (18 months) were enrolled.

15.4 OBSERVATION AND RESULTS

15.4.1 Age distribution

In the present study, a total of 90 male patients were enrolled with an average age of 68.70 ± 6.99 years and median age of 67 years, of this majority of the patients belonged to the age group of 60 to 70 years (66.67%), followed by 71 to 80 year (25.56%) as shown in Table 15.1.

In the current study, majority of the patients presented with inguinal hernia, of these, 33 (36.67%) had direct inguinal hernia, 16 (17.78%) had right direct inguinal hernia, 17 (18.89%) had left direct inguinal hernia, and 2 (2.22%) had bilateral direct inguinal hernia. Similarly, out of 33 patients with indirect inguinal hernia, 21 (23.33%) patients had right, 12 (13.33%) had left indirect inguinal hernia, and 2 (2.22%) had bilateral indirect inguinal hernia (Table 15.2). Patients with umbilical hernia, appendicitis and hydrocele were observed among 11 (12.22%), 5(5.56%), 2 (2.22%) patients, respectively.

15.4.2 Surgical management

In the present study, we observed that hernioplasty was the commonest mode of management (right sided among 41.11%, left sided among 32.22%, bilateral among 6.67% study patients) followed by Mayo's repair in 7(7.78%), open appendicectomy in 5 (5.56%) and Excision & Eversion surgery in 2 (2.22%) patients as shown in Table 15.3.

Table 15.1 Distribution of cases according to their age

Age distribution	*Number of patients*	*Percentage*
60 to 70	60	66.67%
71 to 80	23	25.56%
81 to 90	07	7.77%
More than 90	0	0%
Total	90	100%
Mean age ± SD	68.70 ± 6.99 years	
Median age	67 years	

Table 15.2 Distribution of cases according to their diagnosis

Diagnosis		*Number of patients*	*Percentage*
Inguinal Hernia (Direct)	**Right**	16	17.78%
	Left	17	18.89%
	Bilateral	2	2.22%
Inguinal Hernia (Indirect)	**Right**	21	23.33%.
	Left	12	13.33%
	Bilateral	2	2.22%
Right Indirect and Left Direct Inguinal Hernia		2	2.22%
Umbilical Hernia		11	12.22%
Appendicitis		5	5.56%
Right Hydrocele		1	1.11%
Left Hydrocele		1	1.11%
TOTAL		**90**	100%

Table 15.3 Distribution of cases based on their type management

Surgical management		*Number of surgeries*	*Percentage*
Hernioplasty	**Right**	37	41.11%
	Left	29	32.22%
	Bilateral	06	6.67%
	Hernioplasty	04	4.44%
Mayo's Repair		07	7.78%
Open Appendicectomy		05	5.56%
Excision & Eversion		02	2.22%
TOTAL		**90**	**100%**

In the current study, we assessed the IPSS score among the study patients as mentioned in Table 15.4. The mean IPSS score was 3.79 ± 1.70. Median score was 4 (range 0–7).

Table 15.5 gives the details of patients with urinary retention. There were patients with urinary retention, with a mean age of 78.75 years and a mean

Table 15.4 IPSS score

Parameters	*IPSS score*
Mean	3.79
Standard Deviation	1.70
Median	4
Min	0
Max	7

Table 15.5 Details of patients with urinary retention

Details of patients with urinary retention		*Incidence*
Mean age		78.75 years
Mean IPSS score		5
Diagnosis	Left Indirect Inguinal hernia	2 (2.23%)
	B/L Inguinal hernia	3 (3.34%)
Procedures	Left Hernioplasty	2 (2.23%)
	Bilateral Hernioplasty	3 (3.34%)

IPSS (International Prostate Symptom Score) score of 5. Among these patients, there were 2 cases (2.23%) of left indirect inguinal hernia and 3 cases (3.34%) of bilateral inguinal hernia. Regarding the procedures performed, there were 2 cases (2.23%) of left hernioplasty and 3 cases (3.34%) of bilateral hernioplasty.

It's important to note that inguinal hernia refers to a condition where soft tissue, usually a part of the intestine, protrudes through a weak point or tear in the abdominal muscles, and can be either direct or indirect depending on the location of the protrusion (Table 15.6). The IPSS is a tool used to assess the severity of lower urinary tract symptoms (LUTS) in men.

Table 15.7 gives the incidence of urinary retention in unilateral and bilateral inguinal hernia. The incidence of urinary retention in patients diagnosed with unilateral inguinal hernia was found to be 2.23%, while in patients with bilateral inguinal hernia, the incidence was 3.34%. It's worth noting that for other diagnoses, such as appendicitis, umbilical hernia, and hydrocele, the incidence of urinary retention was found to be 0%.

15.5 SUMMARY OF THE RESEARCH

In our study conducted at Krishna Institute of Medical Sciences, Karad, we assessed the age distribution among study patients. We observed that

Table 15.6 Correlation of patient's age and IPSS in patient with urinary retention

Diagnosis	*Patient age*	*IPSS*
Right Indirect & Left Direct Inguinal Hernia	74	5
Left Indirect Inguinal Hernia	85	7
Left Indirect Inguinal Hernia	76	6
Bilateral Direct Inguinal Hernia	75	4
Bilateral Direct Inguinal Hernia	88	7

Table 15.7 Incidence of urinary retention in unilateral and bilateral inguinal hernia.

Diagnosis	*Incidence of urinary retention*
Unilateral inguinal hernia	2.23%
Bilateral inguinal hernia	3.34%
Others (appendicitis, umbilical hernia, hydrocele)	0%

majority of the patients belonged to the age group of 60 to 70 years (66.67%), followed by 71 to 80 years (25.56%). The mean age of the study subjects was 68.70 ± 6.99 years.

In the present study, combination of Tamsulosin and Dutasteride was given to 90 patients 3 week prior to surgery. We observed the study subjects among which 5 patients had incidents of urinary retention. Among that 5 patients, 3 patients had bilateral inguinal hernia and 2 patients had unilateral inguinal hernia. Most of them age more than 75 years, which explains the role of age-related benign prostatic hyperplasia among the study subjects. We observed that among those 5 patients, the mean age is 68.7 ± 7.06 years and also observed that the median age of patients was 67 years.

In the current study, majority of the patients presented with inguinal hernia, of these 33 (36.67%) had direct inguinal hernia, 16 (17.78%) had right direct inguinal hernia, 17(18.89%) had left direct inguinal hernia, and 2 (2.22%) had bilateral direct inguinal hernia. Similarly, out of 33 patients with indirect inguinal hernia, 21 (23.33%) patients had right, 12 (13.33%) had left indirect inguinal hernia, and 2 (2.22%) had bilateral indirect inguinal hernia. Patients with umbilical hernia, appendicitis, and hydrocele were observed among 11 (12.22%), 5 (5.56%), and 2 (2.22%) patients, respectively.

Five patients had postoperative urinary retention out of 90 patients, and all the patients were diagnosed as inguinal hernia. Among the whole study,

5.56% incidence of urinary retention and 94.44% did not have incidence of urinary retention among study subject, showing that postoperative urinary retention can be avoided by Tamsulosin and Dutasteride combination.

15.6 CONCLUSION

The combination of Tamsulosin and Dutasteride has been found to be effective in preventing postoperative urinary retention in elderly male patients undergoing elective surgery. In our study, we observed that most of the patients belonged to the age group of 60 to 70 years, followed by 71 to 80 years. The majority of the patients presented with inguinal hernia, and among the five patients who had postoperative urinary retention, three had bilateral inguinal hernia and two had unilateral inguinal hernia. The results of our study showed that the incidence of postoperative urinary retention was 5.56% among the study subjects, and all the patients who developed urinary retention were diagnosed with inguinal hernia. This indicates that Tamsulosin and Dutasteride combination can be an effective preventive strategy for postoperative urinary retention in elderly male patients undergoing elective surgery, especially those with inguinal hernia. Overall, our study provides evidence that the use of Tamsulosin and Dutasteride combination prior to surgery can significantly reduce the risk of postoperative urinary retention in elderly male patients, thereby improving their quality of life and reducing healthcare costs.

REFERENCES

1. Shin HW, Kim JH. Comparison of the efficacy and safety of tamsulosin+dutasteride and tamsulosin for the treatment of benign prostatic hyperplasia: a meta-analysis of randomized controlled trials. *BMC Urol.* 2021;21(1):105. doi:10.1186/s12894-021-00887-9
2. Aboumarzouk OM, Agarwal T, Syed NH, et al. Role of alpha-blockers in management of postoperative urinary retention: a systematic review. *Arab J Urol.* 2015;13(4):241–246. doi:10.1016/j.aju.2015.08.003
3. Rajeev TP, Dharwadkar S, Tandon S, Senthilnathan S. Incidence of postoperative urinary retention and evaluation of tamsulosin in its management following elective lower limb orthopaedic surgery under spinal anaesthesia. *Indian J Anaesth.* 2012;56(5):465–469. doi:10.4103/0019-5049.103985
4. Holm-Larsen T, Frost P, Lautrup MD, et al. The impact of anesthesia on urinary retention following total hip arthroplasty: a prospective cohort study. *J Arthroplasty.* 2016;31(6):1277–1282. doi:10.1016/j.arth.2015.12.010
5. Liu L, Li C, Zhu Y, et al. Preventive effect of tamsulosin on postoperative urinary retention after transurethral resection of bladder tumor: a meta-analysis. *Medicine.* 2019;98(37):e16900. doi:10.1097/MD.0000000000016900

6. McConnell JD, Roehrborn CG, Bautista OM, et al. The long-term effect of doxazosin, finasteride, and combination therapy on the clinical progression of benign prostatic hyperplasia. *N Engl J Med*. 2003;349(25):2387–2398.
7. Nickel JC, Sander S, Moon TD. A meta-analysis of the vascular-related safety profile and efficacy of alpha-adrenergic blockers for symptoms related to benign prostatic hyperplasia. *Int J Clin Pract*. 2008;62(10):1547–1559.
8. Roehrborn CG, Siami P, Barkin J, et al. The effects of combination therapy with dutasteride and tamsulosin on clinical outcomes in men with symptomatic benign prostatic hyperplasia: 4-year results from the CombAT study. *Eur Urol*. 2010;57(1):123–131.
9. Gajendran M, Siddiqui T, Ellias E, Jaffe WI. A review of the role of dutasteride in the management of benign prostatic hyperplasia. *Ther Adv Urol*. 2019;11:1756287219843483. doi:10.1177/1756287219843483
10. Yilmaz Y, Kizilay F, Altuntas CZ, et al. Comparison of tamsulosin and tamsulosin plus dutasteride treatment in men with lower urinary tract symptoms/benign prostatic hyperplasia: a prospective study. *Urol J*. 2021;18(4):398–402. doi:10.22037/uj.v18i.6356
11. Kim M, Lee HE, Lee SR, et al. Tamsulosin and dutasteride combination therapy for the management of benign prostatic hyperplasia: a review of the current literature. *Korean J Urol*. 2011;52(9):569–574.
12. Sun Y, Li G, Li H, et al. Tamsulosin and dutasteride combination therapy versus monotherapy for lower urinary tract symptoms due to benign prostatic hyperplasia: a meta-analysis. *Medicine*. 2017;96(19):e6784.
13. Ozcan L, Polat E, Karakus S, et al. Tamsulosin and dutasteride combination therapy for the prevention of postoperative urinary retention after transurethral resection of the prostate: a randomized controlled trial. *Urol Int*. 2019;103(3):316–322.
14. Capogrosso P, Ventimiglia E, Chierigo F, et al. Tamsulosin and dutasteride combination therapy for the management of benign prostatic hyperplasia: a randomized controlled trial. *Int Urol Nephrol*. 2019;51(11):1945–1952.
15. Roehrborn CG. Benign prostatic hyperplasia: an overview. *Rev Urol*. 2005;7(Suppl 9):S3–S14.
16. Lepor H. Medical treatment of benign prostatic hyperplasia. *Rev Urol*. 2006;8(Suppl 4):S9–S15.
17. Montorsi F, Roehrborn C, Garcia-Penit J, et al. The effects of dutasteride or tamsulosin alone and in combination on storage and voiding symptoms in men with lower urinary tract symptoms (LUTS) and benign prostatic hyperplasia (BPH): 4-year data from the Combination of Avodart and Tamsulosin (CombAT) study. *BJU Int*. 2011;107(9):1426–1431.
18. Teng J, Zhang J, Chen Y, et al. The efficacy and safety of combination therapy with tamsulosin and dutasteride for benign prostatic hyperplasia: a systematic review and meta-analysis. *Curr Med Res Opin*. 2018;34(3):477–486.

Chapter 16

Substantiating random forest algorithm for prognosis of various infirmities

S. M. Soundarya, M. Sharanya, Sujey Rajesh Naik, C. Manjunatha Swamy, and B. Meenkashi Sundaram

16.1 INTRODUCTION

Machine learning is an artificial intelligence subfield that involves the development of algorithms and models that can learn from and forecast data.

Machine learning is classified into numerous forms, including supervised learning, unsupervised learning, semi-supervised learning, and reinforcement learning. The model is trained using the data that is labelled and then used to generate predictions on fresh, unseen data in supervised learning. The model is trained on data that is unlabeled and used to uncover patterns and relationships in the data using the unsupervised learning. While in the semi-supervised learning, model is built on a combination of labeled and unlabeled data. In reinforcement learning, the model is trained through trial-and-error interactions with an environment [1].

Machine learning has many practical applications in various fields, including natural language processing, computer vision, speech recognition, and healthcare. In healthcare, machine learning is used to improve diagnosis, treatment planning, and disease management. In this chapter, we have analyzed the accuracies of the models built using the algorithms – Random Forest [2], Logistic Regression, and K Nearest Neighbor.

Random Forest is a machine learning approach that may be applied to both classification and regression. It is a collection of decision trees that are produced at random and then integrated to make predictions [3, 4]. The algorithm is called "Random Forest" because it generates multiple decision trees, or a "forest" of trees, and uses random subsets of the data to train each tree [5]. The final prediction is found by calculating the average of the predictions of all the trees in the forest. It has the ability to handle large amounts of data and high-dimensional data, making it well suited for many real-world applications [1, 2].

Logistic Regression is a simple and widely used algorithm that is easy to implement and interpret [6]. It is also computationally efficient and can handle large amounts of data. One of the strengths of using this algorithm is that it is able to build the relationship between the dependent variables and the independent variables in a linear manner, which makes it well suited

DOI: 10.1201/9781003536352-16

for simple, linear problems [7]. This algorithm is a widely used statistical method for binary classification tasks in machine learning [8]. Thus, its simplicity, efficiency, and ability to handle large amounts of data make it well suited for many real-world applications.

K-Nearest Neighbors (KNN) comes under the branch of supervised learning that is used for classification and issues [9]. The algorithm is based on the idea that similar instances are likely to have similar outcomes and makes predictions contingent to the outcome of the k number of nearest neighbors of the data that is used for training [10]. KNN is simple, easy to implement, and well suited for complex and non-linear problems, making it a popular choice for many real-world applications [11].

This chapter has the conclusions of the implementations of the disease detection models for the diseases, that is, heart [3, 6, 10], diabetes [12], liver [7] [8], kidney [13], breast cancer [2] using the above-mentioned algorithms.

16.2 METHODOLOGY

The methodology used for disease prediction in machine learning can vary depending on the type of disease, the available data, and the specific machine learning algorithm being used. However, the following steps are typically followed for our model's creation:

1. **Data Aggregation.** The initial stride is to gather pertinent data that can be utilized to forecast the condition. This can include demographic information, medical history, symptoms, test results, and other relevant information [3].
2. **Data Preprocessing.** The accumulated data is then cleaned from noise and preprocessed to make sure that it is in a proper composition for use with a machine learning algorithm. This includes removing missing or invalid data, encoding categorical variables and normalizing continuous variables [1, 6].
3. **Feature Selection.** Succeeding stage is to choose the most applicable characteristics from the data that is preprocessed to be utilized in detection. This is done using feature selection techniques, such as feature importance or feature extraction [5, 8].
4. **Model Selection.** Once the data has been preprocessed and the relevant features have been extracted, one of the machine learning algorithms is chosen. Algorithms for disease prediction include Logistic Regression, K-Nearest Neighbors (KNN), and Random Forest [5].
5. **Model Training.** Determined machine learning algorithm is built on the data that is preprocessed using the chosen features. The algorithm is trained to acquire the knowledge of the relationship between the disease outcomes and the features [10].

6. **Model Evaluation.** Estimation of the trained model is evaluated using a suitable evaluation metric, such as accuracy and confusion matrix [1].
7. **Hyperparameter Tuning.** The parameters of the chosen machine learning algorithm that are established before training are known as hyperparameters. Hyperparameter tuning is the mechanism of evaluating the best combination of hyperparameters to achieve optimal performance [3, 11].
8. **Model Deployment.** Finally, if the evaluation of the model is satisfactory, it is deployed for use in a real-world setting.

In conclusion, the methodology used for disease prediction in machine learning typically involves collecting and preprocessing relevant data, selecting relevant features, selecting a machine learning algorithm, training the algorithm, evaluating its performance, and deploying the model if performance is satisfactory.

16.3 ALGORITHMS USED

After reviewing multiple papers, the following are few algorithms which were discussed by the authors to get the desired result.

Some of the mandatory steps that needs to be performed in order to use for the algorithms would be the following:

```
#Import packages
import pandas as pds
import numpy as npy
from sklearn.model_selection import train_test_split
# The data is loaded into a created pandas DataFrame
data1 = pds.read_csv("csvdata.csv")
# The data1 is split into features (X) and target (y)
x = data1.drop("target", axis=1)
y = data1["target"]
# The data1 is split into sets for training and testing
x_trained, x_tested, y_trained, y_tested = train_test_
split(x, y, test_size=0.3)
```

The algorithms used for disease detection in our implementation includes:

1. **Random Forest**

   Random Forest comes under the category of ensemble machine learning methodology that makes predictions by combining decision trees [1]. It is widely used for disease prediction due to its high accuracy and ability to handle large datasets with many features [3].

```
#The package RandomForestClassifier needs to be
imported
from sklearn.ensemble import RandomForestClassifier
# The Random Forest model is skilled using the training
data
clf = RandomForestClassifier(n_estimators=100)
clf.fit(x_trained, y_trained)
#the trained model is used to make predictions on the
test data
y_predicted = clf.predict(x_tested)
# Estimate the model's performance by calculating the
accuracy score
from sklearn.metrics import accuracy_score
accuracy1 = accuracy_score(y_tested, y_predicted)
print ("Accuracy:", accuracy1)
```

2. **Logistic Regression**
   This algorithm is a statistical method used for binary classification problems [6], such as predicting whether a patient has a particular disease or not [7]. It is a simple and interpretable algorithm that is used to build a model which creates a relationship between a binary outcome and predicator variables [8].

```
#import LogisticRegression package
from sklearn.linear_model import LogisticRegression
#the logistic regression model is created using the
data which needs to be trained
clf = LogisticRegression()
clf.fit(x_trained, y_trained)
# Do the predictions on the testing data
y_predicted = clf.predict(x_tested)
# Evaluate the model's accuracy
from sklearn.metrics import accuracy_score
accuracy1 = accuracy_score(y_tested, y_predicted)
print ("Accuracy:", accuracy1)
```

3. **K-Nearest Neighbors (KNN)**
   This is a machine learning method that is non-parametric and instance-based and is used for regression as well as classification tasks [9]. It works by ascertaining the K nearest instances in the training data and relates it to the new instance and using these neighbors to make a prediction [11].

```
#Import KNeighborsClassifier package
from sklearn.neighbors import KNeighborsClassifier
# Fit the k nearest neighbor model to the data that
needs to be trained
clf = KNeighborsClassifier(n_neighbors=7)
clf.fit(x_trained, y_trained)
```

```
# Do the predictions on the testing data
y_predicted = clf.predict(x_tested)
# Evaluate the model's accuracy
from sklearn.metrics import accuracy_score
accuracy1 = accuracy_score(y_tested, y_predicted)
print ("Accuracy:", accuracy1)
```

16.4 HYPERPARAMETER TUNING

A machine learning model's performance in disease detection can be considerably improved by fine-tuning its hyperparameters. The created model's accuracy is calculated by the selection of hyperparameters, and determining the ideal collection of hyperparameters may considerably enhance the model's performance. To enhance the accuracy of our model using hyperparameter tuning, the following steps were taken:

- Defining the hyperparameters to be tuned and their range of values.
- Choosing an evaluation metric to measure the model's performance.
- The data is split into testing and testing sets [3].
- Passing the model, hyperparameter grid, and evaluation metric to a hyperparameter tuning tool, such as GridSearchCV or RandomizedSearchCV.
- The model is created by training using the training data and evaluating its performance on the validation data [7].
- Using the compatible set of hyperparameters found by the hyperparameter tuning tool to re-train the model using the full training data.
- Evaluating the final model's accuracy using the test data.

1. **RandomizedSearchCV**
   RandomizedSearchCV is a tool for hyperparameter tuning in machine learning models for disease detection. It uses a random search strategy to explore different combinations of hyperparameters and finds the compatible set of hyperparameters that maximize a specified performance metric. To improve our model accuracy, we have mainly focused on use of RandomizedSearchCV hyperparameter tuning method [3].

```
import numpy as npy
from sklearn.ensemble import RandomForestClassifier
from sklearn.model_selection import RandomizedSearchCV
# Define the hyperparameter range to be searched
parameter_grid = {
'max_depth': [None, 5, 10, 15],
'min_samples_split': npy.arange(3, 10, 2),
'n_estimators': npy.arange(50, 200, 50),
```

```
'min_samples_leaf': npy.arange(2, 5, 1)}
# Create the RandomForestClassifier and
RandomizedSearchCV objects
rf_model = RandomForestClassifier()
rf_search = RandomizedSearchCV(rf_model, parameter_
grid, n_iter=10, cv=6, scoring='roc_auc')
# Fit the RandomizedSearchCV object using the training
data
rf_search.fit(x_trained, y_trained)
#showcase the best hyperparameters and the score
print ("The best hyperparameters: ", rf_search.
best_params_)
print ("The best score: ", rf_search.best_score_)
```

The scoring argument sets the performance metric used to assess the models. In our case, the ROC-AUC metric is used, which is commonly used for disease detection tasks.

2. **GridSearchCV**

GridSearchCV is another tool for hyperparameter tuning in machine learning models for disease detection [11]. It performs a systematic search in the hyperparameter space by exhaustively trying all combinations of hyperparameters defined in a grid. Unlike RandomizedSearchCV, which uses a random search strategy, GridSearchCV uses a grid search strategy, which can be slower but more precise in finding the optimal hyperparameters [3].

```
import pandas as pds
import numpy as npy
from sklearn.model_selection import GridSearchCV
from sklearn.ensemble import RandomForestClassifier
# The hyperparameter grid is defined to search
parameter_grid = {
'max_depth': [2, 5, 7, 8, 10],
'n_estimators': [15, 20, 50, 100],
'min_samples_leaf': [2, 5, 7, 8],
'min_samples_split': [2, 6, 9, 16]
}
# Create a RandomForestClassifier with default
hyperparameters
clf1 = RandomForestClassifier()
# Perform grid search to find the best hyperparameters
grid_search_model = GridSearchCV(clf1, parameter_grid,
cv=7)
grid_search_model.fit(x_trained, y_trained)
# Print the best hyperparameters found
print ("Best hyperparameters:", grid_search.
best_params_)
# Evaluate the model's accuracy on the testing data
accuracy1 = grid_search.score(x_tested, y_tested)
print ("Accuracy:", accuracy1)
```

16.5 DATASETS USED FOR DATA CREATION

1. **Dataset used for heart disease detection**
   This dataset contains 303 records of patient data and has 14 features listed [5]. The features needed to build the model are listed in the dataset and few of them are trestbps, chol, fbs, restecg, thalach, exang, oldpeak, etc. The dataset is collected and created from the following researchers [3].
   - Hungarian Institute of Cardiology: Andras Janosi, M.D.
   - V.A. Medical Center, Long Beach and Cleveland Clinic Foundation: Robert Detrano, M.D., Ph.D.
   - University Hospital, Basel: Matthias Pfisterer, M.D.
   - University Hospital, Zurich: William Steinbrunn, M.D.
2. **Dataset used for breast cancer detection**
   This dataset consists of 569 records of patient data and has 32 features listed. After correlation few of the attributes were removed and the final count came to 27 features. Few of them are diagnosis, concavity_mean, radius_mean, texture_mean, area_mean, perimeter_mean, compactness_mean, smoothness_mean, etc. The dataset is collected and created from the following researchers.
   - Dr. William H. Wolberg. University of Wisconsin.
   - Olvi L. Mangasarian. University of Wisconsin.
   - W. Nick Street. University of Wisconsin.
3. **Dataset used for liver disease detection**
   This dataset comprises 583 records of patient data and has 11 features listed. Few of the features are Total_Bilirubin, Alamine_Aminotransferase, Direct_Bilirubin [14], Total_Protiens, Alkaline_Phosphotase, Aspartate_Aminotransferase, etc. [15]. The dataset is collected and created from the following researchers [11].
   - Bendi Venkata Ramana, Aditya Institute of Technology and Management.
   - Prof. M. Surendra Prasad Babu, Andhra University College of Engineering.
   - Prof. N. B. Venkateswarlu, Aditya Institute of Technology and Management.
4. **Dataset used for diabetes detection**
   This dataset comprises 768 records of patient data and has nine features listed. Few of the features are BloodPressure, Pregnancies, BMI, Glucose, Insulin, Skin Thickness, etc. [4, 12].
5. **Dataset used for kidney disease detection**
   This dataset consists of 400 records of patient data and has 26 features listed [13]. Few of the features are ba(bacteria), pc (pus cell), bgr(blood glucose random), sc(serum creatinine), pcc(pus cell clumps), bu(blood urea), etc.

16.6 RESULTS

The results include the models trained using the algorithms K Nearest Neighbor, Logistic Regression, and Random Forest. It has been observed that for the above-mentioned diseases, the Random Forest model gave the highest accuracies than the other two after the hyper tuning process for the given dataset. The technique used for hyper tuning is the RandomizedSearchCV and the hyperparameters chosen are the n_estimators, max_features, max_depth, criterion, bootstrap, min_samples_split and min_samples_leaf. All the above-mentioned diseases are integrated using the Flask API and is deployed as a web application.

1. Accuracy of 100% to detect kidney disease built using Random Forest after hyperparameter tuning process
2. Accuracy of 96% to detect breast cancer built using Random Forest after hyperparameter tuning process
3. Accuracy of 88% to detect heart disease built using Random Forest after hyperparameter tuning process
4. The heat map in Figure 16.4 shows the data on the heart disease attributes which is moderately negatively correlated
5. Accuracy of 80% to detect diabetes built using Random Forest after hyperparameter tuning process
6. The heat map in Figure 16.6 shows the data on the diabetes attributes which is highly negatively correlated
7. Accuracy of 79% to detect liver disease built using Random Forest after hyperparameter tuning process
8. The heat map in Figure 16.8 shows the data on the liver disease attributes which is highly negatively correlated
9. The web application's main page deployed using Flask API with all disease modules on the nav bar

Table 16.1 Accuracies of the above-mentioned algorithms for detection of diseases

Diseases	*Algorithms*		
	Logistic regression	*K nearest neighbor*	*Random forest*
Kidney disease	96.88	84.38	100.0
Breast Cancer	96.49	94.25	96.49
Heart disease	86.52	75.41	88.52
Diabetes	74.68	79.87	80.51
Liver disease	74.36	77.97	79.66

```
Accuracy: 100.0%
Confusion matrix:
 [[ 9  0]
 [ 0 23]]
Report:
               precision    recall  f1-score   support

         ckd       1.00      1.00      1.00         9
      notckd       1.00      1.00      1.00        23

    accuracy                           1.00        32
   macro avg       1.00      1.00      1.00        32
weighted avg       1.00      1.00      1.00        32
```

Figure 16.1 Accuracy of 100% to detect kidney disease built using Random Forest algorithm after hyperparameter tuning process.

```
Accuracy: 96.49122807017%
Confusion matrix:
 [[70  1]
 [ 3 40]]
Report:
               precision    recall  f1-score   support

           0       0.96      0.99      0.97        71
           1       0.98      0.93      0.95        43

    accuracy                           0.96       114
   macro avg       0.97      0.96      0.96       114
weighted avg       0.97      0.96      0.96       114
```

Figure 16.2 Accuracy of 96% to detect breast cancer built using Random Forest after hyperparameter tuning process.

```
Accuracy: 88.52459016393%
Confusion matrix:
 [[25  4]
 [ 3 29]]
Report:
               precision    recall  f1-score   support

           0       0.89      0.86      0.88        29
           1       0.88      0.91      0.89        32

    accuracy                           0.89        61
   macro avg       0.89      0.88      0.88        61
weighted avg       0.89      0.89      0.89        61
```

Figure 16.3 Accuracy of 88% to detect heart disease built using Random Forest after hyperparameter tuning process.

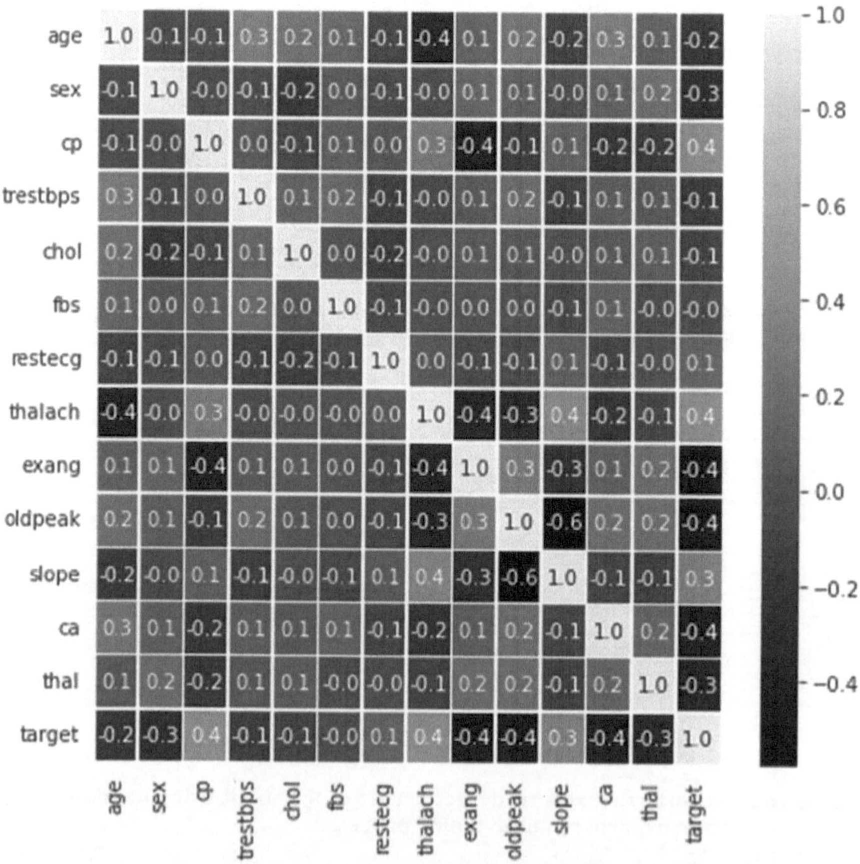

Figure 16.4 The above heat map is showing the data on the heart disease attributes which is moderately negatively correlated.

```
Accuracy: 80.5194805195%
Confusion matrix:
 [[98  9]
 [21 26]]
Report:
              precision    recall  f1-score   support

           0       0.82      0.92      0.87       107
           1       0.74      0.55      0.63        47

    accuracy                           0.81       154
   macro avg       0.78      0.73      0.75       154
weighted avg       0.80      0.81      0.80       154
```

Figure 16.5 Accuracy of 80% to detect diabetes built using Random Forest after hyperparameter tuning process.

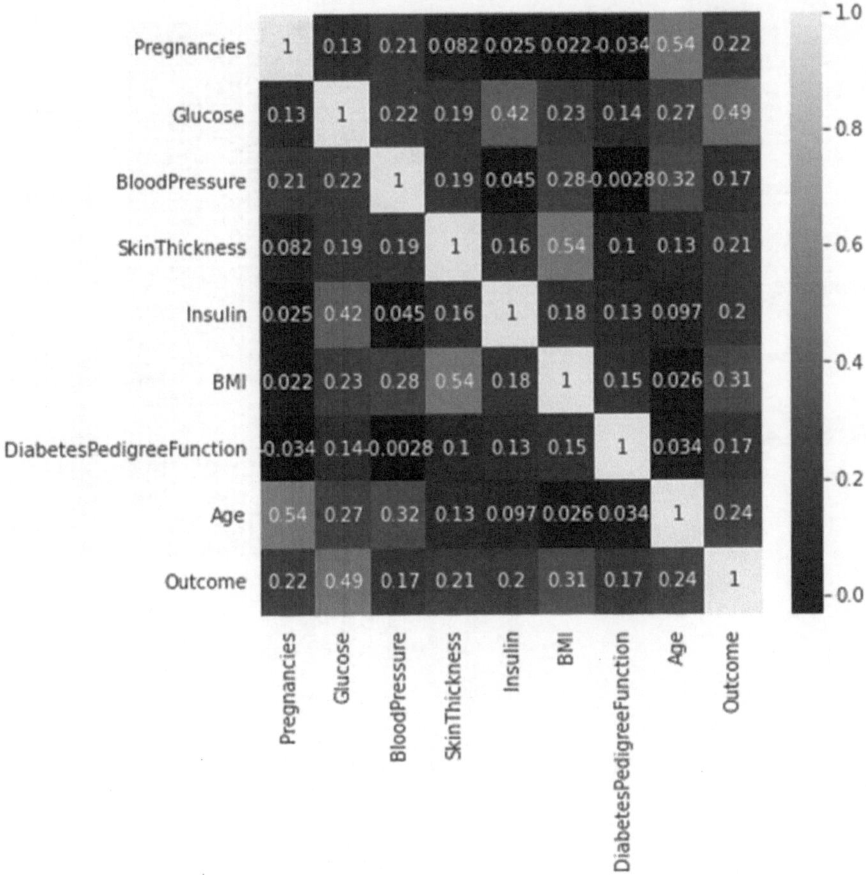

Figure 16.6 The above heat map is showing the data on the diabetes attributes which is highly negatively correlated.

```
Accuracy: 79.6610169492%
Confusion matrix:
 [[42  3]
 [ 9  5]]
Report:
              precision    recall  f1-score   support

           0       0.82      0.93      0.87        45
           1       0.62      0.36      0.45        14

    accuracy                           0.80        59
   macro avg       0.72      0.65      0.66        59
weighted avg       0.78      0.80      0.78        59
```

Figure 16.7 Accuracy of 79% to detect liver disease built using Random Forest after hyperparameter tuning process.

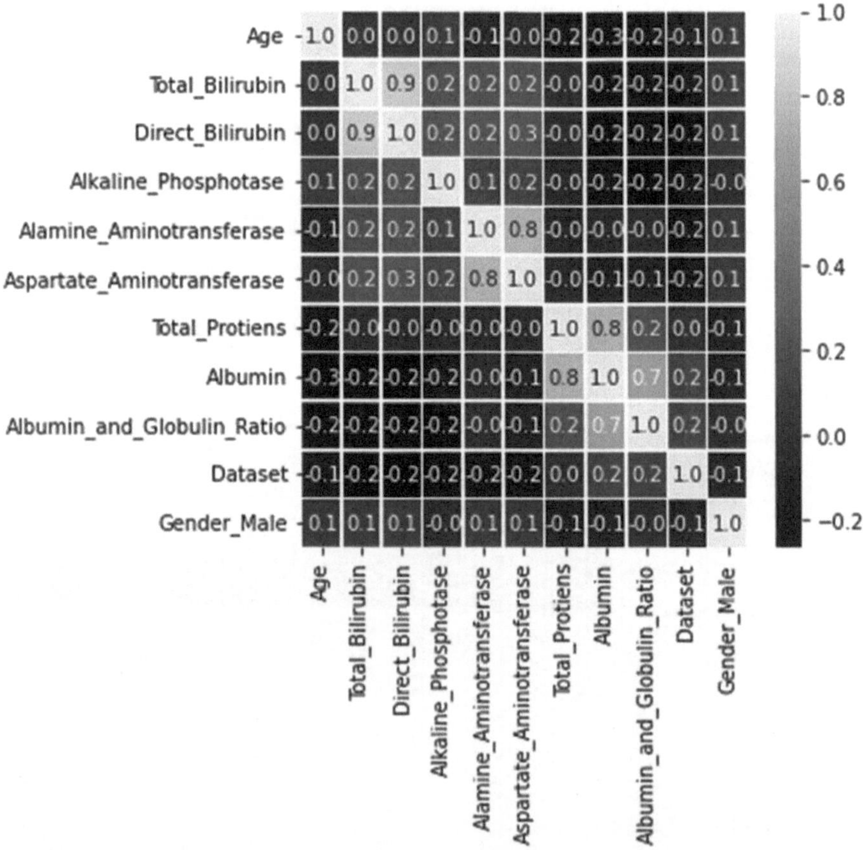

Figure 16.8 The above heat map is showing the data on the liver disease attributes which is highly negatively correlated.

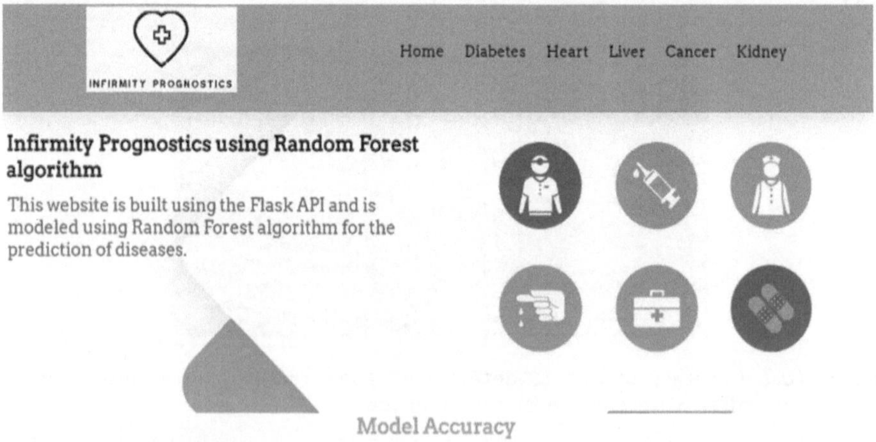

Figure 16.9 The web application's main page deployed using Flask API with all disease modules on the nav bar.

16.7 CONCLUSION

Based on our research model which is detection of various diseases using the algorithms Logistic Regression, K Nearest Neighbor, and Random Forest, we were able to conclude that Random Forest gave the highest accuracies for the above-stated diseases. On the basis of our research, we have used datasets from sources, that is, Cleveland's cardiovascular data records, UCI repository, PIMA dataset, Breast Cancer – Breast Cancer Wisconsin (Diagnostic) Dataset, and are analyzed for training the models.

Different algorithms have different accuracy levels, which have been improved by altering the hyperparameters of the algorithms by choosing appropriate attributes.

16.8 SUGGESTIONS

The future scope of using Random Forest expands through horizon and few of the fields that can be enhanced include

- Precision medicine: Creating personalized medical treatments from data of patient's medical history
- Automated diagnosis: Automating the diagnostic process and improving the speed and accuracy of diagnosis.

The other fields include multi-modal data analysis, high-dimensional data analysis, and early diagnosis, etc.

ACKNOWLEDGMENT

We express our regard to Mr. Manjunatha Swamy C, Senior Assistant Professor, our project guide, and Dr. B. Meenakshi Sundaram, Professor, for continuously monitoring the project's progress and establishing exact timelines. Their insightful counsel served as the driving force behind finishing the task.

NOMENCLATURE

Names	*Description*
Trestbps	Resting blood pressure in mm Hg.
Chol	Serum cholesterol in mg/dl.
Fbs	fasting blood sugar > 120 mg/dl (0 = false, 1=true).
Restecg	resting electrocardiographic results.
Thalach	maximum heart rate
Exang	exercise induced angina (0 = no, 1 = yes)

Names	*Description*
oldpeak	ST depression induced by exercise relative to rest
diagnosis	M = malignant, B = benign
concavity_mean	mean of severity of concave portions of the contour
radius_mean	mean of distances from center to points on the perimeter
texture_mean	mean of standard deviation of gray-scale values
compactness_mean	mean of perimeter^2 / area - 1.0
smoothness_mean	mean of local variation in radius lengths

REFERENCES

1. A. Al-Mousa, N. Abdulhadi "Diabetes Detection Using Machine Learning Classification Methods". IEEE 2021.
2. Wazid, M., Singh, J., Das, A. K., Shetty, S., Khan, M. K., & Rodrigues, J. J. (2022). ASCP-IoMT: AI-enabled lightweight secure communication protocol for internet of medical things. *IEEE Access*, *10*, 57990–58004, 10.1109/ACCESS.2022.3179418
3. A.U. Rehman, T. M. Ghazal, M. Ahmad, M. Saleem, F. Mehmood, S. Ahmad "Intelligent Model to Predict Early Liver Disease using Machine Learning Technique". IEEE 2022.
4. V. H. Sree, A. N. V. K. Swarupa, Y. K. S. Kishore, S. Nookambika, U. R. Teja "Disease Prediction: Smart Disease Prediction System using Random Forest Algorithm". *ICISSGT, IEEE* 2021.
5. C. C "Prediction of Heart Disease Using Different KNN Classifier". *ICICCS, IEEE* 2021.
6. Chieh-Chen Wu, Tahmina Nasrin Poly, Wen-Chun Yeh, Hsuan-Chia Yang, Md. Mohaimenul Islam, Wen-Ding Hsu, Yu-Chuan Li, Yu-Chuan Jack Wang, Phung Anh Nguyen "Prediction of Fatty Liver Disease Using Machine Learning Algorithms". *Computer Methods and Programs in Biomedicine*, 170, 2019, 23–29.
7. Shahadat Uddin, Ibtisham Haque, Haohui Lu, Mohammad Ali Moni, Ergun Gide "Comparative Performance Analysis of K-Nearest Neighbour (KNN) Algorithm and Its Different Variants for Disease Prediction". *Sci Rep*, 12, 2022, 6256.
8. Jagdeep Singh, Ranjodh Kaur, Sachin Bagga "Software-based Prediction of Liver Disease with Feature Selection and Classification Techniques". *Procedia Computer Science*, 167, 2020, 1970–1980, ISSN 1877-0509.
9. Sharma, R., Kim, M., & Gupta, A. (2022). Motor imagery classification in brain-machine interface with machine learning algorithms: Classical approach to multi-layer perceptron model. *Biomedical Signal Processing and Control*, *71*, 103101, 10.1016/j.bspc.2021.103101
10. Madan, P., Singh, V., Singh, D. P., Diwakar, M., & Kishor, A. (2022). Denoising of ECG signals using weighted stationary wavelet total variation. *Biomedical Signal Processing and Control*, *73*, 103478. http://dx.doi.org/10.1016/j.bspc.2021.103478

11. Koppula and PSM Lal, Phalinkar, Riya, Bhanu Prakash Reddy, Keerthana, Nidhi "A Prediction Model of Detecting Liver Diseases in Patients using Logistic Regression of Machine Learning". *ICICC*, IEEE 2020.
12. S. Maini and S. Dhanka "Random Forest for Heart Disease Detection: A Classification Approach", *ICEPES, IEEE* 2021.
13. Pawar, D., Phansalkar, S., Sharma, A., Sahu, G. K., Ang, C. K., & Lim, W. H. (2023). Survey on the Biomedical Text Summarization Techniques with an Emphasis on Databases, Techniques, Semantic Approaches, Classification Techniques, and Similarity Measures. *Sustainability*, *15*(5), 4216. 10.3390/su15054216
14. Rabiei, R., Ayyoubzadeh, S. M., Sohrabei, S., Esmaeili, M., & Atashi, A. (2022). Prediction of breast cancer using machine learning approaches. *Journal of Biomedical Physics & Engineering*, *12*(3), 297.
15. K. V. Kanimozhi and K. S. Kumar Reddy "Intelligent Heart Disease Prediction using Novel Random Forest Algorithm with Enhanced Accuracy over SVM". *ICTACS, IEEE* 2022.

Chapter 17

Assessing the perception of customers towards telehealth systems and intention to adopt with reference to Uttar Pradesh

Amar, Komal Malik, and Namita Srivastava

17.1 INTRODUCTION

Telehealth systems are crucial to the communication of electronic healthcare information between patients and clinicians. These systems have also substantially increased access to care and the quality of care received. Additionally, telehealth has dramatically lowered the cost of healthcare in several nations. In one meta-analysis, telemedicine's effect on treating chronic disorders (e.g., diabetes, hypertension) was largely beneficial. This study of the perception of middle-aged people indicated favourable impacts of telehealth adoption. Due to the effectiveness of telehealth technologies, the American Telemedicine Association estimates that the utilisation of these systems is projected to increase or treble during the next five to ten years.

The patients saw telehealth as a possibility to increase their quality of life, enabling them to live independently at home and assist them in taking and being in greater control over their health status. The outcomes of this research supported telemedicine for the regular management of persons with type 2 diabetes (Lee, 2018).

Telemedicine started in India in 1999, although the government recognised the potential of telemedicine in 2000. The Indian Space Research Organisation launched the first nationwide SATCOM-based telemedicine network in 2001. Figure 17.1 shows the basic infrastructure.

The theoretical framework in this study is based on Technological Acceptance Model (TAM). The TAM implies that adopting a telehealth system is primarily driven by its perceived utility (PU) and perceived ease of use (PEOU). PU and PEOU each have multiple subconstructs linked to telehealth technology adoption, including motivation and behavioural intents. Numerous studies have expanded the TAM by integrating user trust, technological readiness, or perceived danger (i.e., technology will replace a job). Since the TAM was initially presented, it has been quite effective in predicting telehealth acceptability and adoption (variance accounted for ranges from 50% to 70% in most research) across numerous demographics.

 DOI: 10.1201/9781003536352-17

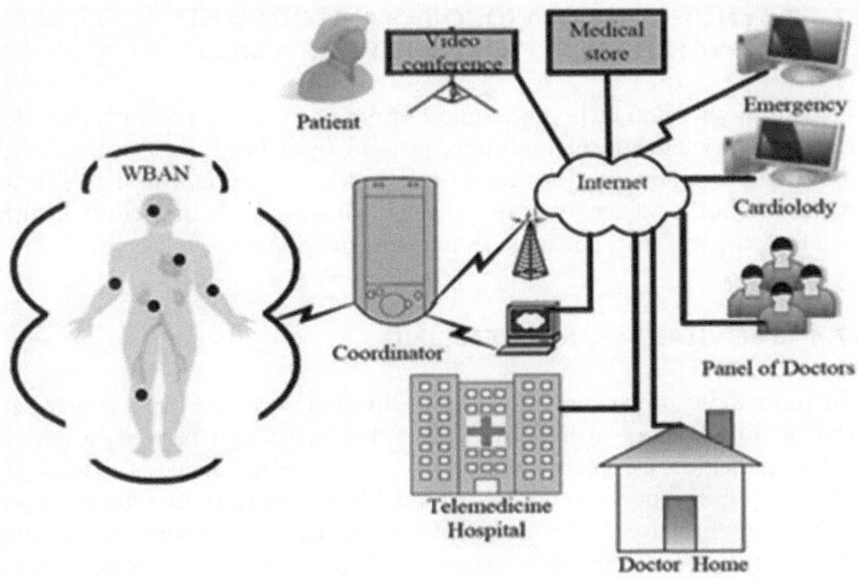

Figure 17.1 Infrastructure of Telemedicine.

Nevertheless, the TAM is not without its problems. For example, more nuanced research on system trust must be undertaken before this element can be included entirely in the TAM since this literature needs consistent findings. Additionally, the TAM does not address or include the severity of diseases or the effect of disease burden into its framework like the HBM. Conversely, the TAM predicts that, regardless of sickness, most users will accept telehealth technologies on the grounds of perceived utility and usability.

During the COVID-19 national emergency, applications like WhatsApp, Facebook Messenger, Google Hangout, Zoom, Practo or Skype, etc. were utilised in good faith to care for patients through telehealth during the lockdown time (Mechanic, 2022).

17.2 MAJOR TYPES OF TELEHEALTH SYSTEMS

While many various forms of telehealth exist, there are four primary categories of telehealth that exist in today's medical market. The advantages of each category vary and may help you and your patients, in various ways depending on what you need to acquire a complete perspective of their health.

17.3 ASYNCHRONOUS VIDEO (AKA STORE-AND-FORWARD) (AKA STORE-AND-FORWARD)

Asynchronous video is the electronic communication of a patient's recorded health history outside of real-time, utilised by a healthcare professional. Often employed in rural locations when doctors are consulting with an expert in another place, this sort of telemedicine also helps deliver healthcare to areas where it, particularly in terms of specialists, is scarce.

17.4 LIVE VIDEO-CONFERENCING

The most well-known sort of telehealth, live video-conferencing is precisely what it sounds like —a live, two-way video-based chat between a patient and their healthcare professional. This sort of telemedicine is extensively utilised by everyone from doctors at local hospitals to those who run their own private practise. Live video-conferencing not only minimises commuting time and stress for both the patient and physician but also helps to bring healthcare to places, generally rural, that don't have nearly as many healthcare alternatives as metropolitan ones.

17.5 MOBILE HEALTH (MHEALTH)

Mobile health is the usage of smart devices (smartphones, tablets, etc.), and the health-based software programmes produced for these devices, that promotes continuing healthcare. Several health-based applications exist today and can track anything from a diabetic patient's blood sugar level to one's regular water consumption. These applications serve to promote healthy living practices and also (if built to) may interact with a patient's personal health information.

In the ever-growing telehealth industry, there are various sorts of telehealth that may enhance your patients' lifestyle choices and raise their overall health. Likewise, telehealth gives you with a complete scope of your patients' daily vitals enabling you to take action and/or alter therapy in order to enhance their health.

17.6 REMOTE PATIENT MONITORING (RPM)

Commonly utilised for seniors or in senior living areas, remote patient monitoring involves collecting a patient's health data from a patient or resident in one place that is then electronically communicated to a healthcare expert (provider, nurse, etc.) for monitoring and evaluation. RPM is essential in senior living facilities to avoid falls and constantly check residents' vitals.

17.7 THE CURRENT STUDY

The current research aims to assess consumers aged 18 to 55 years' opinions of the benefits and drawbacks of telehealth systems. We may better forecast future needs for this demographic and incorporate those needs into the design of future telehealth systems by analysing the current barriers to telehealth adoption in a cohort of UP customers. A theme analysis is one method for examining this cohort's perceived advantages and disadvantages. Two hundred respondents from Uttar Pradesh made up the convenience sampling method sample, which was chosen. While referring to telehealth systems in this research, we included telemedicine, diagnostic, counselling, and telecare.

Demographics of the study:

Item	*No. of respondents*	*Percentage (%)*
Gender		
Female	98	49
Male	102	51
Age		
18–25	84	42
26–35	36	18
36–45	55	27.5
46–55	25	12.5
Health Problems		
Minor (Chronic)	85	42.5
Major (Acute)	65	32.5
None	50	25

17.8 THEORY OF REASONED ACTION (TRA)

The theory of reasoned action (TRA) is one of the three main impact models of psychology. The idea of reasoned action was created by Martin Fishbein and Icek Ajzen in 1967 and was drawn from earlier investigations that began as the concept of the state of mind. The theory aims to elucidate the link between dispositions and practices within human action. TRA forecasts how individuals would continue in light of their prior dispositions and behavioural ambitions. A person's decision to take part in a given behaviour relies on the effects the individual thinks will emerge as a consequence of acting out the conduct.

According to Ajzen and Fishbein, TRA (Theory of Reasoned Action) is a model regarded as the most widely used social psychology platform which demonstrates the components of consciously designed activities.

According to TRA, a person's performance is defined by his behavioural intention (BI) to execute the activity. BI is simultaneously governed by a person's attitude (A) and subjective norm (SN) with relative weights assessed by a regression equation:

$$BI = A + SN$$

17.8.1 Measured variables

Perceived Usefulness: Mobile apps give me complete information to take purchase decisions (like product specification, price, payment mode, etc.), Telehealth system provides virtual experience of product use and assures those services which supports my service consumption, Telehealth systems provide help in analysing which services are best, Suggestions by IT enables benefits me, Telehealth systems give product availability information, advanced availability or exclusivity of the items in Apps, Mobile apps are more user-friendly, Repeated shopping is more accessible, Mobile apps are more comfortable.

Perceived Ease of Use Mobile Apps: Contains Features, clarity in understanding functions, added free applications, simple payment system.

Perceived Value: Experience, value, matching expectations, app advantages.

Intention to use.

17.9 MODEL HYPOTHESISED AND ACHIEVED MODEL FIT (FIGURE 17.2)

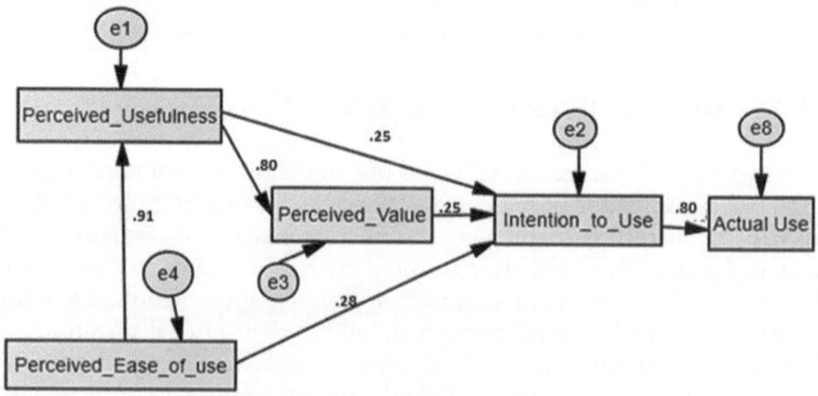

Figure 17.2 Model Hypothesis.

17.9.1 Assessing structural model fitness

Based on Structure Equation Model using SPSS Amos 21, CMIN/DF is the minimum discrepancy, which is 2.2. Wheaton et al. suggested that if the minimum discrepancy is less than five, the model is reasonable to fit.

The following value is found in our study for each parameter to test model fit

Based on numerous research it was indicated that if the Index value is more significant than 0.9 and if RMSEA values are less than 0.08, it shows the model is reasonably fit and accepted.

Consequently, it is determined that the suggested research model fits the data satisfactorily.

17.9.2 Testing structural relationship

The predicted research model strongly matches the observed data described above. The route estimations in the structural model have essential relevance for validity. All the six hypothesised routes are significant with a P-value less than 0.05 and so supported. The standardised regression weights of the output and outcomes of the hypothesis testing giving evidence for hypotheses H1 to H6 are shown in the following tables.

Hypothesis 1 (H1): The Perceived simplicity of use significantly influences Perceived Usefulness.

Hypothesis 2 (H2): Perceived Usefulness considerably influences Perceived value.

Hypothesis 3 (H3): The Perceived value significantly influences the Intention to utilise.

Table 17.1 Parameter value for model fit measures with SPSS Amos

Name of the parameter	*Value*
The goodness of Fit Index (GFI)	0.991
Adjusted Goodness of Fit Index (AGFI)	0.962
Normed Fit Index (NFI)	0.992
Comparative Fit Index (CFI)	0.994
Tucker-Lewis Index (TLI)	0.998
Incremental Fit Index (IFI)	0.992
Relative Fit Index (RFI)	0.981
Root Mean Square Error of Approximation (RMSEA)	0.06

Hypothesis 4 (H4): Perceived Usefulness has a significant impact on the Intention to use

Hypothesis 5 (H5): The Perceived ease of use has a significant influence on the Intention to use

Hypothesis 6 (H6): The Intention to use has a significantly lesser moderate impact on Actual use

1: Perceived ease of use significantly impacts the Perceived Usefulness of Telehealth systems as the p-value is less than 0.05.
2: Perceived Usefulness significantly impacts the Perceived value of Telehealth systems as the p-value is less than 0.05.
3: Perceived Usefulness significantly impacts the Intention to use Telehealth systems, as the p-value is less than 0.05.
4: The Perceived ease of use significantly impacts the Intention to use Telehealth systems, as the p-value is less than 0.05.
5: The Intention to use has a significant impact on Actual use as the p-value is less than 0.05.

Table 17.2 Amos output extract: standardised regression estimates of the hypothesis tested

No	*Hypothesis*	*Path coefficient value*	*P-values*	*Supported/ Not supported*
H1	The Perceived ease of use has a significant impact on Perceived Usefulness	0.911	0.000	Supported
H2	Perceived Usefulness has a significant impact on the Perceived value	0.805	0.000	Supported
H3	The Perceived value has a significant impact on the Intention to use	0.250	0.000	Supported
H4	Perceived Usefulness has a significant impact on the Intention to use	0.220	0.000	Supported
H5	The Perceived ease of use has a significant impact on the Intention to use	0.280	0.000	Supported
H6	The Intention to use has a significantly lesser moderate impact on Actual use	0.801	0.000	Supported

P-value shows the significance of the estimation. If the P-value is less than 0.05, the hypothesis is supported, and we conclude that the independent variable has a significant effect on the dependent variable.

17.10 CONCLUSION

Here the suggested structural equation model says Usefulness is effecting "ease of use" and perceived value, which in turn affects "intention to use" with the following observations based on statistical results impact of "usefulness" on "ease of use" is significant, the impact of "usefulness" on "perceived value" is significant, the impact of "ease of use" on "intention to use" is significant, the impact of "perceived value" on "intention to use" is significant, very high impact of "usefulness" on "ease of use", very high impact of "usefulness" on "perceived value". So, it may be concluded that the SEM model is a fit.

The appropriate coefficient of statistical dispersion value of 2.408 also obtains the mode fit. The RMSEA (default model) value is 0.042 which is less than 0.05; therefore, the error is exceptionally minimal. Hence, it is proven that demonstrated structural equation model is a fit. Hence, because the error is low and goodness of fit is exceptionally high, the suggested structural equation model is fit.

17.10.1 Results concerning telehealth systems usage

Easy to use Applications design is the fundamental and sufficient demand of digital device consumers. Straightforward and user-friendly interface design is a crucial component in producing practical and convenient experiences in Apps.

To a considerable degree, app usefulness is a big incentive in Apps-based service adoption. Because of the necessity of giving customers more efficiency, pleasant interface design and appealing display are also vital in raising customers' attention. Additionally, the ubiquitous features of Telehealth applications should be effectively leveraged. Delivering real-time and up-to-date information is crucial in enhancing the efficiency of the application's purchasing experience.

Straightforward and user-friendly interface design is crucial in producing practical and convenient buying experiences in Apps.

To a considerable degree, Apps usefulness is a big incentive in Telehealth Apps-consumption adoption. Because of the necessity of giving customers more efficiency in Apps and other IOT devices (Internet of Things Devices), telehealth services providers are encouraged to supply a wide variety of service information in precise category categorisation. Apart from a pleasant interface design, an appealing display of applications is also vital in raising customers' attention. Additionally, the ubiquitous features of digital devices should be effectively leveraged.

17.10.2 Limitations

The study is mainly based on consumers' perception of using technology-based services related to Telehealth systems using mainly Smartphones/

Tablets and their applications. The other limitations are that the sample considered was only 200. In contrast, it could be increased, and geographical location was considered Uttar Pradesh districts, so more regions could be covered to gain a more valuable inference. Future research is recommended in other digital devices and can be spread to the entire nation.

BIBLIOGRAPHY

Lee, P. A. (2018, July 13). Patients' perception of using telehealth for type 2 diabetes management: a phenomenological study. Retrieved from bmchealthservres.biomedcentral.com: https://bmchealthservres.biomedcentral.com/articles/10.1186/

Mechanic, O. J. (2022, September 12). www.ncbi.nlm.nih.gov. Retrieved from ncbi: https://www.ncbi.nlm.nih.gov/books/NBK459384/

IJERPH. (n.d.). Use of telemedicine technology among general practitioners during COVID-19: A modified technology acceptance model study in Poland. Retrieved falseMarch 27, 2023, from https://www.mdpi.com/1660-4601/19/17/10937

JMIR (n.d.). Medical informatics—Using an extended technology acceptance model to understand the factors influencing telehealth utilization after flattening the COVID-19 curve in South Korea: Cross-sectional survey study. Retrieved false-March 27, 2023, from https://medinform.jmir.org/2021/1/e25435/

Lee, P. A., Greenfield, G., & Pappas, Y. (2018). Patients' perception of using telehealth for type 2 diabetes management: A phenomenological study. *BMC Health Services Research*, 18(1), 549. https://doi.org/10.1186/s12913-018-3353-x

Mayo Clinic. (n.d.). Managing your health in the age of Wi-Fi. *Mayo Clinic.* Retrieved falseMarch 27, 2023, from https://www.mayoclinic.org/healthy-lifestyle/consumer-health/in-depth/telehealth/art-20044878

Márquez, G., Astudillo, H., & Taramasco, C. (2020). Security in telehealth systems from a software engineering viewpoint: A systematic mapping study. *IEEE Access*, 8, 10933–10950. https://doi.org/10.1109/ACCESS.2020.2964988

Parmanto, B., Pulantara, I. W., Schutte, J. L., Saptono, A., & McCue, M. P. (2013). An integrated telehealth system for remote administration of an adult autism assessment. *Telemedicine and E-Health*, 19(2), 88–94. https://doi.org/10.1089/tmj.2012.0104

Rossow, R. (2018, August 15). The different types of telehealth. *ISalus*. https://isalushealthcare.com/blog/the-different-types-of-telehealth/

Seto, E., Smith, D., Jacques, M., & Morita, P. P. (2019). Opportunities and challenges of telehealth in remote communities: Case study of the Yukon telehealth system. *JMIR Medical Informatics*, 7(4), e11353. https://doi.org/10.2196/11353

Ingenta Connect. (n.d.). The adoption of a telehealth system: The integration of extended .... *Ingenta Connect*. Retrieved falseMarch 27, 2023, from https://www.ingentaconnect.com/contentone/asp/jmihi/2014/00000004/00000003/art00019

Tsai, C.-H. (2014). Integrating social capital theory, social cognitive theory, and the technology acceptance model to explore a behavioral model of telehealth systems. *International Journal of Environmental Research and Public Health*, 11(5), Article 5. https://doi.org/10.3390/ijerph110504905

Wang, C., Lu, W., Narayanan, M. R., Redmond, S. J., & Lovell, N. H. (2015). Low-power technologies for wearable telecare and telehealth systems: A review. *Biomedical Engineering Letters*, 5(1), 1–9. https://doi.org/10.1007/s13534-015-0174-2

Zhou, M., Zhao, L., Kong, N., Campy, K. S., Qu, S., & Wang, S. (2019). Factors influencing behavior intentions to telehealth by Chinese elderly: An extended TAM model. *International Journal of Medical Informatics*, 126, 118–127. https://doi.org/10.1016/j.ijmedinf.2019.04.001

Telemedicine in India. (n.d.). Retrieved falseMarch 28, 2023, from https://www.doconline.com/for-business/blog/telemedicine-india

Chapter 18

The quest for novel drugs against COVID-19: In silico study

Shalini Prajapati, Lubna Zeenat, Satyam Sangeet, Arshad Khan, and Khushhali M. Pandey

18.1 INTRODUCTION

Major Corona Virus (CoV) outbreaks associated with mild to severe human airway infections include (Coelho et al., 2022) the severe acute respiratory syndrome coronavirus (SARS-CoV-1) (Chathappady House et al., 2021) discovered in 2002 (Baxi & Saxena, 2020), Middle East respiratory syndrome coronavirus (MERS-CoV) discovered in 2012 (Zaki et al., 2012) (Antonio et al., 2003), and the other novel coronavirus (2019-nCoV), first diagnosed in 2019 in Wuhan, China (Lan et al., 2020) (Romano et al., 2020) (Voto et al., 2020). In terms of transmission rate and case fatality rate, the 2019-nCoV has already surpassed all previous coronavirus's records (Ong et al., 2020) (Zhou et al., 2020). It later infected 32.4 million people in the world till August 2021 (*Coronavirus Update (Live): 131,384,646 Cases and 2,859,657 Deaths from COVID-19 Virus Pandemic – Worldometer*, n.d.). The evolutionary studies have assisted in building advanced techniques for diagnostic as well as improved therapeutic drugs and vaccines for researchers (Agarwal et al., 2020). SARS-CoV-2 is a positive sense RNA virus composed of four major infective components: spike protein (S), membrane protein (M), nucleocapsid protein(N), envelope protein (E) (Lan et al., 2020) (Mittal et al., 2020) (Chathappady House et al., 2021).

The S proteins are considered to use the ACE2 (Angiotensin Converting Enzyme-2) membrane-bound receptor of the host's cell and many proteases for the activation of the S1 subunit (Mittal et al., 2020; Omolo et al., 2020). The spike protein's receptor binding domain (RBD) is mainly responsible for binding with its host receptors, Angiotensin Converting Enzyme 2 (ACE2). Much unlike SARS-CoV-1, LYS417 in SARS-CoV-2 interacts with ACE2's ASP30. This contributes to the electrostatic potential on the RBD surface (Lan et al., 2020; Tian et al., 2020; Walls et al., 2020), thus preventing 2019-nCoV spike protein from binding to human ACE2 receptors which are the most promising target for developing a novel therapeutic drug. Potential drugs such as nelfinavir, rupintrivir, lopinavir, remdesivir, indinavir, cobicistat, caspofungin acetate, lopinavir, atazanavir, etc. (Rismanbaf, 2020) with effective records (against SARS and MERS) are also being used in the treatment. Interestingly,

 DOI: 10.1201/9781003536352-18

several approved drugs against hepatitis C virus (HCV), another enveloped (-) ssRNA virus (paritaprevir, simeprevir, grazoprevir, and velpatasvir) as well as drugs against transmissible diseases, cancer, or other diseases have also been identified as candidates against SARS-CoV-2 (Nand et al., 2020).

All the commercial drugs after repurposing are effective against SARS-COV-2, but these drugs too have the potential to cause several side effects especially to patients already suffering from life-threatening diseases. Bioactive substances called phytochemicals are present in plants and are well-known for having a variety of pharmacological characteristics, such as antiviral activity. Numerous investigations have concentrated on determining if phytochemicals can prevent important viral proteins from being involved in the entrance and reproduction of SARS-CoV-2, the virus that causes COVID-19. In silico research offers insightful information on possible interactions between phytochemicals and viral proteins, which are eventually added into in vitro and in vivo tests and are necessary to confirm these results. In addition, a comprehensive assessment of the pharmacokinetic characteristics, safety profile, and bioavailability of phytochemicals is necessary to determine their eligibility as possible COVID-19 treatments. Among other reasons, the pathophysiology of lung damage involves inflammation, which makes phytochemicals desirable options for novel compounds to combat coronaviruses. Several chemicals, including gallic acid, quercetin, naringin, capsaicin, and psychotrine, which were isolated from medicinal plants using GC/MS and HPLC, have been discovered in a recent study as important reservoirs for prospective antiviral medicines targeting COVID-19. Quercetin, kaempferol, myricetin, apigenin, and resveratrol have been shown in another study to be beneficial against coronaviruses. Furthermore, alkaloids have antiviral qualities against coronaviruses; lycorine, an indolizidine alkaloid that was extracted from *Lycoris radiata* (L'Hér) Herb, which is one such alkaloid that shows remarkable effectiveness. Literature studies have reported several phytochemicals such as the extract of *Ocimum sanctum* being effective against the main protease protein, isoflavone extract (plant: *Psorothamnus arborescens*) against 3-chymotrypsin-like protease (Tahir Ul Qamar et al., 2020) and *Alpinia galanga* and *Caesalpinia sappan* extracts against both protease and RBD of S-protein (Basu et al., 2020). Another study reported on the review that focuses on herbal preparation and different beneficial aspects of herbal medicine with antiviral activity, and these herbal drugs are proposed to be used for the treatment of Coronavirus disease (Biradar & Tyagi, 2021). Yet another literature study suggested that in a molecular docking investigation with its human receptor ACE2, five phytochemicals, which are from a flavonoid and anthraquinone subclass, were chosen for SARS-CoV2, spike protein (Basu et al., n.d.). An additional literature study of plant-based product reported against the three protein targets of corona virus which showed best binding affinity between glucoraphanin: spike protein, alpha amyrin: hemagglutinin, and beta-sitosterol: nucleocapsid (Biradar & Tyagi, 2021).

The major question that this work targets is to explore the binding affinity of natural phytochemicals with the RBD domain and to examine the important residue involved in the binding process. In silico studies evaluate the mechanism of phytochemical interaction to explore the potential antiviral candidates. Another question that the current work focuses on is to evaluate the pharmacological characteristics of the selected phytochemicals to analyze whether they are on par with the current medication being administered to the patients.

18.2 MATERIAL AND METHOD

18.2.1 Preparation of protein and ligands

The 3D structure of spike protein (PDB ID: 6VSB) was retrieved using Protein Data Bank (Burley et al., 2021) and visualized using PyMol (PyMOL | Pymol.Org, n.d.) (Figure 18.1.). The structures of five approved synthetic drugs (Standard drug) and 20 phytochemicals were retrieved from PubChem (Kim et al., 2021) Databases (Table 18.1). The 2D structures were converted into 3D (PDB format) using Open Babel (O'Boyle et al., 2011). Further, all the 3D structures were energy minimized using Chimera (http://www.cgl.ucsf.edu/chimera) (Pettersen et al., 2004) by keeping the default parameters same (steepest descent steps: 100, steepest descent step size (Å), conjugate gradient steps: 10 conjugate gradient steps size (Å): 0.02 update interval: 10).

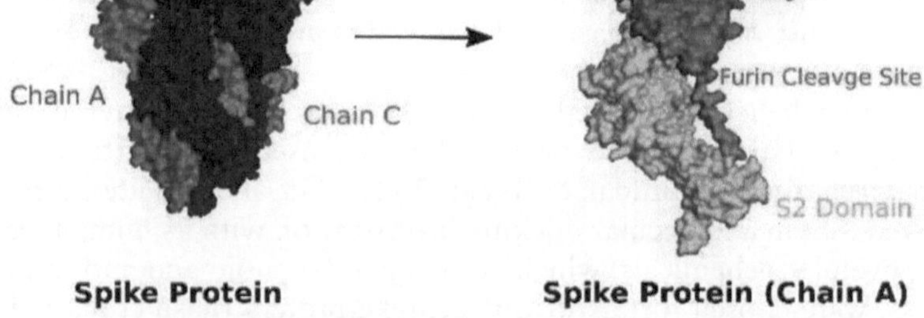

Figure 18.1 Molecular surface representation of trimeric spike protein of SARS-CoV-2 (1 up 2 down state) showing (a) three chains (A, B, C) and (b) single chain showing different regions of spike protein. The regions are color-coded according to their labelling.

18.2.2 Molecular docking

Docking of minimized protein and ligands was done using a Patchdock server (Duhovny et al., 2002; Sangeet & Khan, n.d.; Schneidman-Duhovny et al., 2005) and parameters such as clustering RMSF (4.0) and complex type were set at default. The results obtained consisted of a list of potential complexes sorted by shape complementarity criteria followed by visualization

Table 18.1 Molecular weight, the structure of standard drugs, and top hit phytochemicals used in the current study

Name	*Molecular weight (g/mol)*	*Structure*
Standard drugs		
Simeprevir	749.9	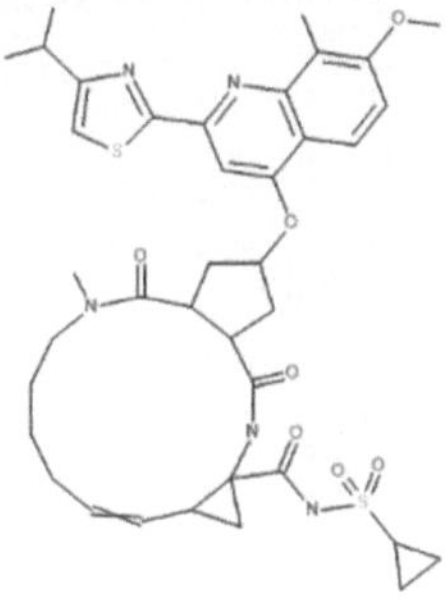
Paritaprevir	765.9	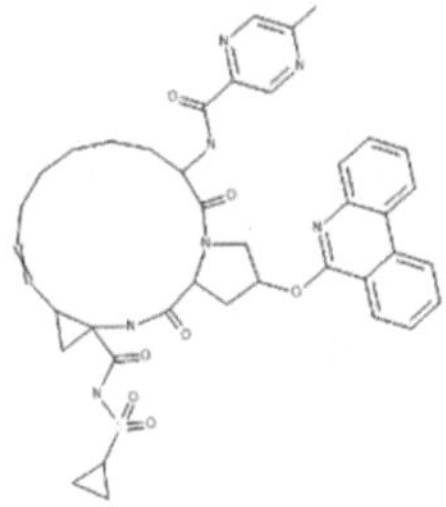
Grazoprevir	766.9	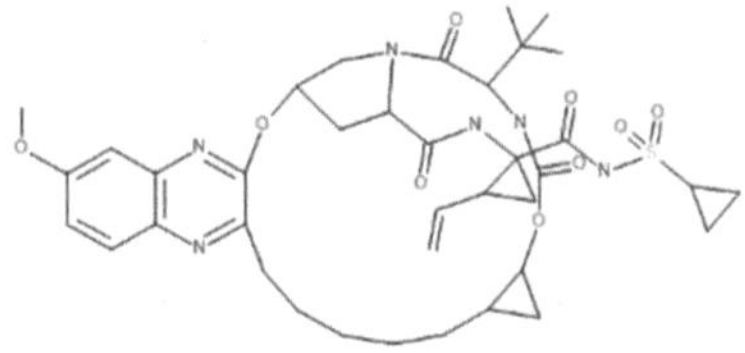
Teniposide	656.7	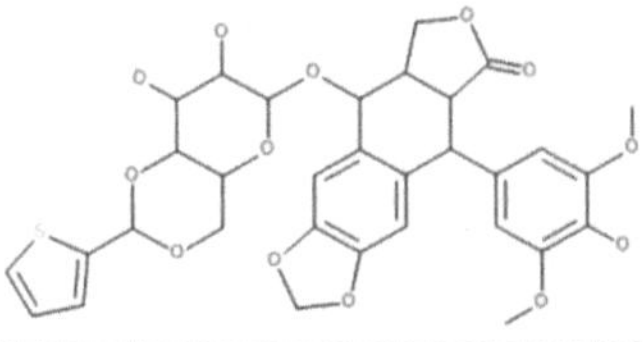

(Continued)

Table 18.1 (Continued)

Name	*Molecular weight (g/mol)*	*Structure*
Velpatasvir	883	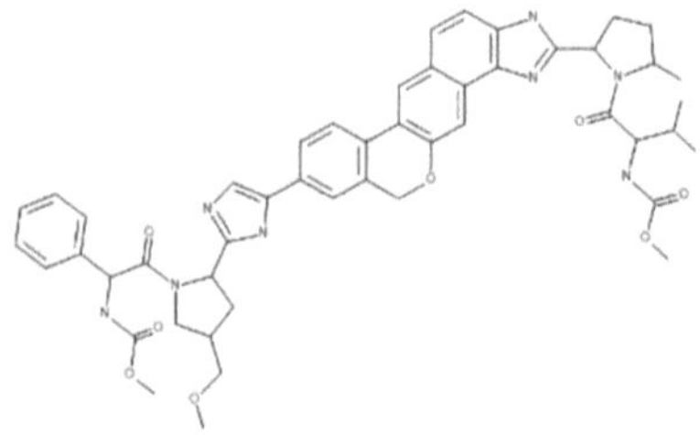
Phytochemicals		
Hexadecanoic Acid	256.42	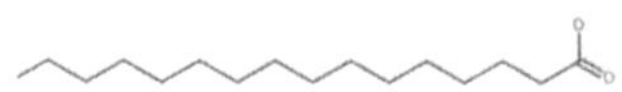
Caryophyllene oxide	220.35	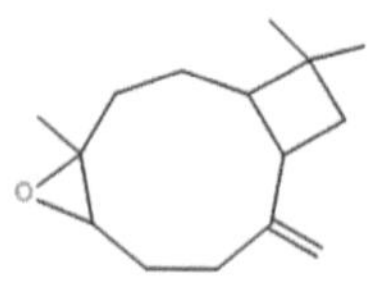
Menthol	156.26	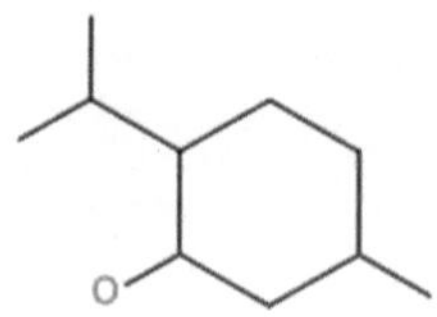
Methyleugenol	178.23	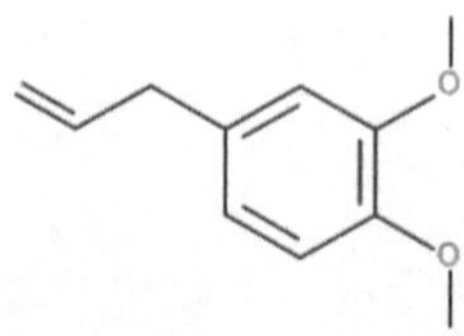
Sitosterol	414.7	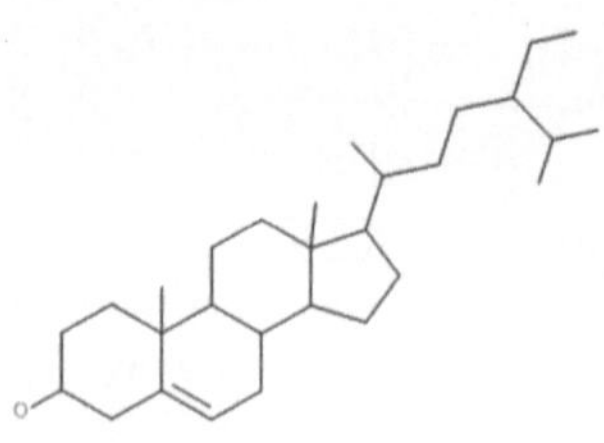

in Ligplot (Daina et al., 2017; Das et al., 2022). The values were tabulated based on molecular interaction with the key active residues.

18.2.3 Molecular dynamic simulation

Molecular dynamic simulation of the docked protein-ligand complex was carried out using CABS-flex 2.0 (http://biocomp.chem.uw.edu.pl/

CABSflex2) (Kuriata et al., 2018; Sangeet et al., 2022). The values were set to the default parameters. The results obtained were downloaded as an Excel file. Jupyter Notebook and Matplotlib Python programs were used for plotting the RMSF (root mean square fluctuation) curves.

18.2.4 Drug likeness of phytochemicals

The phytochemicals were screened against the drugs by analyzing their Lipinski's value (http://www.scfbio-iitd.res.in/software/drugdesign/lipinski.jsp). Lipinski's rule of five (RO5) is a set of parameters that allows early screening of drug-like properties of the phytochemicals and commercial drugs.

18.2.5 ADME/T analysis

Absorption, digestion, metabolism, excretion, and toxicity studies were performed using SWISS-ADME server (http://www.swissadme.ch/) (Daina et al., 2017). The structures of the drug and the phytochemicals were uploaded, and the corresponding drug likeness features such as lipophilicity, solubility, and drug likeness score were obtained.

18.3 RESULTS

18.3.1 Molecular docking

The binding affinity between the receptor and ligand was determined based on the PatchDock score. High PatchDock score represents a better binding affinity. The active site residue interaction of RBD with ACE2 is communicated via Leu455, Phe486, Glu493, and Ser494. The commercial drugs were docked with the RBD of spike protein. All the standard drugs showed similar binding affinity with the RBD domain, but none showed interactions with the active site residues. Among 20 phytochemicals, sitosterol was identified as the major phytochemical with a docking score of 4800 and an ACE value of −199.28 kcal/mol. Sitosterol showed hydrogen bonding with Lys458 and Glu471 along with hydrophobic interactions with Pro479, Val483, Gly482, Cys480, Ile472, Gln474, Tyr473, and Arg457 (Figure 18.2). The interaction of other residues is represented in Table 18.2.

18.3.2 Molecular dynamic simulation

The docked complex of top hit phytochemicals and the standard drugs were subjected to 10 ns of molecular dynamic simulation with default parameters of simulation trajectory in CABS-Flex 2.0 (http://biocomp.

chem.uw.edu.pl/CABSflex1/index). The RMSF values obtained were plotted for each docked complex to analyze the residual fluctuation. Most of the interaction of RBD with synthetic drugs as well as phytochemicals was found in the range of 450–500 amino acids. Analyzing the RMSF curve of phytochemicals with respect to synthetic drugs, the results indicated a stable binding affinity of methyleugenol with its RMSF fluctuation being lowest. The RMSF characteristic of methyleugenol resembles the behavior of velpatasvir (Figure 18.3).

18.3.3 Lipinski's analysis

Drug-likeness characteristic is significant in testing the ability of a molecule to act as a drug. With Lipinski's analysis, synthetic drugs and screened phytochemicals were analyzed for drugable properties. Approved drugs showed a maximum of four violations in velpatasvir, three violations in teniposide, and one violation in simeprevir, paritaprevir, and grazoprevir. On the other hand, among the best three phytochemicals, only a single violation was identified in hexadecanoic acid and the rest of phytochemicals followed all the parameters (Table 18.3).

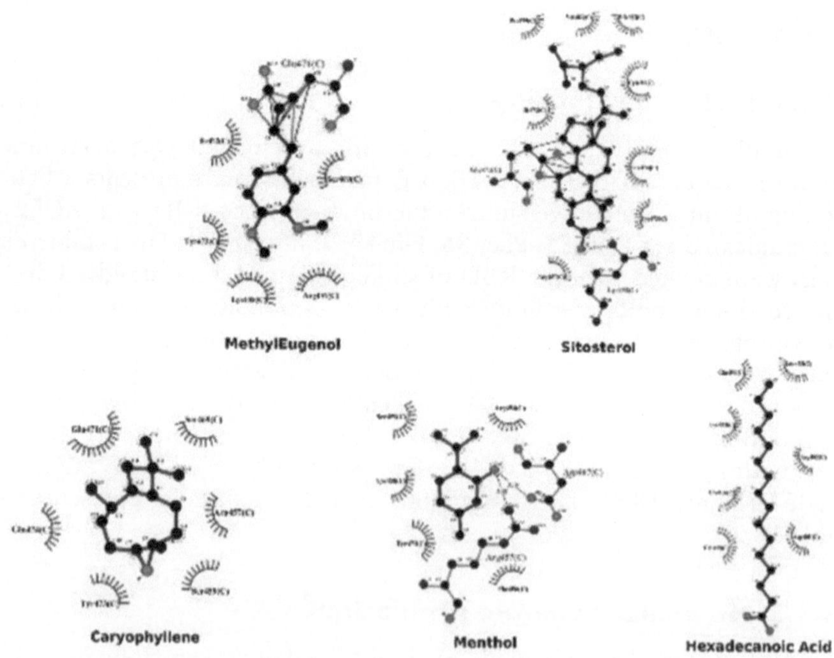

Figure 18.2 Interaction of phytochemicals with the residues of the RBD domain of the spike protein.

Table 18.2 Molecular docking results of protein-drug and protein-phytochemical interactions

Ligand	*Patchdock score*	*ACE (atomic contact energy) (kcal/mol)*	*Interacting residues*
Standard drugs			
Simeprevir	6212	−195.29	Phe347,Thr345,Tyr451, Leu441,Asp442,Arg509, Lys444,Asn448,Asn450, Arg346, Leu452,Ala352, Ser349,Asn354,Ala348
Paritaprevir	6246	−264.74	Arg346,Thr345, Leu441, Asn440, Ser443, Lys444, Asp442,Tyr449,Asn448, Phe347,Tyr451
Grazoprevir	5412	−150.78	Glu471, Gln474, Cys480, Ile472, Asn460,Tyr473,Tyr421, Arg457, Ser469
Teniposide	5130	−137.28	Tyr473, Glu471, Ile472, Ser459, Lys462,Arg457,Tyr421
Velpatasvir	6730	−205.23	Ile468,Arg466,Asp467,Arg457, Lys458,Tyr473, Ile472, Gln474, Glu471,Arg454, Ser469
Phytochemicals			
Hexadecanoic acid	4214	−1.80	Leu455, Gln493,Tyr453,Arg403, Glu406, Gln409,Asp405
Caryophyllene oxide	3260	−92.42	Ser469, Glu471, Gln474,Tyr473, Ser459,Arg457
Menthol	2768	−34.81	Arg454, Ser459, Lys458,Tyr473, Phe456,Arg457,Asp467
Methyleugenol	3118	−89.26	Glu471, Ile472,Tyr473, Lys458, Arg457, Ser469
Sitosterol	4800	−199.28	Gly482,Val483, Pro479, Ile472, Glu471,Arg457, Lys458, Tyr473, Gln474, Cys480

Notes: The table summarizes the docking results of standard drugs and top hit phytochemicals in terms of patchDock score and ACE value.

18.3.4 ADME/T analysis

ADME/T analysis was performed to identify the absorption, distribution, metabolism excretion, and toxicity of the screened phytochemicals because Lipinski's rule of five is not that strict a parameter. All synthetic drugs showed many violations in drug likeness properties Such as Lipinski's rule of five (RO5), Ghose filter rule, Veber rule, Egan rule, and Muegge rule.

On the other hand, the phytochemicals showed maximum drug likeness properties. Lipophilicity (Log P) is an important parameter that defines the absorption of a drug, higher the Log P value lower the absorption, among the five commercial drugs, three have lower values of Log P as compared to phytochemicals. Molecular weight and TPSA (topological polar surface area) values define the oral bioavailability and optimal cell permeability of a compound. Lower these physiochemical properties better the bioavailability and cell permeability. As opposed to synthetic drugs, selected phytochemicals have lower values for these parameters. Synthetic accessibility (SA) is a part of medicinal chemistry, which confirms the feasibility of the chemical synthesis of the phytochemicals, SA value = 1; denotes synthesis, SA = 10; denotes challenging synthesis (Table 18.3).

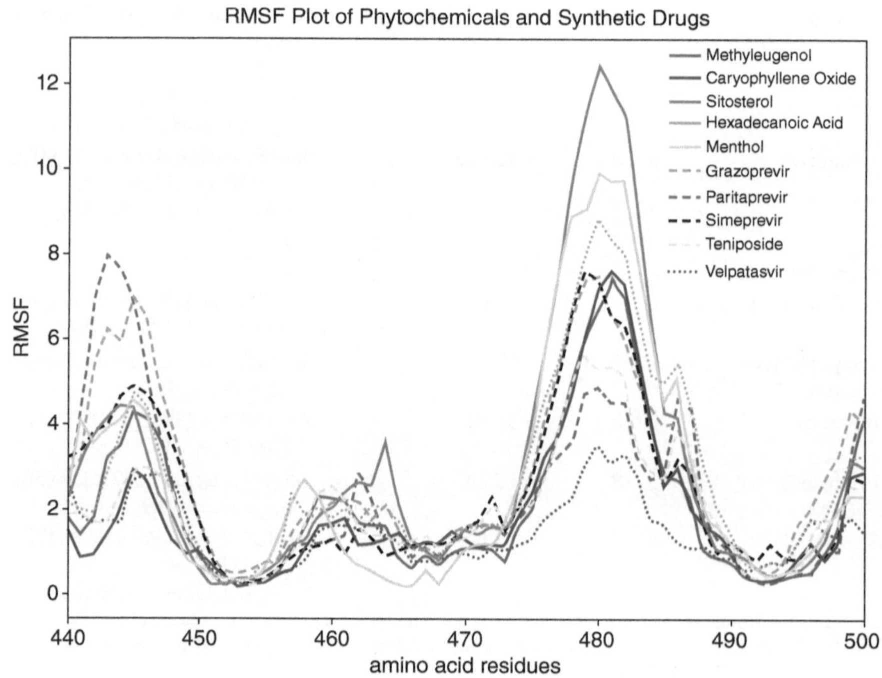

Figure 18.3 Root mean square fluctuation (RMSF) graph plot to analyze the residual fluctuation in between (450–500) amino acid residues of top hit phytochemicals and synthetic drugs.

18.4 DISCUSSION AND CONCLUSION

The continuous spread of the coronavirus and emergence of new mutants, development of novel drug candidates to inhibit the spread of the virus garners utmost attention in recent times (Sinha et al., 2023). The interaction of spike proteins of coronavirus with the human ACE2 protein (hACE2) governs the way coronavirus spreads its infectivity (Benton et al., 2020). Understanding the mechanism of coronavirus infectivity helps us to target different potential sites in order to inhibit the viral spread (Sangeet & Khan, 2022). RBD domain being one of them. Various drugs are being targeted at RBD domain considering the mutation rate of RBD and its major involvement with ACE2 attachment. These commercial drugs, being good candidates for their inhibiting properties, pose some serious threat in the form of side effects to the terminally ill patients. Thus, a new and novel approach is required to compensate for the shortcomings of the commercial drugs. Phytochemicals from natural plant sources can act as a substitute for the commercial drugs because of their natural antiviral properties. Medicinal plants have long seen the usage for treating different viral and bacterial diseases. The current investigation explored the properties of the natural medicinal plants to examine their potential as potent antiviral candidates. Molecular docking studies revealed the binding affinity of the top hit phytochemicals with the active residue region of RBD domain of the spike protein of SARS-CoV-2. The binding affinity of velpatasvir showed the highest interaction in terms of PatchDock score and ACE value. Although the interaction was not observed with the key residues, but the commercial application of the drug suggests a positive response function in terms of inhibition of RBD and ACE2 interaction. Sitosterol showed the highest binding affinity with the RBD domain along with other top hit phytochemicals and resembled a similar binding pattern as that of the standard drugs. Based on the docking examinations, molecular simulation studies suggested a stable interaction of the phytochemicals which is represented in the RMSF plot. RMSF plot shows a residual fluctuation which is a more specific understanding of the stability of the ligand with the protein. RMSF fluctuations of the top hit phytochemicals also resembled a similar pattern as that of the standard drugs. Based on these results, it becomes evident that the selected phytochemicals do have a potential to act as a potent inhibitor of RBD and ACE2 interaction. Clinical relevance is important for any kind of drug before it becomes available for the general public. ADMET studies revealed the drug likeness relevance of these phytochemicals where the phytochemicals perform better than the standard drugs by following the Lipinski's rule of five and showing a better ADMET analysis than the standard drugs. Thus, from the current study, it becomes relevant that natural medicinal plants provide useful phytochemicals that can be synthesized and used as a better alternative as compared with standard drugs which are chemically synthesized. This ethnobotanical approach shows the diverse characteristics of these phytochemicals acting as antiviral and antibacterial agents. With the current global situation, it becomes more relevant to find and develop novel drug candidates to target emerging viral and bacterial diseases.

Table 18.3 Lipinski's and ADMET analysis of the standard drugs and the top hit phytochemicals

Property	*SP*	*PP*	*GP*	*TP*	*VP*	*HA*	*CO*	*MT*	*ME*	*SS*
Molecular Mass	312	312	312	656	882	256	220	156	178	414
H-bond donor	5	5	5	3	4	1	0	1	0	1
H-bond acceptor	6	6	6	13	14	2	1	1	2	1
Log P	4.24	2.76	3.17	1.97	5.02	5.20	3.68	2.58	2.58	7.19
GI absorption	Low	Low	Low	Low	Low	High	High	High	High	Low
BS	0.17	0.17	0.17	0.17	0.17	0.85	0.55	0.55	0.55	0.55
SA	7.16	6.97	8.31	6.48	7.49	2.31	4.35	2.63	1.71	6.30
Skin Permeation	−7.46	−7.67	−7.61	−9.43	−7.31	−2.77	−5.12	−4.84	−5.60	−2.20

Notes: SP – Simeprevir; PP – Paritaprevir; GP – Grazoprevir; TP – Teniposide.
VP – Velpatasvir; HA – Hexadecanoic Acid; CO – Caryophyllene Oxide.
MT – Menthol; ME – Methyleugenol; SS – Sitosterol.
BS – Bioavailability score; SA – Synthetic Accessibility.

ACKNOWLEDGMENT

We would like to thank the Department of Biological Science and Engineering, MANIT, Bhopal, for providing us the infrastructure to carry out the in silico studies.

CONFLICT OF INTEREST

The authors declare no conflict of interest.

REFERENCES

Agarwal, K. M., Mohapatra, S., Sharma, P., Sharma, S., Bhatia, D., & Mishra, A. (2020). Study and overview of the novel corona virus disease (COVID-19). *Sensors International*, *1*, 100037. https://doi.org/10.1016/j.sintl.2020.100037

Antonio, G. E., Wong, K. T., Hui, D. S. C., Lee, N., Yuen, E. H. Y., Wu, A., Chung, S. S. C., Sung, J. J. Y., & Ahuja, A. T. (2003). Imaging of severe acute respiratory syndrome in Hong Kong. *American Journal of Roentgenology*, *181*(1), 11–17. https://doi.org/10.2214/ajr.181.1.1810011

Fan, J., Fu, A., & Zhang, L. (2019). Progress in molecular docking. *Quantitative Biology*, *7*, 83–89.

Basu, A., Sarkar, A., & Maulik, U. (2020). Molecular docking study of potential phytochemicals and their effects on the complex of SARS-CoV2 spike protein and human ACE2. *Scientific Reports*, *10*(1), 17699. https://doi.org/10.1038/s41598-020-74715-4

Baxi, P., & Saxena, S. K. (2020). Emergence and reemergence of severe acute respiratory syndrome (SARS) coronaviruses. In S. K. Saxena (Ed.), *Coronavirus disease 2019 (COVID-19): Epidemiology, pathogenesis, diagnosis, and therapeutics* (pp. 151–163). Springer. https://doi.org/10.1007/978-981-15-4814-7_13

Benton, D. J., Wrobel, A. G., Xu, P., Roustan, C., Martin, S. R., Rosenthal, P. B., Skehel, J. J., & Gamblin, S. J. (2020). Receptor binding and priming of the spike protein of SARS-CoV-2 for membrane fusion. *Nature*, *588*(7837), 327–330. https://doi.org/10.1038/s41586-020-2772-0

Biradar, S. K., & Tyagi, C. K. (2021). Immunomodulatory activity of alcoholic extracts of Tinospora cordifolia stem. *Research Journal of Pharmacognosy and Phytochemistry*, *13*(2), 73–77. https://doi.org/10.52711/0975-4385.2021.00012

Burley, S. K., Bhikadiya, C., Bi, C., Bittrich, S., Chen, L., Crichlow, G. V., Christie, C. H., Dalenberg, K., Di Costanzo, L., Duarte, J. M., Dutta, S., Feng, Z., Ganesan, S., Goodsell, D. S., Ghosh, S., Green, R. K., Guranovic, V., Guzenko, D., Hudson, B. P., … Zhuravleva, M. (2021). RCSB protein data bank: Powerful new tools for exploring 3D structures of biological macromolecules for basic and applied research and education in fundamental biology, biomedicine, biotechnology, bioengineering and energy sciences. *Nucleic Acids Research*, *49*(1), D437–D451. https://doi.org/10.1093/nar/gkaa1038

Chathappady House, N. N., Palissery, S., & Sebastian, H. (2021). Corona viruses: A review on SARS, MERS and COVID-19. *Microbiology Insights*, *14*, 117863612110024. https://doi.org/10.1177/11786361211002481

Coelho, R. M., Periolo, N., Duhalde, C. P., Alonso, D. O., Bellomo, C. M., Corazza, M., Iglesias, A. A., & Martinez, V. P. (2022). Hantavirus pulmonary syndrome in a COVID-19 patient, Argentina, 2020. *Emerging Infectious Diseases*, *28*(4), 876–878. https://doi.org/10.3201/eid2804.211837

Coronavirus Update (Live): 131,384,646 Cases and 2,859,657 Deaths from COVID-19 Virus Pandemic—Worldometer. (n.d.).

Daina, A., Michielin, O., & Zoete, V. (2017). SwissADME: A free web tool to evaluate pharmacokinetics, drug-likeness and medicinal chemistry friendliness of small molecules. *Scientific Reports*, *7*(1), 42717. https://doi.org/10.1038/srep42717

Das, S. K., Deka, S. J., Paul, D., Gupta, D. D., Das, T. J., Maravi, D. K., Tag, H., & Hui, P. K. (2022). *In-silico* based identification of phytochemicals from *Houttuynia cordata* Thunb. As potential inhibitors for overexpressed HER2 and VEGFR2 cancer genes. *Journal of Biomolecular Structure and Dynamics*, *40*(15), 6857–6867. https://doi.org/10.1080/07391102.2021.1891136

Duhovny, D., Nussinov, R., & Wolfson, H. J. (2002). Efficient unbound docking of rigid molecules. In R. Guigó & D. Gusfield (Eds.), *Algorithms in bioinformatics* (Vol. 2452, pp. 185–200). Springer Berlin Heidelberg. https://doi.org/10.1007/3-540-45784-4_14

Kim, S., Chen, J., Cheng, T., Gindulyte, A., He, J., He, S., Li, Q., Shoemaker, B. A., Thiessen, P. A., Yu, B., Zaslavsky, L., Zhang, J., & Bolton, E. E. (2021). PubChem in 2021: New data content and improved web interfaces. *Nucleic Acids Research*, *49*(D1), D1388–D1395. https://doi.org/10.1093/nar/gkaa971

Kuriata, A., Gierut, A. M., Oleniecki, T., Ciemny, M. P., Kolinski, A., Kurcinski, M., & Kmiecik, S. (2018). CABS-flex 2.0: A web server for fast simulations of flexibility of protein structures. *Nucleic Acids Research*, *46*(W1), W338–W343. https://doi.org/10.1093/nar/gky356

Lan, J., Ge, J., Yu, J., Shan, S., Zhou, H., Fan, S., Zhang, Q., Shi, X., Wang, Q., Zhang, L., & Wang, X. (2020). Structure of the SARS-CoV-2 spike receptor-binding domain bound to the ACE2 receptor. *Nature*, *581*(7807), 215–220. https://doi.org/10.1038/s41586-020-2180-5

Mittal, A., Manjunath, K., Ranjan, R. K., Kaushik, S., Kumar, S., & Verma, V. (2020). COVID-19 pandemic: Insights into structure, function, and hACE2 receptor recognition by SARS-CoV-2. *PLOS Pathogens*, *16*(8), e1008762. https://doi.org/10.1371/journal.ppat.1008762

Nand, M., Maiti, P., Joshi, T., Chandra, S., Pande, V., Kuniyal, J. C., & Ramakrishnan, M. A. (2020). Virtual screening of anti-HIV1 compounds against SARS-CoV-2: Machine learning modeling, chemoinformatics and molecular dynamics simulation based analysis. *Scientific Reports*, *10*(1), 20397. https://doi.org/10.1038/s41598-020-77524-x

O'Boyle, N. M., Banck, M., James, C. A., Morley, C., Vandermeersch, T., & Hutchison, G. R. (2011). Open Babel: An open chemical toolbox. *Journal of Cheminformatics*, *3*(1), 33. https://doi.org/10.1186/1758-2946-3-33

Omolo, C. A., Soni, N., Fasiku, V. O., Mackraj, I., & Govender, T. (2020). Update on therapeutic approaches and emerging therapies for SARS-CoV-2 virus. *European Journal of Pharmacology*, *883*, 173348. https://doi.org/10.1016/j.ejphar.2020.173348

Ong, J. S. M., Tosoni, A., Kim, Y., Kissoon, N., & Murthy, S. (2020). Coronavirus disease 2019 in critically ill children: A narrative review of the literature*. *Pediatric Critical Care Medicine*, *21*(7), 662–666. https://doi.org/10.1097/PCC.0000000000002376

Pettersen, E. F., Goddard, T. D., Huang, C. C., Couch, G. S., Greenblatt, D. M., Meng, E. C., & Ferrin, T. E. (2004). UCSF Chimera—A visualization system for exploratory research and analysis. *Journal of Computational Chemistry*, *25*(13), 1605–1612. https://doi.org/10.1002/jcc.20084

PyMOL | pymol.org. (n.d.). Retrieved May 23, 2024, from https://pymol.org/

Rismanbaf, A. (2020). Potential treatments for COVID-19; a narrative literature review. *Archives of Academic Emergency Medicine*, *8*(1), e29.

Romano, C. M., Chebabo, A., & Levi, J. E. (2020). Past, present, and future of COVID-19: A review. *Brazilian Journal of Medical and Biological Research*, *53*(9), e10475. https://doi.org/10.1590/1414-431x202010475

Mitra, S., Anjum, J., Muni, M., Das, R., Rauf, A., Islam, F., ... & Wilairatana, P. (2022). Exploring the journey of emodin as a potential neuroprotective agent: novel therapeutic insights with molecular mechanism of action. *Biomedicine & Pharmacotherapy*, *149*, 112877. https://doi.org/10.1016/j.biopha.2022.112877

Sangeet, S., & Khan, A. (2022). Exploratory data analysis of genomic sequence of variants of SARS-CoV-2 reveals sequence divergence and mutational localization. *Bioinformatics and Biology Insights*, *16*, 117793222211262. https://doi.org/10.1177/11779322221126294

Sangeet, S., Pawar, S., Nawani, N., Junnarkar, M., & Gaikwad, S. (2022). Computational approach to attenuate virulence of pseudomonas aeruginosa through bioinspired silver nanoparticles. *3 Biotech*, *12*(11), 317. https://doi.org/10.1007/s13205-022-03367-0

Schneidman-Duhovny, D., Inbar, Y., Nussinov, R., & Wolfson, H. J. (2005). PatchDock and SymmDock: Servers for rigid and symmetric docking. *Nucleic Acids Research*, *33*(Web Server), W363–W367. https://doi.org/10.1093/nar/gki481

Sinha, A., Sangeet, S., & Roy, S. (2023). Evolution of sequence and structure of SARS-CoV-2 spike protein: A dynamic perspective. *ACS Omega*, *8*(26), 23283–23304. https://doi.org/10.1021/acsomega.3c00944

Tahir Ul Qamar, M., Alqahtani, S. M., Alamri, M. A., & Chen, L.-L. (2020). Structural basis of SARS-CoV-2 3CLpro and anti-COVID-19 drug discovery from medicinal plants. *Journal of Pharmaceutical Analysis*, *10*(4), 313–319. https://doi.org/10.1016/j.jpha.2020.03.009

Tian, X., Li, C., Huang, A., Xia, S., Lu, S., Shi, Z., Lu, L., Jiang, S., Yang, Z., Wu, Y., & Ying, T. (2020). Potent binding of 2019 novel coronavirus spike protein by a SARS coronavirus-specific human monoclonal antibody. *Emerging Microbes & Infections*, *9*(1), 382–385. https://doi.org/10.1080/22221751.2020.1729069

Voto, C., Berkner, P., & Brenner, C. (2020). Overview of the pathogenesis and treatment of SARS-CoV-2 for clinicians: A comprehensive literature review. *Cureus*. https://doi.org/10.7759/cureus.10357

Walls, A. C., Park, Y.-J., Tortorici, M. A., Wall, A., McGuire, A. T., & Veesler, D. (2020). Structure, function, and antigenicity of the SARS-CoV-2 spike glycoprotein. *Cell*, *181*(2), 281–292.e6. https://doi.org/10.1016/j.cell.2020.02.058

Zaki, A. M., Van Boheemen, S., Bestebroer, T. M., Osterhaus, A. D. M. E., & Fouchier, R. A. M. (2012). Isolation of a novel coronavirus from a man with pneumonia in Saudi Arabia. *New England Journal of Medicine*, *367*(19), 1814–1820. https://doi.org/10.1056/NEJMoa1211721

Zhou, P., Yang, X.-L., Wang, X.-G., Hu, B., Zhang, L., Zhang, W., Si, H.-R., Zhu, Y., Li, B., Huang, C.-L., Chen, H.-D., Chen, J., Luo, Y., Guo, H., Jiang, R.-D., Liu, M.-Q., Chen, Y., Shen, X.-R., Wang, X., ... Shi, Z.-L. (2020). A pneumonia outbreak associated with a new coronavirus of probable bat origin. *Nature*, *579*(7798), 270–273. https://doi.org/10.1038/s41586-020-2Basu012-7

Chapter 19

Graph convolutional network for COVID-19 detection from X rays: Advancing accurate diagnosis

Pratyush Puri, Pawan Kumar Tiwari, Hritik Dubey, Prafull Pandey, Mohit Narayan Gupta, and Amit Kumar Tiwari

19.1 INTRODUCTION

One of the most important areas of research in the fight against the global pandemic brought on by the Novel Coronavirus 2019 is getting to know about Corona Virus utilising X-ray imaging [1, 2]. Since the disease spreads quickly and has disastrous impacts on public health, it is imperative that swift and accurate detection procedures be used. Because they can show distinctive patterns linked to the disease in the lungs, chest X-rays (CXRs) are now frequently used in the diagnosis of COVID-19 [3, 4]. However, the increased demand for CXR interpretations creates difficulties for labour-intensive and time-consuming diagnoses, which has led to the investigation of novel strategies to improve and expedite the detection process.

Deep Learning, a subfield of artificial intelligence, has demonstrated significant promise in improving medical imaging and diagnosis, notably the ability to identify the SARS Corona Virus from chest images [5–7]. Deep learning techniques can use advanced neural networks and machine learning algorithms to automate and speed up the detection of COVID-19 patterns in CXR. This could alleviate the workload on healthcare systems and frontline medical practitioners. Current research efforts are mostly focused on developing lightweight neural networks specifically designed for COVID-19 detection in CXR pictures, with the goal of balancing diagnostic accuracy with computing economy [8, 9]. The use of X-ray imaging in SARS-COVID-19 prediction is a crucial intersection between medical imaging and artificial intelligence that might have a significant impact on the efficacy and accuracy of this infectious illness diagnosis.

Due of the ongoing pandemic's worldwide effects, there is an increasing need for accurate and dependable diagnostic equipment. By examining complex patterns, deep learning algorithms provide a potential method for automating the identification of COVID-19 from chest X- ray pictures. For the checking of SARS-COVID-19, radiological characteristics on X-rays such as consolidation and ground-glass opacities are essential. Through the successful customisation of deep learning models to identify these patterns, researchers hope to improve both the speed and accuracy of detection [10, 11].

DOI: 10.1201/9781003536352-19

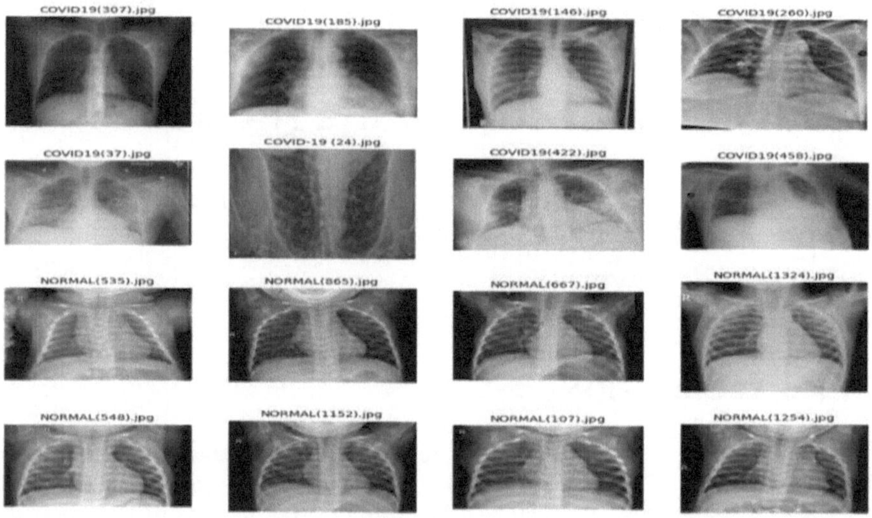

Figure 19.1 Different X-ray images in the dataset.

To balance computational efficiency with diagnostic accuracy, researchers are fine-tuning network architecture, kernel sizes, and pruning criteria. The objective is to develop a reliable method for correctly recognising COVID-19 from chest X-ray pictures by means of extensive testing on a variety of datasets, thereby offering a useful instrument for medical practitioners fighting the epidemic [12–14].Since asymptomatic people might unintentionally spread the virus, early detection is essential. New testing techniques, such as medical imaging such as X-rays, are being developed to overcome the shortcomings of existing diagnostics. Because COVID-19 affects the lungs, chest X-rays are important for identifying the virus.

19.2 RELATED WORKS

Several studies have recently used Machine Learning (ML) tools to fight the COVID-19 pandemic, demonstrating creative methods for early diagnosis and detection [15, 16]. To quickly predict SARS-COVID-19 pictures from X-ray (CXR) images, for instance, researchers have investigated integrating multi-level thresholding approaches with different classifiers [17]. SVM classifiers were able to detect COVID-19 patients from contrast-enhanced CXR pictures with up to 97% accuracy, according to these research' outstanding classification accuracies [18–20]. Furthermore, improved SVM classifiers, Random Forest, XG Boost, and Graph Convolutional Network for increased SARS-COVID-19 checking accuracy have been developed as a result of ML algorithm development [21–23].

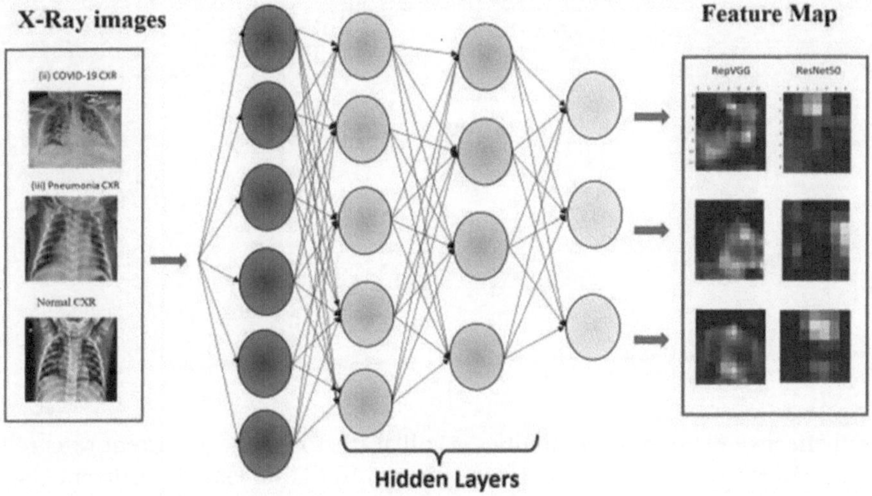

Figure 19.2 CNN—Network for image processing.

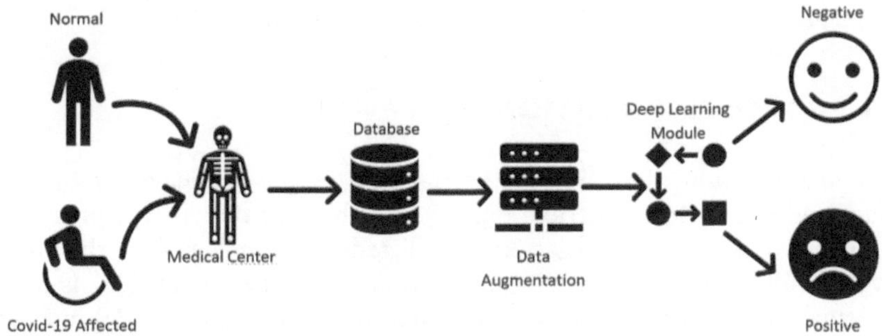

Figure 19.3 Architecture of the proposed system.

More complex models and strategies, such as ensemble models that combine CNN and long-short-term memory (LSTM) and Deep Learning (DL) architectures like Capsule Networks and EfficientNet, have emerged as ML methodologies for COVID-19 detection. These models demonstrate the potential of deep learning (DL) to transform medical imaging and illness diagnosis. They have been painstakingly constructed and optimised to analyse X-ray pictures with remarkable accuracy [14, 24]. Moreover, the successful diagnosis of COVID-19 from X-ray pictures through the integration of Generative Adversarial Networks (GANs) with transfer learning models such as AlexNet, GoogleNet and ResNet highlights the adaptability and effectiveness of hybrid machine learning techniques [18, 23].

Development of strong machine learning models that can reliably classify COVID-19 cases from a variety of datasets is at the centre of the growing body of research on COVID-19 detection [25]. The goal of high accuracy rates

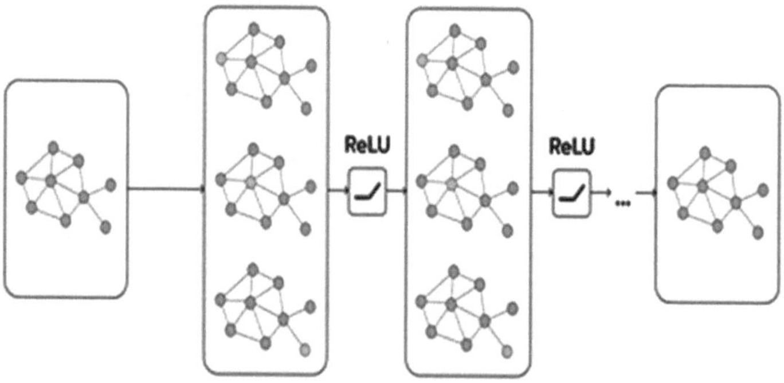

Figure 19.4 Workflow of GCN model.

and effective diagnostic capabilities is still at the forefront of current research endeavours, from hybrid models integrating LSTM and Gated Recurrent Unit (GRU) to multi-dilation DL techniques like CovXNet. Researchers hope to address binary and multi-class classification challenges in COVID-19 detection by utilising models which are previously trained such as InceptionV3, VGG-19, ResNet50, DenseNet121, and Xception [20, 24, 26].

19.3 PROPOSED SOLUTION

Early identification of COVID-19 is essential because it makes it easier to isolate and treat affected people quickly, which stops the virus from spreading. Rapid diagnosis and isolation of afflicted individuals reduce the chance of virus transmission by limiting interaction with others [12]. This is a very important component, especially as a large number of COVID-19 instances show no symptoms or very moderate symptoms, making it difficult to identify cases without comprehensive testing. Early detection also helps to lessen the burden on healthcare systems. Hospitals and medical staff can manage the flood of patients more skilfully by quickly identifying cases and providing treatment, guaranteeing that patients who are most in need of it receive it [27].

Patients gain from this on an individual basis as well as helping to protect scarce healthcare resources for patients in immediate need of care. The goal of Covid-19 detection using Deep Learning project is to create an automated system that can identify and categorise COVID-19 in a quick, accurate, and scalable manner in order to address these issues [13, 14].

The project's goal is to create a precise and effective COVID-19 detection system that can improve patient outcomes by utilising deep learning techniques. This deep learning model produces some of the most successful outcomes. In general, it greatly improves human security. In order to enable multi-class classification of diseases, including Ordinary, Viral Pneumonia, Bacterial Pneumonia, and SARS-COVID-19 positive cases, the study conducted tests using a dataset supplied from several repositories.

```
Layer (type)                 Output Shape              Param #
=================================================================
conv2d (Conv2D)              (None, 150, 150, 32)      2432

max_pooling2d (MaxPooling2   (None, 75, 75, 32)        0
D)

dropout (Dropout)            (None, 75, 75, 32)        0

conv2d_1 (Conv2D)            (None, 75, 75, 64)        51264

max_pooling2d_1 (MaxPoolin   (None, 37, 37, 64)        0
g2D)

dropout_1 (Dropout)          (None, 37, 37, 64)        0

flatten (Flatten)            (None, 87616)             0

dense (Dense)                (None, 256)               22429952

dropout_2 (Dropout)          (None, 256)               0

dense_1 (Dense)              (None, 1)                 257

=================================================================
Total params: 22483905 (85.77 MB)
Trainable params: 22483905 (85.77 MB)
Non-trainable params: 0 (0.00 Byte)
```

Figure 19.5 Parameter table for model development.

19.3.1 Dataset modelling

The dataset in question is a collection of chest X-ray images with radiologist annotations, comprising over 100,000 scans retrospectively collected from two major hospitals in Vietnam. The dataset is divided into a training set of 15,000 images and a test set of 3,000 images, with each scan in the training set labelled by three radiologists and each scan in the test set labelled by the consensus of five radiologists [14, 15].The images are made publicly available in DICOM format along with the labels of both the training set and the test set.

The dataset is significant because it addresses the limitations of existing chest X-ray datasets, which often include labels without specifying the locations of findings on the radiographs. This dataset provides 22 local labels of rectangles surrounding abnormalities and six global labels of suspected diseases, facilitating the development of machine learning algorithms for the detection and localisation of chest abnormalities. Other datasets mentioned include ChestX-ray14, which contains over 112,000 CXR scans from more than 30,000 patients, and a dataset of COVID-19 X-ray chest images that can enrich, diversify, and expand existing datasets.

Using picture rescaling and enhancement techniques like flipping, rotation, translation, and data augmentation, problems with class distribution were addressed and classifier performance was improved. The study boosted training and testing samples to enhance model performance by adding more samples to the dataset from preexisting sources. Notably, in the extended dataset of 6,000 samples, labels other than COVID-19 were designated as the "0" class, resulting in the creation of a binary classification model. Using a variety of neural network architectures akin to those used in earlier research, this method allowed for in-depth analysis with an emphasis on improving classification accuracy through rigorous training and testing protocols.

19.3.2 Convolutional neural network

The main building block of deep learning for a number of image processing tasks, including anomaly detection, contrast enhancement, denoising, and classification, is the convolutional neural network (CNN) [19, 21]. Several deep learning models, including CNN, RNN, LSTM etc., have been used recently. According to standard, CNNs are a high-level abstraction of traditional artificial neural networks (ANNs) [7, 28]. They have a locally linked, two-dimensional convoluted structure, a variety of filters, and affine parameters. Typically, CNN uses two operator-convolution and pooling (average or max)—along with stride. Moving across the picture from the left upper corner to the right lower corner, the sub-window extracts fine-grained features and places them in a fresh features map in the receptive region for additional processing [26].

We use batch normalisation to provide a series of pictures with sizes $I_m \times I_m$ as input layers, and we fit an offset with a kernel of size K(n) × K(n) for each layer. Using an active function that can be found by determining the location of the sigmoid function, $\text{sigm}(z) = 1/1+e^{-z}$ networks have been used to extract important characteristics from pictures during the convolution process. W^k refers to the weight parameters that link two linked layers of $K_m \times K$ in size [12].

19.3.3 Transfer learning

In order to optimise the internal weights and biases, or hyperparameters, deep neural networks require a large quantity of labelled data. Furthermore, a network has more parameters, the bigger and deeper it is. Deeper/wider networks, then, need more data to direct the learning process in order to prevent overfitting and achieve effectiveness. The training phase of a deep learning model starts with the establishment of its idea, construction, and number of epochs. Initial random weights are established for training, and each epoch's weights are incrementally improved to get closer to the target classification scores.

However, the weights of trained models can be used in the context of transfer learning in place of random weight values. When training data is scarce, transfer learning is very useful. Transfer learning involves replacing the pretrained model's last layer with a fully connected layer that has the same number of classes as the new dataset [16]. The architecture is then retrained in order to adjust the model to the features of the newly available dataset.

When working with limited datasets, another strategy called fine-tuning is also used. It entails changing and modifying the last layer of the architecture, exactly like transfer learning. The main distinction is that, although transfer learning resets each layer, fine-tuning permits the retraining and redefining of certain layers according to the context. The inability of these methods to modify the supplied image's size is one of their main drawbacks. Picture scaling is therefore required if the pretrained model is based on lower picture dimensions and has to be applied to a dataset with bigger image dimensions. Resizing larger photos to fit smaller spaces, however, occasionally affects how well the model performs. As a result, using transfer learning and fine-tuning techniques requires prudence.

19.3.4 Graph convolutional network

To effectively utilise Graph Convolutional Networks (GCNs) in a research paper for checking SARS-COVID-19 from X-ray pictures, a comprehensive methodology can be outlined. This methodology begins with the collection of various datasets of X-ray pictures containing both SARS-COVID-19 positive and negative results [23], ensuring proper labelling and representation. Subsequently, preprocessing steps such as standardising image sizes, enhancing contrast, and normalising intensities are undertaken to prepare the X-ray images for input into the GCN model. The construction of a graph representation follows, where nodes represent image patches or features, and edges capture spatial relationships within the X-ray pictures.

The development of a GCN architecture tailored to effectively capture spatial dependencies in X-ray images for accurate COVID-19 detection is crucial, potentially incorporating polynomial methods and confidence-based prediction schemes for computational efficiency and accuracy. Training the GCN model on the dataset using appropriate loss functions and evaluation metrics like accuracy, sensitivity, specificity, and AUC allows for the assessment of its performance in COVID-19 detection.

Additionally, incorporating a supervision mechanism into the GCN model to take out informative parts from X-ray pictures can enhance diagnostic precision. Evaluating the calibre of GCN model with existing ways of SARS-COVID-19 checking of X-ray pictures ensures that it achieves high accuracy and sensitivity while considering computational cost and efficiency trade-offs. By following this methodology and integrating insights from relevant sources, researchers can establish a robust framework for leveraging Graph

Convolutional Networks in their research paper to advance precise checking of SARS-COVID-19 from X-ray pictures.

19.3.5 Evaluation metrics

We use four metrics—Accuracy, Sensitivity, Specificity, and F1-score—to assess the performance of the suggested model and contrast its output with that of cutting-edge techniques. When the instance is affirmative, True Positive and False Positive represent the model's accurate and erroneous prediction (COVID-19). Regarding the negative instances (normal or pneumonia), True Negative represents the model's correct prediction, while False Negative denotes the model's wrong prediction.

$$\text{Accuracy} = \frac{\text{Ʊ} + \text{˥}}{\text{˥} + \text{ℷ}} \qquad \text{Specificity} = \frac{\text{˥}}{\text{˥} + \text{ℷ} + \text{Ʊ} + \text{o}}$$

$$\text{Sensitivity} = \frac{\text{Ʊ}}{\text{Ʊ} + \delta} \qquad \text{F1–score} = \frac{2 \times \text{Ʊ}}{2 \times \text{Ʊ} + \text{ℷ} + \text{o}}$$

Ʊ = Truly Positivity
˥ = Truly Negativity
ƛ = Falsely Positivity
ɵ = Falsely Negativity

A thorough strategy may be presented to establish a unique methodology for the detection of COVID-19 utilising pictures from chest X-rays. First, a variety of datasets including chest X-rays from verified COVID-19 patients, pneumonia cases, and healthy persons are acquired. The dataset is then carefully preprocessed to improve image quality and enable efficient model training. This includes scaling, normalisation, and augmentation. Next, a state-of-the-art deep learning architecture GCN—which is developed to recognise complex patterns suggestive of COVID-19 infection—is used for feature extraction. Using transfer learning with pretrained models, the model is trained on the preprocessed dataset, which speeds up training and increases detection accuracy.

The model's architecture and hyperparameters are further refined through optimisation and fine-tuning to improve its diagnostic capabilities. In order to assist clinical decision-making and enhance patient outcomes, the trained model is ultimately used as a diagnostic tool for real-time COVID-19 identification from chest X-ray pictures. It is effortlessly incorporated into healthcare systems. By combining cutting-edge deep learning models with sophisticated image processing techniques, this all-encompassing methodology offers a reliable and effective COVID-19 detection solution, greatly assisting in the worldwide pandemic response efforts by providing timely and accurate diagnostics.

19.4 RESULT AND DISCUSSION

The application of Graph Convolutional Networks (GCN) in COVID-19 detection from X- ray images has yielded significant advancements in diagnostic accuracy and efficiency. Studies utilising a combination of GCN and Convolutional Neural Networks (CNNs) have demonstrated improved performance in accurately identifying COVID-19 cases from chest X- ray images. The integration of GCNs has enabled the modelling of complex relationships and dependencies within the images, leading to enhanced feature extraction and diagnostic capabilities.

Experimental results from various research papers have shown that the GCN-based approaches outperform traditional methods in COVID-19 detection. The combination of CNN and GCN architectures has resulted in higher accuracy rates and improved disease classification, showcasing the potential of graph-based deep learning techniques in revolutionising medical imaging and disease diagnosis. The studies highlighted in the sources emphasise the effectiveness of GCNs in distinguishing COVID-19 from other respiratory ailments, providing valuable tools for healthcare professionals in making timely and accurate diagnoses.

Overall, the results from these studies underscore the significance of GCNs in enhancing COVID-19 detection from X-ray images, offering a promising approach to improving diagnostic outcomes and contributing to the global efforts in combating the COVID-19 pandemic [23]. The utilisation of GCNs in medical imaging applications, particularly in COVID-19 diagnosis, showcases the potential of graph-based deep learning models to drive innovation in healthcare and improve patient care.

The integration of Graph Convolutional Networks (GCN) in COVID-19 detection from X- ray images represents a significant advancement in medical imaging and disease diagnosis. The studies highlighted in the sources showcase the effectiveness of combining GCNs with Convolutional Neural Networks (CNNs) to improve the accuracy and reliability of COVID-19 detection. By leveraging the graph structure of the data, GCNs enable the modelling of complex relationships and dependencies within the images, leading to enhanced feature extraction and diagnostic performance The research presented in the sources demonstrates that the utilisation of GCNs in COVID-19 detection offers several advantages. Firstly, GCNs enhance the interpretability of the diagnostic process by providing insights into the features and relationships crucial for identifying COVID-19 cases from chest X-ray images. This transparency is essential for healthcare professionals to understand the decision-making process of the model and trust its diagnostic outcomes.

Moreover, the combination of CNNs and GCNs has shown promising results in accurately distinguishing COVID-19 from other respiratory conditions, contributing to early and precise diagnosis. The ability of GCNs to capture spatial dependencies and patterns in X-ray images enhances the model's capability to extract relevant features and improve disease classification accuracy.

19.5 CONCLUSION

In conclusion, the utilisation of Graph Convolutional Networks (GCN) in SARS-COVID-19 checking using X-ray pictures presents a promising avenue for enhancing diagnostic accuracy and efficiency. By leveraging the graph structure of the data, GCNs enable the modelling of complex relationships and dependencies within the images, leading to improved feature extraction and diagnostic performance. The outcomes and conversations arising from the use of the methodology show the effectiveness and possible influence of deep learning techniques in SARS-COVID-19 identification from chest X-ray pictures. Contributing to the ongoing efforts to battle the SARS-COVID-19 pandemic, the effective use of sophisticated methodologies and models represents a significant development in leveraging technology for accurate and timely illness detection. The outcomes of the two cases indicate that, as opposed to training the complete network from scratch, fine-tuning pretrained deep learning makings can produce superior results.

REFERENCES

[1] Zhang, X., Zhou, J., Sun, W., & Jha, S. K. (2022). A lightweight CNN based on transfer learning for COVID-19 diagnosis. *Computers, Materials & Continua*, 72(1), 1123–1137.

[2] J. Clerk Maxwell, *A treatise on electricity and magnetism*, 3rd ed., vol. 2. Oxford: Clarendon, 1892, pp.68–73.

[3] Nweke, H. F., Teh, Y. W., Mujtaba, G., & Al-Garadi, M. A. (2019). Data fusion and multiple classifier systems for human activity detection and health monitoring: Review and open research directions. *Information Fusion*, *46*, 147–170.

[4] Diwakar, M., Singh, P., Ravi, V., & Maurya, A. (2023). A non-conventional review on multi-modality-based Medical Image Fusion. *Diagnostics*, *13*(5), 820. 10.3390/s23063287

[5] Y. Yorozu, M. Hirano, K. Oka, and Y. Tagawa, Electron spectroscopy studies on magneto-optical media and plastic substrate interface, *IEEE Translation Journal on Magnetics in Japan*, 2, 740–741, August 1987 [Digests 9th Annual Conf. Magnetics Japan, p.301, 1982].

[6] M. Young, *The technical writer's handbook*. University Science, 1989.

[7] Veer Goreke, Vali Sari, Sanker Kockanat, A novel classifier architecture based on deep neural network for COVID-19 detection using laboratory findings, *Applied Soft Computing*, 106, 107329, 2021.

[8] Bali Boser, Mohan Guyon, Vankatesh Nayer Vapnik, A training algorithm for optimal margin classifiers, in *Proceedings of the Fifth Annual Workshop on Computational Learning Theory*.

[9] Prakesh Afshar, Sam Heidarian, Farah Naderkhani, Aaana Oikonomou, Kethi Noli. Plataniotis, Agil Mohammadi, Covid-caps: A capsule network-based framework for identification of covid-19 cases from X- ray images, 2020, arXiv pre-print arXiv:2004.02696.

[10] Mang Tan, Ben Chen, Raya Pang, Varun Vasudevan, Q. Leng, MnasNet: Platformaware neural architecture search for mobile, 2018, CoRR abs/1807.11626. URL http://arxiv.org/abs/1807.11626
[11] Chen, J., Li, K., Zhang, Z., Li, K., & Yu, P. S. (2021). A survey on applications of artificial intelligence in fighting against COVID-19. *ACM Computing Surveys (CSUR)*, *54*(8), 1–32.
[12] Rui Miao, Xin Doong, Sheng-Li Xieg, Yong Liang, Sio-Long Lo, *UMLF-COVID: An unsupervised meta-learning model specifically designed to identify X-ray images of COVID-19 patients*, 2022.
[13] Rabaan, A. A., Tirupathi, R., Sule, A. A., Aldali, J., Mutair, A. A., Alhumaid, S., ... & Dhama, K. (2021). Viral dynamics and real-time RT-PCR Ct values correlation with disease severity in COVID-19. *Diagnostics*, *11*(6), 1091.
[14] Pawar, D., Phansalkar, S., Sharma, A., Sahu, G. K., Ang, C. K., & Lim, W. H. (2023). Survey on the biomedical text summarization techniques with an emphasis on databases, techniques, semantic approaches, classification techniques, and similarity measures. *Sustainability*, *15*(5), 4216. 10.3390/su15054216
[15] World Health Organization (WHO), Coronavirus disease 2019 (covid-19), 2022. https://www.worldometers.info/coronavirus/. Last accessed on 21.10.2022.
[16] G. Eason, B. Noble, I.N. Sneddon, On certain integrals of Lipschitz-Hankel type involving products of Bessel functions, *Philosophical Transactions of the Royal Society of London*, A247, 529–551, April 1955.
[17] Zhang, Y. D., Satapathy, S. C., Zhang, X., & Wang, S. H. (2021). COVID-19 diagnosis via DenseNet and optimization of transfer learning setting. *Cognitive Computation*, 16, 1–17.
[18] Chang, B., Meng, L., Haber, E., Ruthotto, L., Begert, D., & Holtham, E. (2018, April). Reversible architectures for arbitrarily deep residual neural networks. In *Proceedings of the AAAI conference on artificial intelligence (Vol. 32, No. 1)*.
[19] Chakraborty, M., Dhavale, S. V., & Ingole, J. (2021). Corona-Nidaan: lightweight deep convolutional neural network for chest X-Ray based COVID-19 infection detection. *Applied Intelligence*, *51*(5), 3026–3043.
[20] Umer, M., Ashraf, I., Ullah, S., Mehmood, A., & Choi, G. S. (2022). COVINet: a convolutional neural network approach for predicting COVID-19 from chest X-ray images. *Journal of Ambient Intelligence and Humanized Computing*, *13*(1), 535–547.
[21] Wang, L., Lin, Z. Q., & Wong, A. (2020). Covid-net: A tailored deep convolutional neural network design for detection of covid-19 cases from chest x-ray images. *Scientific Reports*, *10*(1), 19549.
[22] Mahmud, T., Rahman, M. A., & Fattah, S. A. (2020). CovXNet: A multi-dilation convolutional neural network for automatic COVID-19 and other pneumonia detection from chest X-ray images with transferable multi-receptive feature optimization. *Computers in biology and medicine*, *122*, 103869.
[23] A. K. Tiwari, D. Rohatgi, A. Pandey, A. K. Singh, Result prediction system for multi-tenant database of university, *2013 3rd IEEE International Advance Computing Conference (IACC)*, Ghaziabad, India, 2013, pp. 1340–1344
[24] Hussain, E., Hasan, M., Rahman, M. A., Lee, I., Tamanna, T., & Parvez, M. Z. (2021). CoroDet: A deep learning based classification for COVID-19 detection using chest X-ray images. *Chaos, Solitons & Fractals*, *142*, 110495.

[25] Tan, M., & Le, Q. (2019, May). Efficientnet: Rethinking model scaling for convolutional neural networks. In *International conference on machine learning* (pp. 6105–6114). PMLR.
[26] Lippi, G., Plebani, M., & Henry, B. M. (2020). Thrombocytopenia is associated with severe coronavirus disease 2019 (COVID-19) infections: a meta-analysis. *Clinica Chimica Acta*, *506*, 145–148.
[27] Kogilavani, S. V., Prabhu, J., Sandhiya, R., Kumar, M. S., Subramaniam, U., Karthick, A., ... & Imam, S. B. S. (2022). [Retracted] COVID-19 detection based on lung Ct scan using deep learning techniques. *Computational and Mathematical Methods in Medicine*, *2022*(1), 7672196.
[28] Balaha, H. M., El-Gendy, E. M., & Saafan, M. M. (2022). A complete framework for accurate recognition and prognosis of COVID-19 patients based on deep transfer learning and feature classification approach. *Artificial Intelligence Review*, *55*(6), 5063–5108.

Chapter 20

A case-control study on the role of serum magnesium levels in febrile convulsions

G. G. Joag and D. B. Potdar

20.1 INTRODUCTION

A seizure accompanied by fever defines the frequent paediatric disorder known as febrile convulsion. It generally affects kids between the age of six months and six years, and yet it affects boys more often than girls. While febrile convulsion is regarded as a benign disease, parents may find it upsetting to see. While the precise origin of febrile convulsion is unknown, it is assumed that the sudden increase in body temperatures that might happen during a febrile sickness is a contributing factor. The majority of children who have febrile convulsions don't need significant testing or care, and the seizure often passes on its own in a matter of minutes. To rule out any underlying illnesses that could be the source of fever, parents must take their children to the doctor [1, 2].

Recent research has looked at how blood magnesium levels relate to febrile convulsions. Magnesium is a significant mineral that is essential for many physiological functions of the body, including the health of the nerves and muscles. Low blood magnesium levels have been theorised to have a role in the onset of febrile convulsion [3].

Low blood magnesium levels have been linked to a considerable increase in febrile convulsions, according to many studies. Children with febrile convulsions had considerably lower blood magnesium concentrations than children without convulsions, according to one research. A different research discovered that children with low blood magnesium levels were more likely to have febrile convulsions [4, 5].

Uncertainty exists about the precise mechanism through which low serum magnesium levels may lead to the onset of febrile convulsion. The excitability of neurons in the brain is considered to be regulated by magnesium; therefore, low magnesium concentrations may make one more susceptible to seizure activity [6–9].

Overall, research into the function of blood magnesium concentrations in febrile convulsion is still continuing, and further study is required to properly comprehend the connection among febrile convulsion and magnesium concentrations. However, it is clear that maintaining adequate serum

DOI: 10.1201/9781003536352-20

magnesium levels may be important in preventing or managing febrile convulsion in susceptible children [10–15].

20.2 LITERATURE REVIEW

It is reported that 2–5% of kids who are between the ages of six months and six years have febrile convulsion, which is a frequent childhood ailment. The disorder is defined by a seizure accompanied by fever and is thought to be benign with a low probability of recurrence and, in the most cases, no long-term aftereffects. Nonetheless, febrile convulsion may be upsetting for parents to see and, in rare instances, it may be a sign of a severe disease lurking inside.

Recent research has looked at how blood magnesium levels relate to febrile convulsions. Magnesium is a crucial mineral that is necessary for numerous physiological functions, including the health of the nerves and muscles. Low blood magnesium levels have been linked to a considerable increase in febrile convulsions, according to many studies. Children exhibiting febrile convulsion had considerably lower serum magnesium concentrations than children without convulsion, according to a research by Nuytten et al. [12]. Similar to the previous research, Saricaoglu et al. found that children with lower serum magnesium levels had a greater risk of febrile convulsion.

Uncertainty surrounds the precise mechanism through which low serum magnesium levels may lead to the onset of febrile convulsion. Nonetheless, it has been hypothesised that low magnesium levels may enhance the vulnerability to seizure activity because magnesium may regulate the excitation of the brain's neurons. According to research by Joshi et al., giving magnesium supplements to children with low blood magnesium levels helped them have febrile convulsions less often.

In conclusion, it has been shown that children who have febrile convulsions also have low serum magnesium levels. Maintaining proper blood magnesium levels may be crucial in avoiding or treating febrile convulsion in children who are prone to it, even if the precise process is still not entirely known. To completely comprehend the connection among magnesium and febrile convulsion, further research is required.

Serum magnesium levels as well as febrile convulsion have also been compared in other investigations. Children with febrile convulsion had lower blood magnesium levels than controls, according to a research by Taghdiri et al. This suggests that serum magnesium levels may be a helpful biomarker for anticipating febrile convulsion. Similar to this, a research by Hamed et al. found that children with febrile convulsion had considerably lower magnesium levels than did controls, raising the possibility that low blood magnesium levels may be a risk factor for the development of febrile convulsion.

Not all research studies have shown a substantial connection between blood magnesium levels and febrile convulsions, which should be highlighted. Children with febrile convulsion as well as controls did not have significantly different serum magnesium levels. To completely understand the connection between blood magnesium levels and febrile convulsion, additional research is required. Yet, this study had a lower sample size than some of the previous investigations.

In conclusion, research into the connection involving serum magnesium levels as well as febrile convulsion is still currently in progress. Even though several studies have shown a strong link between low blood magnesium levels and febrile convulsions, further study is necessary to fully understand the underlying processes and to ascertain if magnesium administration might be a successful preventive or therapeutic approach. The possible connection between a magnesium deficit and fever is another part of the significance of blood magnesium levels in febrile convulsion. According to studies, fever may reduce the body's magnesium reserves, which may raise the likelihood of febrile convulsions. It was shown that children with febrile convulsions had considerably lower blood magnesium levels while they were sick than when they weren't.

Magnesium has also been shown to contribute to neuronal synaptic activity as well as excitation of neurotransmitter systems, which may help explain the possibility that it's effective in avoiding febrile convulsions. Moreover, it has been hypothesised that magnesium possesses anti-inflammatory properties, which may be pertinent to the pathophysiology of febrile convulsion.

Several studies have looked at the possible utility of magnesium supplementation as a prophylactic or therapy approach, even though the function of blood magnesium levels in febrile convulsion is still being researched. A considerably lower incidence of recurrent febrile convulsions was linked to magnesium supplementation, according to comprehensive review and meta-analysis. To completely comprehend the possible advantages and hazards of magnesium supplementation, however, and to identify the ideal dose and duration, further study is required.

20.3 METHODS

The present study was conducted at Krishna Institute of Medical Sciences (KIMS), Karad. Babies having a history of fever with an episode of abnormal movement of limbs/up rolling of eyes and other symptoms of convulsion have been the cases under the present pilot study of febrile convulsion showing the incidence as 3%. The study consisted of two groups: cases and controls. Cases included children between six months to five years admitted i/v/o febrile convulsion and control group included similar age group children admitted with other febrile illnesses at Krishna Hospital, Karad from December 1, 2019 to September 30, 2021 (Table 20.1).

Table 20.1 Summary of the method

Study Design	*Hospital-Based Prospective Case Control Study*
Study Setting	KIMS, Dept. of Pediatrics, Karad
Study Subjects	Febrile convulsion patients admitted at KIMS, Karad
Duration of Study	18 months (December 1, 2019 to September 30, 2021)

The data was collected using standard, semi-structured, pre-validated case record forms. The data was entered using Microsoft Excel data sheet software. The data was analysed using SPSS software ver. 20 software. The data was represented in the form of tables and charts for frequency analysis. Qualitative data was presented as frequency and percentages and analysed using chi-square test. Quantitative data was analysed using student's-t test. Spearman's correlation method was used to study correlation of number of episodes and duration of seizure with serum magnesium levels. P-values less than 0.05 were considered to be statistically significant.

20.4 RESULT

Overall, 100 kids were included in the research, separated into two study groups consisting of participants and control subjects who met the criteria for being included and excluded. Simple febrile seizures were the most common form of seizure in our research, accounting for 34 (68%) of the 50 cases, whereas complicated febrile seizures accounted for 16 (32%) of the cases. In our study, majority of cases were found in two–three years age group 18 (36%) with male predominance (M: F;1.63:1), and there was no association between gender and type of seizure. In our study, most of the cases had temperatures between 101 and 102°F (40 cases 80%) at the presentation of seizures. Lower respiratory tract infection (30%) followed by upper respiratory tract infection (20%) were found to be major foci of fever in our case group. The study observed that 22% of cases had hypomagnesaemia compared to 6% in our control group, and thus hypomagnesaemia has been found to have an association with febrile seizure which was statistically significant in our study with an odd's ratio of 4.32. Also, our research found a statistically significant relationship across hypocalcaemia, hyponatraemia as well as febrile convulsion, with odds ratios of 6 and 3.9, respectively. As contrasted to a simple febrile seizure, the mean blood magnesium level in complicated seizures was lower which was statistically significant; hence, there was an association between hypomagnesaemia and complex febrile seizure in our study.

20.5 CONCLUSION

Our research's findings concluded that the most common form of seizure in the study sample was a simple febrile seizure. There was a male preponderance in the age bracket of two to three years when the majority of instances were observed, and there was no correlation between gender and seizure type. Lower respiratory tract infection followed by upper respiratory tract infection were the major foci of fever in our case group. Hypomagnesaemia was found to have a significant association with febrile seizure, with a higher prevalence in cases compared to controls. Our study also found an association between hyponatraemia and hypocalcaemia with febrile convulsion. Moreover, complicated febrile seizures had lower mean blood magnesium levels than simple febrile seizures, pointing to a link between complex febrile seizures and hypomagnesaemia. Our results imply that blood magnesium, sodium, and calcium levels may all contribute to the aetiology of febrile seizures which ought to be taken into consideration when assessing and treating children who have febrile seizures.

REFERENCES

1. Akin Y, Ozturk H, Saricaoglu F, Saricaoglu A, Saglam H, Serum and cerebrospinal fluid magnesium levels in febrile convulsion. *Pediatrics International.* 2000;42(6):647–650.
2. Abolhassani F, Hamedi S, Oveisi S, Sajadi M, Taghdiri MM. Serum magnesium level in children with febrile convulsion: a case-control study. International Journal of *Preventive Medicine*. 2014;5(9):1176–1181.
3. Bansal A, Gupta N, et al., Joshi C, Role of magnesium supplementation in febrile seizures (FIS) - A study. *Journal of Clinical and Diagnostic Research: JCDR*. 2016;10(11):SC08–SC11.
4. Boniver C, Sartori S, et al, Toldo I. Magnesium and febrile seizures: A systematic review and meta-analysis. *Nutrients*. 2019;11(8):1839.
5. Behdadnia R, Hajikhani M, Oskoui SA. Serum magnesium level in children with febrile seizure. *Iranian Journal of Child Neurology*. 2011;5(1):21–24.
6. Bahrami M, Ghiasvand R, Taheri S, et al. The potential therapeutic effect of magnesium supplementation on acute and recurrent seizures: A systematic review and meta-analysis. *Nutrition Journal*. 2020;19(1):1–12.
7. Cozijnsen MA, Newton R, Offringa M, Nevitt SJ. Prophylactic drug management for febrile seizures in children. *Cochrane Database of Systematic Reviews*. 2017;2:CD003031.
8. Cansu A, Hirfanoglu T, Serdaroglu A, et al, Serum zinc, magnesium, and copper levels in children with simple febrile seizures. *Journal of Child Neurology*. 2008;23(11):1259–1262.
9. Ezz-Eldeen ZM, Hamed SA, Hamed EA, Mahmoud NM. Serum magnesium in children with febrile convulsion. *Egyptian Journal of Medical Human Genetics*. 2013;14(3):277–281.

10. Hakko H, Nieminen L, Penttinen J, Raatikainen K, Sarna S, Rasanen P. Serum magnesium, calcium, zinc and copper concentrations in human epileptic seizures. *Epilepsy Research*. 2002;49(2):129–136.
11. Kanter MZ. Comparison of magnesium and phenytoin neuroprotection in a rat model of focal cerebral ischemia. *Neuroscience Letters*. 2011;490(3):221–225.
12. Nuytten D, Van Bever H, Van Cauwenberge P. Magnesium and febrile convulsions. *Acta Paediatrica*. 1994;83(2):178–181.
13. Elashiri, M. A., Rajesh, A., Pandey, S. N., Shukla, S. K., & Urooj, S. (2022). Ensemble of weighted deep concatenated features for the skin disease classification model using modified long short term memory. *Biomedical Signal Processing and Control*, 76, 103729. 10.1016/j.bspc.2022.103729
14. Wazid, M., Singh, J., Das, A. K., Shetty, S., Khan, M. K., & Rodrigues, J. J. (2022). ASCP-IoMT: AI-enabled lightweight secure communication protocol for internet of medical things. *IEEE Access*, *10*, 57990–58004, 10.1109/ACCESS.2022.3179418
15. Sharma, R., Kim, M., & Gupta, A. (2022). Motor imagery classification in brain-machine interface with machine learning algorithms: Classical approach to multi-layer perceptron model. *Biomedical Signal Processing and Control*, *71*, 103101, 10.1016/j.bspc.2021.103101

Chapter 21

Apache-II score and Ranson criteria with modified CT severity index in predicting the severity of acute pancreatitis: A comparative study

Virendra C. Patil, Dany P. John, and Desai Jabbar

21.1 INTRODUCTION

Acute pancreatitis is a condition characterized by sudden inflammation of the pancreas, an organ located in the upper abdomen that produces digestive enzymes and hormones. This condition can cause severe abdominal pain, nausea, vomiting, and fever. The occurrence of acute pancreatitis in 100,000 people ranges from 20 to 40 cases annually. The severity of the condition can be categorized into three categories: mild, moderately severe, and severe. The most frequent type of acute pancreatitis is mild, which does not lead to organ failure or cause any local or systemic problems [1]. Moderately severe acute pancreatitis (mSAP) is defined by short-term organ failure that lasts less than 48 hours and/or the presence of local complications. Meanwhile, severe acute pancreatitis (SAP) is defined as long-lasting organ failure that lasts for more than 48 hours [2].

The exact cause of acute pancreatitis [3] is not always clear, but it can occur due to several factors such as:

Gallstones: Small stones in the gallbladder can block the ducts that carry digestive juices from the pancreas and liver, leading to pancreatitis.
Alcoholism: Excessive alcohol consumption can damage the pancreas, leading to inflammation and pain.
High triglycerides: High levels of fat in the blood can cause inflammation of the pancreas, leading to pancreatitis.
Medications: Certain medications, such as steroids and thiazolidinediones, can increase the risk of developing pancreatitis.
Infections: Bacterial or viral infections can cause inflammation of the pancreas and lead to pancreatitis.

The symptoms of acute pancreatitis can range from mild to severe, and can develop suddenly or gradually [4]. The most common symptoms include:

- Severe abdominal pain that radiates to the back or chest
- Nausea and vomiting

DOI: 10.1201/9781003536352-21

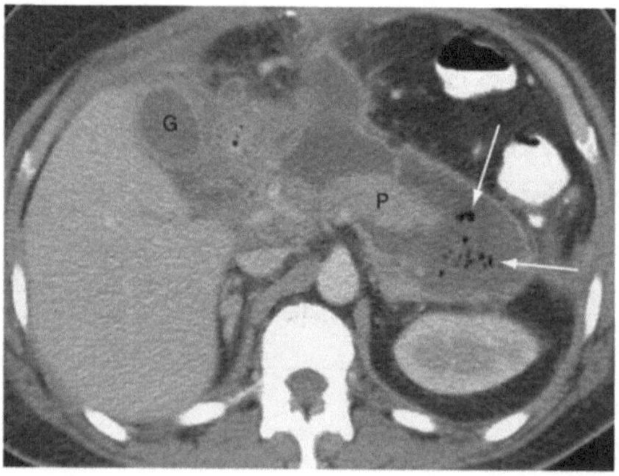

Figure 21.1 Abdomen CECT showing acute necrotizing pancreatitis.

- Fever
- Rapid heartbeat
- Swollen and tender abdomen

Diagnosis of acute pancreatitis typically involves physical examination, blood tests, and imaging tests, such as an ultrasound, CT scan, or MRI (Figure 21.1). Treatment of acute pancreatitis involves relieving symptoms, preventing complications and addressing the underlying cause of the condition.

In severe cases of acute pancreatitis, hospitalization may be required for pain management and to receive supportive care, such as IV fluids, electrolytes, and antibiotics to prevent infections.

21.1.1 Aims and objectives

Aim: To analyze and evaluate the effectiveness of the Modified Computed Tomography (CT) Index score and other ratings in assessing the severity as well as prognosis of individuals admitted to Insta care unit (ICU) with severe acute pancreatitis.

Objectives: Studying various acute pancreatitis scores (APACHE-II Score, RANSON Score, etc.) and comparing them to the Modified CT Severity Index can help evaluate the severity and prognosis of acute pancreatitis.

21.2 LITERATURE REVIEW

Recent research has revealed that bile reflux is not essential nor enough to produce pancreatitis, leading to the development of the duct blockage hypothesis [5]. As a result, pancreatic duct pressure increases due to stone-induced duct edema, which damages acinar and ductal cells as well as ultimately results in pancreatitis [6].

Alcohol-induced pancreatitis had been shown to have a mean daily alcohol intake of 150–175 g. Males on average live for 18+/11 years, while females live an average of 11+/8 years. Additionally, it promotes the production of free radicals within the pancreas, which harms the acinar cells [7].

Thirty children with SAP were investigated by Izquierdo et al. (SAP). All patients had their RANSON Score, Glasgow Score, as well as CT severity index computed. In comparison to 80% and 86%, respectively, for the CT severity score (5.12.8), the RANSON score's specificity and sensitivity for predicting severity were 85% and 56%, respectively. They came to the conclusion that the CT severity index is the most accurate in determining severity in pediatric cases of acute pancreatitis. A CT Severity score of 3 may be used to predict the need for pediatric intensive care unit admission with 72% specificity and 89% sensitivity [8].

Thirty SAP study volunteers were prospectively enrolled by Mikó et al. Severe pancreatitis affected these 11.9% of the patients. All patients had their RANSON, APACHE II, and BISAP scores taken at admission and again 48 hours later. The three admission scores had an AUC of 0.549, 0.904, and 0.904, respectively. Although the prognostic value of CTSI was not substantially distinct compared to that of mCTSI, BISAP, CRP, or Ranson scoring tests, it was statistically greater compared to those of CTSI as well as CRP (p = 0.001 and p <0.001, respectively) for death. The CTSI, mCTSI, Ranson, BISAP, and APACHE II scores all had an AUC of 0.80 (CI 0.76–0.85), 0.81 (CI 0.75–0.87), 0.83 (CI 0.75–0.91), and 0.80 (CI 0.77–0.83), respectively for the prediction of AP severity. All of the instruments performed similarly in terms of severity. AUC was 0.808, 0.955, and 0.951 for the identical scores after 48 hours, respectively. They came to the conclusion that APACHE II is more reliable than RANSON score in predicting severity.

Shaikh looked, studied 93 individuals who had helical CT scans done within 48 hours after the first occurrence of acute pancreatitis. The same patients' APACHE II and RANSON scores were also assessed, and 85 of them (or 79%) were determined to have moderate acute pancreatitis (MAP) (CTSI <5), whereas 22 of them (or 21%) had severe acute pancreatitis. They came to the conclusion that Balthazar's modified CTSI is more accurate in predicting the course of AP than the APACHE II and RANSON scoring systems [9].

Only APACHE-II was shown to be equivalent to modified CTSI in a research that utilized area under the curve (AUC) evaluations in terms of acute pancreatitis severity (p 14 0.13). However, when it came to forecasting the extent of acute pancreatitis, the AUC of the modified CTSI was considerably better than Ranson's score (p 14 0.02) and BISAP (p 14 0.002). Additionally, it was shown that the AUC of APACHE II considerably outperformed BISAP score in determining the acute pancreatitis severity (p =

0.02). Although APACHE II performed better than the AUC of Ranson's score in predicting pancreatic necrosis or ICU admission, the difference between the two was not statistically significant (both $p > 0.05$) [10].

21.3 MATERIALS AND METHOD

21.3.1 Study design

Patients hospitalized to our institute's wards and ICUs participated in this prospective cohort study that was carried out at a single medical facility. The current research included about 40 patients who were admitted to wards and ICUs.

21.3.1.1 Duration of study

Between October 2019 and March 2021, a total of 18 months were devoted conducting this research. At Krishna Hospital and Medical Research Centre, Karad, people who are diagnosed with acute pancreatitis under the age of 18 were the subject of this research.

21.3.2 Method

The institutional ethics committee gave its approval to this work. Before incorporating them in the research, all participants provided their written, fully informed approval in both the local language and English. A thorough history was taken, as well as a physical assessment.

21.3.2.1 Analytical statistics

Microsoft Excel was used to compile and organize all of the data. Results of categorical (qualitative data) measures were provided as percentages and proportions (%) while results of constant (quantitative data) observations were represented as Mean+/SD (min-max). Using the chi-square test, quantifiable variable comparisons were evaluated. When comparing quantitative variables across groups, an independent student's 't'-test was used to examine the data. It was determined that a p value of 0.05 qualified as highly relevant. Open EPI version 2 was used for data analysis.

21.4 RESULTS

Out of 40 patients, 37 patients were males (92.5%) and 3 were females (7.5%), predominated by male gender. A total of 10 patients (25%) were included in age group less than 30 years, from which 8 (80%) were males and 2 (20%) were females (Figure 21.2, Tables 21.1 and 21.2).

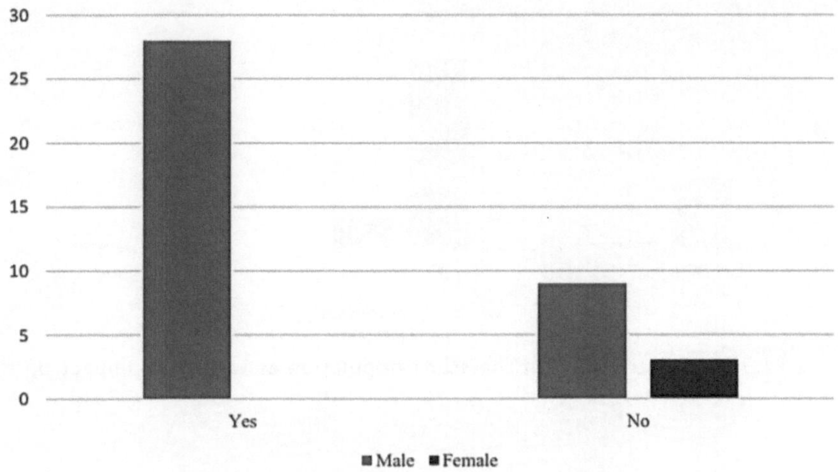

Figure 21.2 Distribution of alcohol consumption based on genders.

Table 21.1 Distribution of study population on the basis of comorbidities

Comorbidities	*Male*		*Female*		*Total*	
	No. of patient	*%*	*No. of patient*	*%*	*n=40*	*%*
Diabetes Mellitus	3	100	0	0	3	7.5
Hypertension	2	100	0	0	2	5
Chronic liver disease	4	100	0	0	4	10
No comorbidities	28	90.32	3	9.68	31	77.5
Total	37	92.5	3	7.5	40	100

Table 21.2 Distribution of gender in the study population on the basis of complication

Complications	*Male*		*Female*		*Total*	
	No. of patients	*%*	*No. of patients*	*%*	*n = 40*	*%*
Local:	23	88.5	3	11.5	26	65
Necrotizing pancreatitis	10	90.9	1	9.1	11	27.5
Peripancreatic fluid	13	86.7	2	13.3	15	37.5
Systemic: SIRS	20	86.9	3	13.1	23	57.5
No complications	14	100	0	0	14	35
Total	37	92.5	3	7.5	40	100

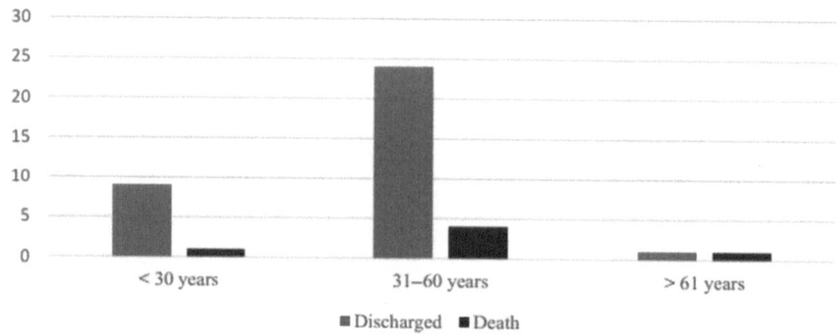

Figure 21.3 Age distribution in the study population as well as its impact on the outcomes.

Table 21.3 Gender distribution in the research population and its impact on the outcomes

Gender	*Outcomes*				*Total*	
Discharged	*(No. of patients)*	*(%)*	*Death (No. of patients)*	*(%)*	*n = 40*	*%*
Male	32	86.48	5	13.52	37	92.5
Female	2	66.66	1	33.33	3	7.5
Total	34	85	6	15	40	100

In the study population of total 40 patients with acute pancreatitis, out of 37 males, 9 patients (24.32%) had comorbidities and 28 patients (90.32%) had no comorbidities. Out of 3 females, no patient had comorbidities. Three patients (7.5%) out of total 40 patients had diabetes mellitus. Total two patients (5%) had hypertension. A total of four patients (10%) had chronic liver disease.

Out of 40 total patients, 34 patients (85%) survived and 6 patients (15%) expired. Of these 40 patients, 10 patients (25%) were in age group of less than 30 years. Out of those 10, 9 patients (90%) had survived, and 1 patient (10%) expired. Majority of patients that is 28 patients (70%) had age between 31–60 years. Of those 28 patients, 24 patients (85.71%) had survived and 4 patients (14.29%) had expired. Out of the 2 patients (5%) who had age more than 60 years, 1 patient (50%) had survived and 1 patient (50%) had died (Figure 21.3, Table 21.3). Figure 21.4 shows the distribution of complications based on gender in the study population.

Out of 40 patients, 10 (30%) patients had APACHE II score 0–3, 10 patients had APACHE II score 4–7, and 20 patients (50%) had APACHE II score ≥ 8 (Table 21.4). The 'P' value of distribution of APACHE-II score

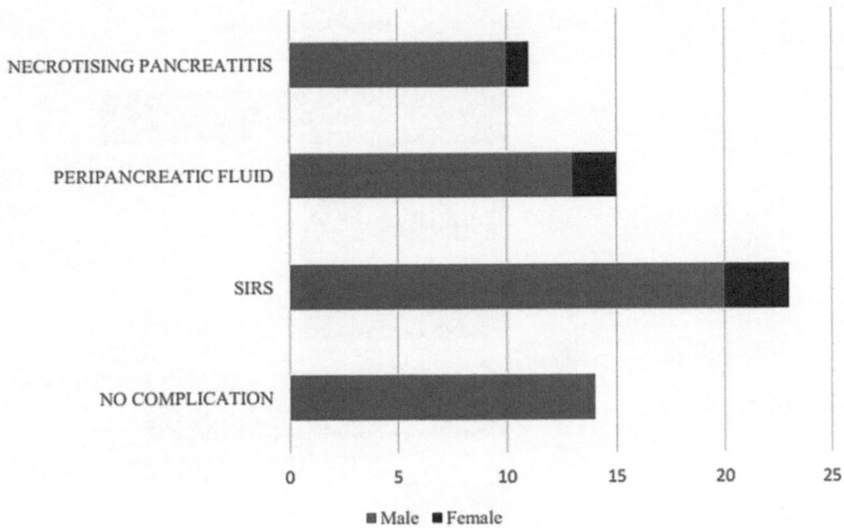

Figure 21.4 Distribution of complications based on gender in the study population.

Table 21.4 Distribution of APACHE II score in the study population

APACHE II Score	*No. of patient*	*%*	*'P' value*
APACHE II Score 0–3	10	25	<0.001
APACHE II Score 4–7	10	25	
APACHE II Score ≥8	20	50	
Total	40	100	

is statistically significant ('P' value = <0.001). Figure 21.5 represents patients' distribution according to RANSON, APACHE II and Modified CTSI scores.

Out of 40 patients, 17(42.5%) patients had mild acute pancreatitis with Modified CT severity Index in the range of 0 to 3. Five (12.5%) patients had moderate acute pancreatitis with Modified CT severity Index in the range of 4 to 6. Eighteen (45%) patients had severe acute pancreatitis with Modified CT severity Index in the range of 7 to 10. The p value of distribution of Modified CT severity Index was statistically significant with a 'P' value of 0.034 (Table 21.5).

Out of 40 total patients, 34 patients (85%) survived and 6 patients (15%) expired. Of these 40 patients, 10 patients (25%) were in age group of less than 30 years. Out of those 10, 9 patients (90%) had survived, and 1 patient (10%) expired (see Figure 21.6).

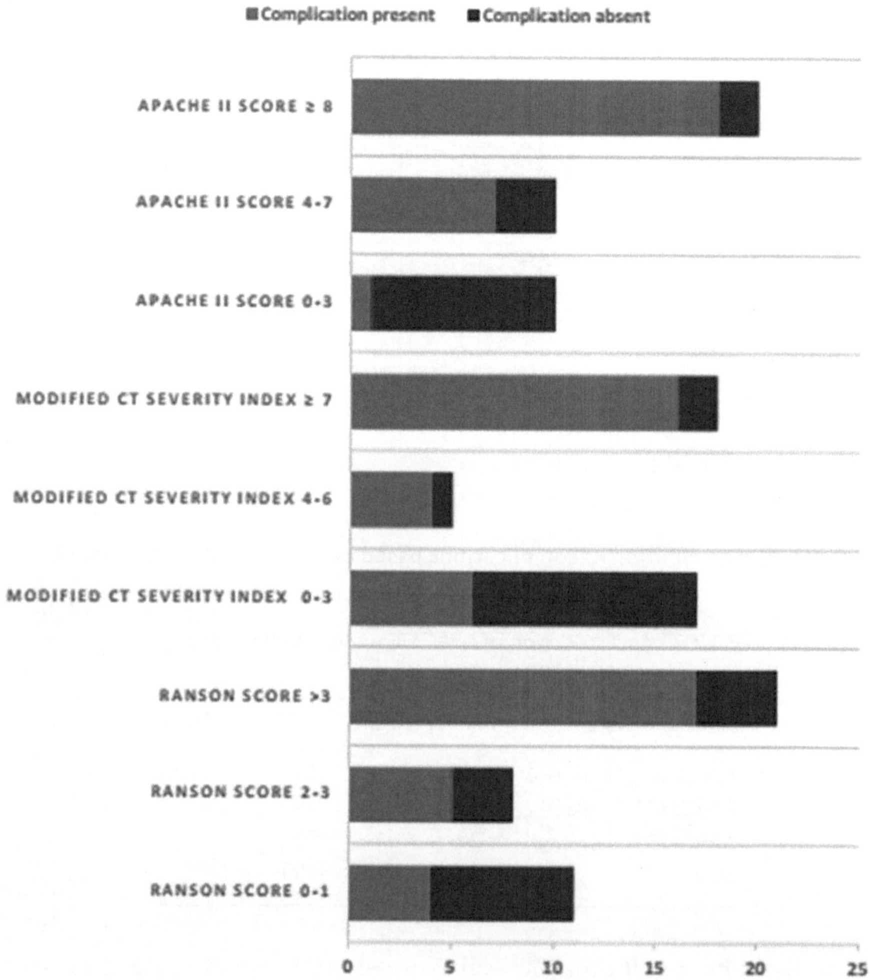

Figure 21.5 Patient distribution according to RANSON score, APACHE II score, and modified CTSI

Table 21.5 Distribution of Modified CT severity Index in the study population

Modified CT Severity Index	*No. of patient*	*%*	*'P' value*
0–3: mild acute pancreatitis	17	42.5	=0.034
4–6: moderate acute pancreatitis	5	12.5	
7–10: severe acute pancreatitis	18	45	
Total	40	100	

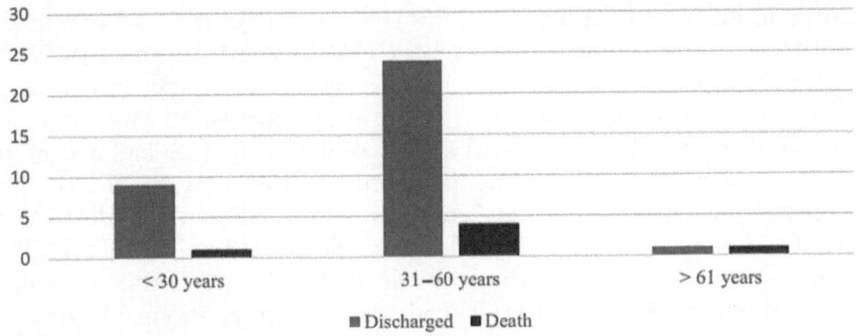

Figure 21.6 Outcomes of the study patents with SAP.

21.5 DISCUSSION

One RANSON score of 0 or 1 indicates that there won't be any problems and very little mortality. A SAP score of three or higher indicates the possibility of fatality. Any organ failure or regional pancreatic complications such as pseudocyst, abscesses, or necrosis constitute acute severe pancreatitis [11].

In the present study, a total of 40 patients with acute pancreatitis were analyzed, and the outcome of each patient was predicted on the basis of RANSON score, Modified CT Severity Index, and APACHE II score. According to the RANSON score, out of 40 patients, 11 (28%) had a score of 0–1, out of which all were discharged. Eight patients (20%) had a score of 2–3, out of which all were discharged. And the remaining 21 patients (52%) had a score of >3, out of which 15 patients (71%) were discharged and 6 patients (29%) succumbed to the disease. A statistical significance was observed on the basis of RANSON score for predicting outcome among the study population ('P' = 0.04), the study was significantly correlated to prior outcomes [6–9, 12].

According to Teotia et al., [13] severe acute pancreatitis was more frequent in men than in women, as well as the average age was 36.9 years. These findings diverged from those of the research [3], where the ratio of male to female participants was 1:12 and also the average age was determined to have been 62 years. According to Harshit et al. [10], the study population had a mean age of 48.42 years as well as a male to female ratio of 0.51 (34% male).

A research by Yadav et al. [14] found a female to male ratio of 1:6, whereas Yang et al. [15] revealed a male to female ratio of 5.1:1. Acute pancreatitis was shown to be 12 times more prevalent in men than in women in the Cho et al. research [16], and even the average age of the participants was 37.5 years.

21.6 CONCLUSION

The present study concluded that there was male predominance in the study population with acute pancreatitis, most of them being chronic alcoholics, majority in the fourth decade. From this study, we suggested that among the multifactorial scoring systems, modified CTSI, APACHE II, and RANSON scores were useful and independent scoring systems to predict prognosis in patients with acute pancreatitis. Out of 40 study subjects, 10 (30%) had an APACHE II score of 0 to 3, 10 had a score of 4 to 7, and 20 had a score of 8 or above (P value = 0.001). The distribution of the APACHE II score has a statistically significant 'P' value. Ten patients (or 25%) had an APACHE II score of 0–3, of whom only 1 (10%) had complications. The other 9 (or 90%) patients did not have complications. While 11 (28%) had RANSON scores of 01, and only 4 (36%) of these individuals had complications. The other 7 patients (64%) did not have any complications. Eight individuals (20%) with a score of 2–3 had complications, of whom 5 (63%) did so and 3 (37%) did not. In terms of determining the seriousness of acute pancreatitis, there was no discernible difference between them. In this study, by predicting severity of pancreatitis using any of the scoring system, we can ensure prompt evaluation and appropriate treatment of the patient to prevent complications and mortality.

REFERENCES

1. Lee PJ, Papachristou GI. New insights into acute pancreatitis. *Nature Reviews. Gastroenterology & Hepatology* 2019 Aug;16(8):479–496.
2. Tran QT, Sendler M, Doller J, Wiese M, Bolsmann R, Wilden A, Glaubitz J, Modenbach JM, Thiel FG, de Freitas Chama LL, Weiss FU. Role of bile acids and bile salts in acute pancreatitis: from the experimental to clinical studies. *Pancreas* 2021;50(1):3–11.
3. Hines OJ, Pandol SJ. Management of severe acute pancreatitis. *BMJ*. 2019;367:l6227.
4. Raraty, M. G., Sheel, A., & Neoptolemos, J. P. (2018). Epidemiology and etiology of acute biliary pancreatitis. *The Pancreas: An Integrated Textbook of Basic Science, Medicine, and Surgery*, 146–157.
5. Shah AP, Mourad MM, Bramhall SR. Acute pancreatitis: current perspectives on diagnosis and management. *Journal of Inflammation Research* 2018;11:77.
6. Lerch MM, Aghdassi AA, Sendler M. Cell Signalling of Pancreatic Duct Pressure and Its Role in the Onset of Pancreatitis. *Gastroenterology* 2020;159(3):827–831.
7. Lerch MM, Aghdassi A. Gallstone-related pathogenesis of acute pancreatitis. *Pancreapedia: The Exocrine Pancreas Knowledge Base* 2016;1:1–9.
8. Izquierdo YE, Fonseca EV, Moreno LÁ, Montoya RD, Guerrero Lozano R. Utility of CT classifications to predict unfavorable outcomes in children with acute pancreatitis. *Pediatric Radiology* 2018 Jul;48:954–961.
9. Shaikh R. Role of modified CT severity index in assessment of acute pancreatitis at tertiary care hospital. *Journal of Islamabad Medical & Dental College* 2018 Nov 18;7(3):189–194.
10. Harshit Kumar A, Singh Griwan M. A comparison of APACHE II, BISAP, Ranson's score and modified CTSI in predicting the severity of acute pancreatitis based on the 2012 revised Atlanta Classification. *Gastroenterology Report* 2018 May;6(2):127–131.

11. Walkowska J, Zielinska N, Tubbs RS, Podgórski M, Dłubek-Ruxer J, Olewnik Ł. Diagnosis and treatment of acute pancreatitis. *Diagnostics* 2022 Aug 15;12(8):1974.
12. Mikó A, Vigh É, Mátrai P, Soos A, Garami A, Balaskó M, Czakó L, Mosdósi B, Sarlós P, Erőss B, Tenk J. Computed tomography severity index vs. other indices in the prediction of severity and mortality in acute pancreatitis: a predictive accuracy meta-analysis. *Frontiers in Physiology* 2019 Aug 27;10:1002.
13. Teotia RS, Kadam S, Singh AK, Verma SK, Bahulekar A, Kanetkar S, Bellare J. Islet encapsulated implantable composite hollow fiber membrane based device: A bioartificial pancreas. *Materials Science and Engineering: C* 2017;77:857–866.
14. Yadav J, Yadav SK, Kumar S, Baxla RG, Sinha DK, Bodra P, Besra RC, Baski BM, Prakash O, Anand A. Predicting morbidity and mortality in acute pancreatitis in an Indian population: a comparative study of the BISAP score, Ranson's score and CT severity index. *Gastroenterology Report* 2016 Aug 1;4(3):216–220.
15. Yang, L., Liu, J., Xing, Y., Du, L., Chen, J., Liu, X., & Hao, J. (2016). Comparison of BISAP, Ranson, MCTSI, and APACHE II in predicting severity and prognoses of hyperlipidemic acute pancreatitis in Chinese patients. *Gastroenterology research and practice*, *2016*(1), 1834256.
16. Cho JH, Kim TN, Chung HH, Kim KH. Comparison of scoring systems in predicting the severity of acute pancreatitis. *World Journal of Gastroenterology* 2015;21(8):2387–2394.

Chapter 22

Comparative study between spot urine protein to creatinine ratio and 24-hour urine protein in type 2 diabetic patients with nephropathy

Sujata R. Kanetkar, Nanda J. Pati, and Divya R. Brahmbhatt

22.1 INTRODUCTION

When the blood sugar level is excessively high, a condition known as hyperglycemia, or high blood glucose, develops. Decreased insulin (the hormone that carries glucose into the body's bloodstream) secretion, reduced glucose utilization, and increased glucose generation may all be causes of hyperglycemia. A collection of common metabolic illnesses with the phenotype of hyperglycemia are referred to together as diabetes mellitus (DM). A complicated interplay of genetic and environmental variables results in the development of many unique forms of DM [Fatrinawati and Sianipar, 2017]. Type 1 and type 2 diabetes-related problems may be separated into vascular and nonvascular issues. Microvascular (retinopathy, neuropathy, and nephropathy) and macrovascular (coronary heart disease [CHD], peripheral artery disease [PAD], as well as cerebrovascular disease) consequences of DM are further divided into groups [Sudhakar, 2021; Arachchige et al., 2018; Dymicka-Piekarska et al., 2020].

Up to 30% of people with insulin-dependent diabetes mellitus and 25% of those with non-insulin-dependent diabetes mellitus have diabetic nephropathy. When diagnosed too late, diabetic nephropathy causes permanent renal failure due to a steady and ongoing decline in glomerular function [Kamath et al., 2021]. A key factor contributing to morbidity and death is diabetic nephropathy.

Microalbuminuria (excess secretion of albumin) has long been regarded as the gold standard for DN early detection. Due to several limitations, it is not a good enough predictor of DN, though [Bhaisare *et al.*, 2020]. Microalbuminuria does not have the sensitivity or specificity to identify DN in its early stages. Moreover, not all T2DM patients with microalbuminuria will develop end-stage renal disease (ESRD); in fact, 30% among them might have normoalbuminuria. According to some reports, diabetes may have been present for up to six years prior to diagnosis. At the time of diagnosis, individuals often have microalbuminuria due to the varying length of the condition. However, in terms of pathophysiology, sensitivity to therapies like glucose management

DOI: 10.1201/9781003536352-22

and anti-angiotensin II medication, as well as progression to CKD, however, diabetic nephropathy in T2DM is comparable to nephropathy in type 1 DM. Table 22.1 represents urinary albumin excretion in microalbuminuria and clinical nephropathy.

Measurement of 24-hour urine protein excretion is the gold standard approach for diagnosing diabetic nephropathy, although this procedure is often time-consuming, impractical for outpatient departments, uncomfortable, and difficult. It is thought to be unreliable in patients who are uncooperative. There is a chance that measurements may be taken incorrectly due to under- or over-collection. In general, patient compliance is low.

This research aims to evaluate the utility of the random spot urine specimen protein to creatinine ratio in predicting the excretion of protein in the urine and early diagnosis of diabetic nephropathy in patients. Determining spot urine protein-creatinine ratio, one of the most recent techniques, is quick and equivalent to gold standard techniques [Bhaisare *et al.*, 2020]. The great degree of fluctuation in the urine protein content during the day may be related to changes in nutrition, activity, recumbency, water consumption, and the pace of diuresis.

22.2 REVIEW OF LITERATURE

To explore the subclinical rise in urinary albumin excretion rate (AER), also known as micro-albuminuria, which may be the early sign of the onset of diabetic renal dysfunction, Keen and Chlouvervakis created a sensitive, specific radioimmunoassay in 1963 [Brissón *et al.*, 2018]. According to some reports, hyperglycemia has a negative impact on plasma lipids and may speed up atherosclerosis in people with diabetes. Hypertriglyceridemia may be brought on by poor diabetes management because of decreased lipoprotein lipase activity.

Diabetes is the main factor in 44% of new occurrences of kidney failure and 65% of fatalities in patients with stroke and cardiovascular disease. About 73% of people with diabetes have blood pressure more than or equal to 130/80 mm/Hg or use prescription drugs for hypertension, and their

Table 22.1 Urinary albumin excretion in microalbuminuria and clinical nephropathy

Term	*Synonym*	*Urinary albumin level*
Normoalbuminuria	—	< 20 mcg/min (<30 mg/day)
Microalbuminuria	Incipient nephropathy	20–200 mcg/min (30–300 mg/day)
Macroalbuminuria	Clinical nephropathy/Overt nephropathy	> 200 mcg/min (>300 mg/day)

mortality rates from heart disease are 2 to 4 times higher than those of persons without diabetes [Lövestam et al., 2019].

Recent research has shown that AGE products attach to particular AGE receptors found on endothelial cells, macrophages, as well as mesangial cells. This causes cytokines like interleukin-1 (IL-1) a powerful inflammatory and immune-stimulating cytokine that is primarily generated by macrophages in response to infections, as well as insulin-like growth factor-1 to be produced and secreted (IGF-1). This could promote mesangial cell growth and Type IV collagen production in the glomeruli [Baccara-Dinet et al., 2019]. On the other hand, in cultivated endothelium cells, advanced glycation seems to lessen the mitogenic activities of basic fibroblast growth factors (b-FGF) [Emanuelsson *et al.*, 2020].

More thorough analyses of nephropathy in both type 1 and type 2 diabetes have been provided by a variety of population-based cohort studies as well as data from clinical institutions. In summary, the frequency of macroalbuminuria in type 2 diabetes mellitus facilities ranges from 5% to 48% (median is 14%), while it ranges from 8% to 22% (median 15%) in type 1 diabetes centers. Corresponding to this, a median of 13% as well as 20% of people with type 1 and type 2 diabetes, however, had microalbuminuria [Koye *et al.*, 2018]. Yet, it's worth noting that the most recent report from the US National Health and Nutrition Examination Survey (NHANES) indicates a steady decline in albuminuria in the country, which might be due to more targeted multivariate therapy during the past few decades [Jitraknatee *et al.*, 2020].

22.3 MATERIALS AND METHOD

22.3.1 Design of study and time period

This is a cross-sectional study of 100 patients of diabetes mellitus type 2 with diabetic nephropathy admitted to tertiary care hospital, from January2020 to May 2021.

22.3.2 Data collection

Written informed consent was taken from all the cases included in the study for utilizing their data for presentation and/or publication. The patients were taken from the medical wards of tertiary care hospital based on random selection. Patients were considered to be having diabetic nephropathy who met American Diabetes Association (ADA) criteria for the diagnosis of diabetes mellitus and have proteinuria.

Inclusion Criteria: (1) Patients of Diabetes Mellitus II with proteinuria on treatment. (2) Newly detected Patients of Diabetes Mellitus II with proteinuria.

Exclusion Criteria: (1) Hypertension (primary/secondary). (2) Congestive cardiac failure. (3) Urinary tract infection. (4) Primary renal disease. (5) Ketonuria. (6) Pregnant women. (7) Febrile illness. (8) Type 1 diabetic patient.

The selected patients were studied in detail with history and physical examination as per proforma:

Patient's age, sex, age of onset, and duration of diabetes were noted.

All details regarding the presenting complaints were noted.

The drugs the patient was taking, along with the dosages, were noted.

Personal history regarding smoking, alcohol consumption, bowel and bladder habits, and drug (other than anti-diabetic medications) intake were noted.

The regularity of the treatment and the control of diabetes as assessed by blood sugar measurement were also noted. The family history regarding diabetes was taken.

A complete clinical examination was done in each patient with particular reference to the complications of diabetes like neuropathy, nephropathy, ischemic heart disease, peripheral vascular disease, retinopathy, and cerebrovascular accident.

22.3.3 Estimation of spot urine protein-creatinine and 24-hour urine protein

One hour of rest was given to all patients before collecting their urine, and they were all afebrile during the process.

The patients were told to start the 24-hour urine collection as soon as the first emptiness of the day was finished, collecting all pee for 24 hours, which included the final void at the end of the period of 24 hours (8 a.m. to 8 a.m.). The jar includes 5 ml of 10% thymol in isopropanol as a 24-hour preservative.

Random urine sample was taken either before starting or after completing the 24-hour urine collection for urine protein–creatinine ratio.

22.3.4 Esbach's albuminometer

U-Urine and R-Reagent are two marks on urine protein that last for 24 hours. The tube is graded from base to the marking "U" from 0 to 12 g. The most common use for this is the quantitative measurement of protein in urine. Picric acid mixed with citric acid in water makes up the reagent. 500 ml of water is mixed with 5 g of picric acid and 10 g of citric acid to make this. A precipitate that can be quantitatively quantified is created when urine protein reacts with picric and citric acid.

As protein precipitates better in acidic urine, we must ensure that the urine is acidic. Add a few drops of 10% acetic acid to the sample of urine if the liquid is not acidic. The albuminometer tube is filled with the ready urine up to the "U" marker.

The tube is then filled with reagent until it reaches the marking "R." A rubber stopper is used to seal the tube, after which the contents are gently inverted several times to stir them.

The tube is then left to rest for around 24 hours in an upright posture, after which the scale is examined to determine the quantity of sediments (see Figure 22.1).

22.3.5 Spot urine protein to creatinine ratio

a. The amount of urine protein was measured utilizing dye binding, chemical, as well as turbidimetric techniques. The results were given in milligrams per deciliter and were calibrated using a calibrator supplied with the kit.
b. Creatinine concentration was calculated and used an enzymatic technique that reported in milligrams per deciliter after calibration with a serum-based XL multical calibrator.
c. Urinary protein concentration (in mg/dL) was divided by urinary creatinine (in mg/dL) to get the urine protein creatinine ratio.
d. Cobas C311 turbidimetric inhibition immunoassay in hemolyzed complete blood was used to determine HbA1c levels.

Other biochemical tests including blood urea, serum creatinine, and blood lipids were also estimated.

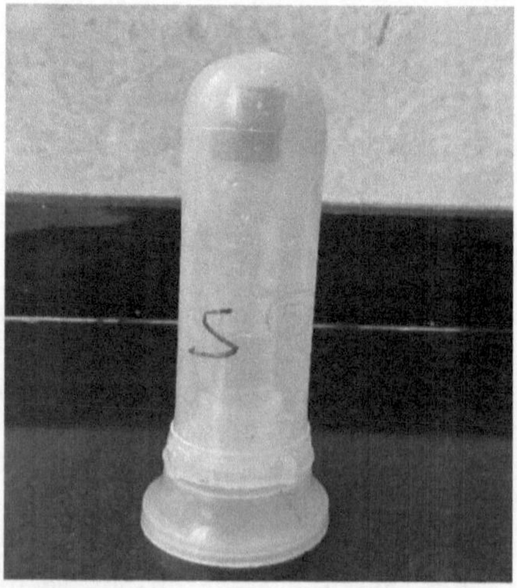

Figure 22.1 Esbach's albuminometer.

Table 22.2 24-Hour urinary protein and spot urinary protein-creatinine ratio in study patients

Variables	*Proteinuria (Mg/24 Hours)*		
	30–299	*300–3499*	*≥3500*
Number (n)	42	46	12
24-Hour proteinuria (average)	211.11	1625.79	6782.5
Spot P/C ratio (average)	214.33	1675.82	4508.08

22.4 RESULT

The present study had 55 male patients and 45 female patients with type 2 diabetes mellitus.

Intraclass Correlation Coefficient (ICC) of total study sample was 0.614 (confidence interval 95%) with Spearman Correlation Coefficient (SCC) being $r = 0.93$. The resulting p was <0.05 which indicates a statistically significant correlation.

After identifying and classifying by levels of proteinuria, the relationship among spot P/C ratio as well as 24-hour urinary protein per 24-hour period remained in the range of proteinuria less than 3500 mg/24-hour period, but this correlation was not seen in the range of proteinuria in the nephrotic frequency band (≥3500 mg/24-hour period). Figure 22.2 represents correlation of severity of diabetic nephropathy with duration of diabetes.

Average 24-hour urinary protein was 172.18 mg in patients with duration of diabetes ≤3 years, which increased to 8320.1 mg in patients with duration of diabetes of >9 years. A steep rise in proteinuria was found in patients with a disease duration of >8 years.

Calculated ICC in patients with proteinuria between 30–299 mg/24 hours was 0.432 and SCC was $r = 0.460$ with $p < 0.001$.

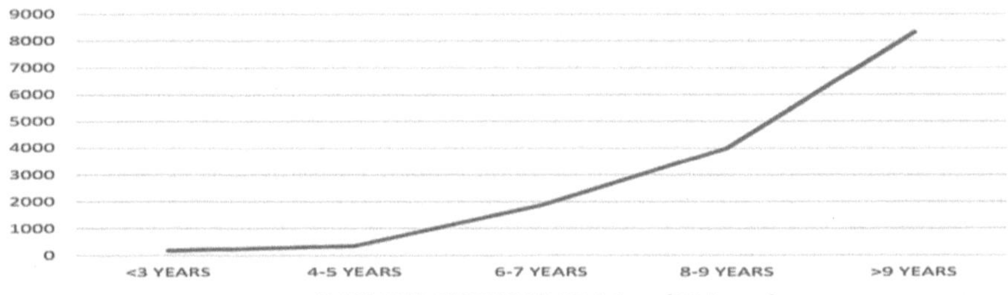

Figure 22.2 Correlation of severity of diabetic nephropathy with duration of diabetes.

Table 22.3 The data for 24-hour urine protein as well as the spot protein/creatinine ratio were correlated using the intraclass correlation coefficient (ICC) with Spearman correlation coefficient (SCC), respectively

24- Hour Urinary Protein (Mg/24 Hour)	*All*	*30–299*	*300–3499*	*≥3500*
N	100	42	46	12
Intraclass correlation coefficient (Icc) (Confidence interval – 95%)	0.614	0.432	0.686	0.314
Spearman correlation coefficient (Scc [R])	0.93	0.460	0.882	0.170
P-value	˂0.05	˂0.001	˂0.001	0.380

ICC of patients with proteinuria of ≥3500 mg/24 hours was 0.314 and SCC was r = 0.170 with p = 0.380 which was not significant [NS] statistically.

The degree of concordance among 24-hour urinary proteins as well as spot urinary protein/creatinine ratio was calculated using Bland and Altman method. It showed that for proteinuria levels <3500 mg/24 hour, the concordance was good, while for proteinuria of >3500 mg/24 hour, the concordance partially disappeared.

Results suggest that there is an acceptable correlation between 24-hour urinary protein and spot urinary protein/creatinine ratio when proteinuria is <3500 mg/24 hour. In the current research, individuals with a HbA1c of 7% had an average proteinuria of 196.7 mg/24 hours, whereas those with a HbA1c of 7.1–8.5% had an average proteinuria of 544.68 mg/24 hours (see Figure 22.3).

As HbA1c rises over 10%, there is a sharp increase in 24-hour proteinuria, which averages 6709.1 mg.

22.4.1 Presenting symptom of diabetic nephropathy

Most common presenting symptom was pedal edema (72%), due to hypoproteinemia secondary to proteinuria in diabetic nephropathy. Puffiness of face were seen in 18% of patients. 22% of patients had decreased urine output suggestive of impending renal failure.

Diabetic retinopathy as a complication of diabetes was most commonly associated (42%) with diabetic nephropathy, 22% had proliferative retinopathy and 20% had non-proliferative retinopathy on fundoscopy examination. The second most common complication observed was ischemic heart disease (34%). Twenty-two patients in the study group had a history of cerebrovascular stroke and 14 patients had peripheral vascular disease upon examination.

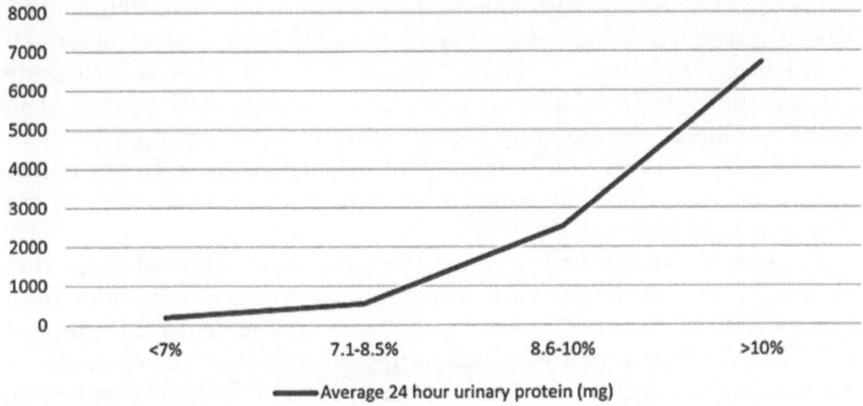

Figure 22.3 Correlation between HbA1c levels and average24-hour urinary protein (mg).

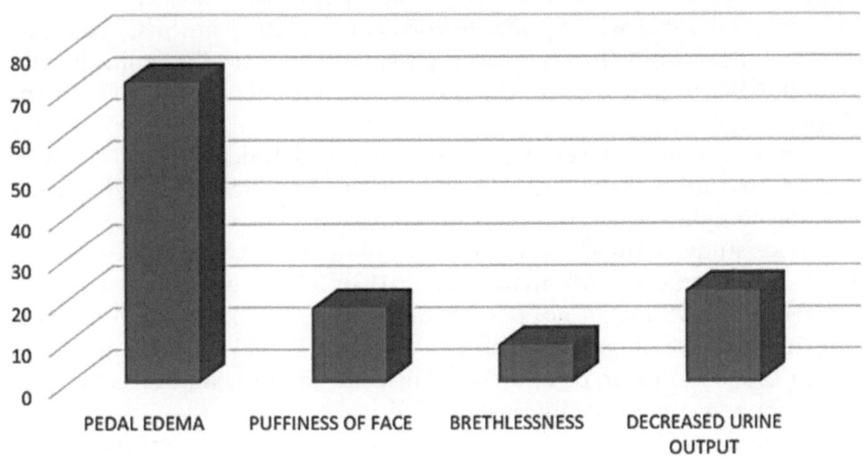

Figure 22.4 Presenting patients with symptoms of diabetic nephropathy in this study.

22.5 DISCUSSION

A sustained increase in albuminuria (>300 mg/d or >200 g/min), proven at least twice during a period of three months, a steady decline in GFR, and an increased arterial blood pressure of 20 mm Hg are all symptoms of DN [Chang et al., 2018]. Microalbuminuria has long been regarded as the gold standard for DN early detection. Due to several restrictions, it is not a good enough predictor of DN [Khunti et al., 2020]. Microalbuminuria does not have the sensitivity or specificity to identify DN in its early stages. Moreover, not all T2DM patients with microalbuminuria will develop end-stage renal disease (ESRD); in fact, 30% among them might have normoalbuminuria. Current research suggests that microalbuminuria occurs after substantial renal damage [Khunti et al., 2020; Thipsawat, 2021]. Thus, it is urgently necessary to find biomarkers that are more sensitive and focused than microalbuminuria for the early identification of DN. Increased levels of some urine biomarkers may be utilized as early indicators of DN in T2DM patients since they can be identified prior to the actual start of severe microalbuminuria [Montero *et al.*, 2013].

The current research had been an 18-month cross-sectional study that was conducted in a tertiary care hospital's department of pathology from January 2020 to May 2021. Around 42% of patients had proteinuria of 30–299 mg/24 hours, that is, incipient nephropathy and 58% of patients had proteinuria of ≥300 mg/24 hours, that is, overt nephropathy suggesting a higher prevalence of overt proteinuria at the time of presentation. An average 24-hour urinary protein excretion was 1650.25 mg.

The average spot urinary protein/creatinine ratio was 1401.89. Intraclass correlation coefficient (ICC) of total study population was 0.614 (confidence interval 95%) with Spearman correlation coefficient (SCC) being $r = 0.93$, and the resulting p was <0.05 suggestive of statistically significant correlation. 65% of patients had duration of diabetes between 4 and 7 years [Koye *et al.*, 2018].

The most common presenting symptom was pedal edema (72%) followed by decreased urine output (22%) and puffiness of face (18%). The most common complication in the study group was diabetic retinopathy (42%).

Present study showed predominance of males compared to females (1.2:1). In the study of Montero et al. (2013), 37.7% of patients had proteinuria of 30,299 mg/24 hours with an average of 163.33 mg/24 hours as compared to 42% of patients with an average of 211.11 mg/24 hours in the present study. However, there are similar results in both studies as both are significant at a confidence interval of 95%.

Compared to 65% of patients in the present study, the study by Boloor et al., (2014) had 62.6% patients with duration of diabetes between 4 and 7 years.

Diabetic retinopathy was the predominant complication which coexisted with diabetic nephropathy in both studies, respectively, 42% and 50.60%. Moreover, ischemic heart disease was present in 29% of patients, while cerebrovascular stroke in 22% of patients in the study by Anastasiou et al. (2019).

22.6 CONCLUSION

In participants with diabetic nephropathy, there had been a significant positive connection among spot protein creatinine ratio as well as 24-hour urine protein. In our investigation, a statistically significant link among spot urine protein/creatinine ratio and 24-hour urinary protein was more often seen in early pre-nephrotic to early nephrotic stages than in overt nephropathy.

Most of the patients had proteinuria ≥300 mg/24 hour, that is, overt nephropathy, at the time of presentation suggesting a long asymptomatic period of diabetic nephropathy. There is a significant increase in the amount of proteinuria with increasing duration of diabetes. As measuring 24-hour urinary protein is time-consuming, inconvenient as well as cumbersome in patients with diabetic nephropathy, Spot urine protein to creatinine ratio may be preferred because it is dependable, simple to repeat, reasonably quick, increases patient compliance as only one urine sample is needed, and has a good correlation with the gold standard of 24-hour urinary protein excretion. Moreover, in our study, diabetic retinopathy was found to be the most prevalent diabetes outcome linked to chronic kidney disease. Thus, it can be concluded that categorization of the spot urine protein to creatinine ratio may be more accurate, sensitive, as well as reliant for the early diagnosis of DN than microalbuminuria.

REFERENCES

Anastasiou I, Eleftheriadou I, Grigoropoulou P, Kokkinos A, Katsilambros N, Perrea D, Tentolouris A, Tsilingiris D, Tentolouris N. The association of diabetic microvascular and macrovascular disease with cutaneous circulation in patients with type 2 diabetes mellitus. *Journal of Diabetes and its Complications* 2019;33(2): 165–170.

Arachchige NS, Bandara SN, Dayarathna RK, Jayasekara KB, Kulasooriya PN, Karunarathna C, Priyadarshani C, Rathnayaka M, Ranaweera I. Prediction of microalbuminuria by analysing total urine protein-to-creatinine ratio in diabetic nephropathy patients in rural Sri Lanka. *The Ceylon Medical Journal* 2018;63(2):72–77.

Baccara-Dinet M, Bhatt DL, Bittner VA, Budaj AJ, Colhoun HM, Diaz R, Goodman SG, Hanotin C, Harrington RA, Ray KK, Szarek M,. Effects of alirocumab on cardiovascular and metabolic outcomes after acute coronary syndrome in patients with or without diabetes: a prespecified analysis of the Odyssey Outcomes randomised controlled trial. *The Lancet Diabetes & Endocrinology* 2019 Aug 1;7(8):618–628.

Bhaisare SD, Jog AS, Kolapkar HU, Rao AK,. Clinical Study of Urine Albumin Creatinine Ratio as an Earlier Predictor of Diabetic Nephropathy. *Journal of Evolution of Medical and Dental Sciences* 2020;9(9):598–603.

Boloor A, Mutneja A, Rao JP. Correlation between spot urine protein creatinine ratio to 24-hour proteinuria in assessing diabetic nephropathy in type 2 diabetes mellitus. *Journal of Pharmaceutical and Biomedical Sciences* 2014;4(07):633–637.

Brissón C, Bonifacino-Belzarena R, Brissón ME, Cuestas V, Denner S, Fernández V, Marsili S, Prono-Mineila P. Cut-off value of proteinuria/creatininuria ratio predictor of proteinurias 150 mg/24 h in a sample of argentinean students. Its utility in proteinuria categorization. Revista Colombiana de Nefrología 2018;5(2):179–189.

Chang CT, Chen CC, Chang YW, Chen CJ, Lee WJ, Lin SY, Liao HY, Liao WL, Tsai FJ, Wu CM. Urinary proteomics for the early diagnosis of diabetic nephropathy in Taiwanese patients. *Journal of Clinical Medicine* 2018 Nov 26;7(12):483.

Dymicka-Piekarska V, Kamińska J, Koper-Lenkiewicz OM, Matowicka-Karna J, Tomaszewska J. Diagnostic utility of protein to creatinine ratio (P/C ratio) in spot urine sample within routine clinical practice. *Critical Reviews in Clinical Laboratory Sciences* 2020;57(5):345–364.

Emanuelsson F, Marott S, Tybjærg-Hansen A, Nordestgaard BG, Benn M. Impact of glucose level on micro-and macrovascular disease in the general population: a Mendelian randomization study. *Diabetes Care* 2020;43(4):894–902.

Fatrinawati W, Sianipar O. Sensitivity of total protein creatinine ratio in urine for diagnosis diabetic nephropathy. *Journal of Medical Sciences* 2017 Apr;49(2):64–71.

Jitraknatee J, Nochaiwong S, Ruengorn C. Prevalence and risk factors of chronic kidney disease among type 2 diabetes patients: a cross-sectional study in primary care practice. *Scientific Reports* 2020 Apr 10;10(1):6205.

Kamath AR, Kamath SJ, Kamath G, Mujeeb S, Nayak RR, Rodrigues GR. Urine protein: Urine creatinine ratio correlation with diabetic retinopathy. *Indian Journal of Ophthalmology* 2021;69(11):3359.

Khunti K, Majeed A, Millett C, Palladino R, Tabak AG, Valabhji J, Vamos EP. Association between prediabetes and microvascular and macrovascular disease in newly diagnosed type 2 diabetes. *BMJ Open Diabetes Research & Care* 2020;8(1):e001061.

Koye DN, Magliano DJ, Nelson RG, Pavkov ME. The global epidemiology of diabetes and kidney disease. *Advances in Chronic Kidney Disease* 2018 Mar 1;25(2):121–132.

Lövestam, Pearce I, Simó R, Adrian M, Wong DT, Evans M. Association between diabetic eye disease and other complications of diabetes: implications for care. A systematic review. *Diabetes, Obesity & Metabolism* 2019;21(3):467–478.

Montero N, Mojal S, Pascual J, Soler MJ. Protein/creatinine ratio in spot urine versus 24-hour urine protein. *Nefrología (English Edition)* 2013;33(1):134–135.

Sudhakar M. A study on correlation of spot urine protein-creatinine ratio with 24 h urinary protein in type 2 diabetes mellitus patients. *International Journal of Scientific Study* 2021;8(12):165–170.

Thipsawat S. Early detection of diabetic nephropathy in patient with type 2 diabetes mellitus: A review of the literature. *Diabetes & Vascular Disease Research* 2021 Nov 9;18(6):14791641211058856.

Chapter 23

The role of electrocardiogram in localizing culprit vessel occlusion in ST-segment elevation myocardial infarction

V. E. Redkar and Nitin Jadhav

23.1 INTRODUCTION

Stroke and cardiovascular disease (CVD) account for around 30% of all death toll worldwide every year. About 80% of these fatalities have occurred in underdeveloped nations. In fact, CVD is the main cause of death in practically every country and region in the globe [1]. More than half of acute myocardial infarction (AMI) fatalities occur before the patient arrives at the hospital, with a 30-day early mortality rate from AMI of 30% [1, 2].

In cases of myocardial infarction, electrocardiogram (ECG) has served as both a preliminary screening tool and one of the most helpful diagnostic tests. Myocardial infarction acute risk assessment continues to be based on straightforward clinical characteristics, lab markers, as well as a 12-lead ECG [3–5]. The only test that can accurately diagnose and predict an acute ST-segment elevated myocardial infarction is the ECG (STEMI). Peaked (hyperacute) T-waves, ST-segment elevation, Q wave development, and T wave inversion are the traditional stages of transformation. From a few hours to many days, this might happen. Although the development of new Q waves (> 30 milliseconds in length and 25% of the R-wave signal amplitude) is informative, 30–50% of acute infarctions do not have Q-waves (non-Q wave infarctions). Based on the characteristics and severity of ST-segment deviation, patients are classified as having an inferior, anterior, or lateral cardiomyopathy [6–8].

A thorough examination of ST-segment elevation might aid in the selection of revascularization therapy. The portion of the myocardium that is at risk may be predicted with the aid of early and precise diagnosis of the infarct-related artery, which can also assist in determining how urgently revascularization should be performed. An important indicator of microvascular flow of blood as well as related prognosis is the ECG reperfusion symptoms [9–11]. The electrophysiology of the myocardial infraction during acute ischemia is reflected by the ECG, while the vascular architecture is identified by coronary angiography (CAG) 6 [12, 13].

This research only compares a 12-lead ECG to coronary angiography to determine which artery is responsible for acute STEMI. However, a lot of

DOI: 10.1201/9781003536352-23

emergency rooms including clinics for chest discomfort have computers that can do uninterrupted ST-segment monitoring [14, 15].

23.2 LITERATURE REVIEW

For ST-segment depressive episodes in lead II, III, as well as aVF in obstruction close to S1 in AWMI, studies by Sponder et al. [7] reported sensitivity to be 48% and specificity to be 83%, whereas studies by Manjunath et al. reported sensitivity to be 93% and specificity to be 79%.

According to a research by Salunke et al., [9] proximal to S1 occlusion affected 52.9% of patients, proximal to D1 occlusion affected 17.6% of patients, and distal to S1 occlusion affected 20.5% of patients. In the vicinity of the S1 occlusion, ST-elevation in lead V1 > 2.5 mm was detected with specificity of 87% and sensitivity of 66% ($P = 0.0019$), complete RBBB was detected with sensitivity of 11.11% as well as specificity of 100% ($P = 0.61$), ST-segment elevation in lead V5 was detected with specificity of 93.75% and sensitivity of 38.89%, ST depression in lead II, III, and aVF was detected with sensitivity.

According to a research by Sanaani et al. [10], RCA blockage was the sole time that lead I and aVL showed ST-segment depression. ST-segment depression in lead aVL was shown to be an early, sensitive ECG indication of RCA blockage, according to a research by Birnbaum et al. [5]. Similar to this, a research by Abhishek et al. 11 found that 22% of their LCX subjects and 59% of their RCA subjects had ST-segment depression in lead I, while in a study, Patil et al. [13] found that 28% of their LCX patients as well as 58% of their RCA participants had the same finding.

A high specificity and sensitivity for RCA occlusion was discovered in a research by Kamal et al. [12] that found that ST-segment elevation in lead III was greater than that in lead II, or that a ratio of elevation in lead III/lead II >1. RCA involvement was detected with a sensitivity of 87%, specificity of 73%, 93.2% of confidence value (positive diagnostic), as well as a negative diagnostic accuracy of 75% in 39 (97.6%) of patients with RCA blockage compared to just 3 (2.4%) of patients with LCX lesion.

23.3 MATERIALS AND METHODS

Type of Study: This was a single-center hospital-based prospective, observational, cohort study.

Sample Size: A total of 100 patients with STEMI were included in the study according to the given formula.

$$\text{Sample size}(N) = Z^2pq / l^2$$

where Z = Standard constant value at 95% CI (confidence interval) = 1.96,

p = Proportional rate of ST-segment elevation MI in Indian population = 0.61,
q = No proportion (1 – p) = 1 0.61 = 0.39 l = Absolute error = 10%,
N = (1.96) 2 (0.61) (0.39) / (0.1) 2 = 3.84 x 0.2379 / 0.01 = 384 x 0.2379 = 91.38
N = 91.38, rounding the figure up to ~100.

Ethics: This study was approved by Institutional Ethics Committee (IEC).

Study Design: The research comprised 100 patients with AMI who were recommended for coronary angiography after being hospitalized to Krishna Hospital, KIMS DU, Karad, with the use of an elevated ST-segment in their ECG. After receiving information about the study's protocols and providing their written agreement, patients who satisfied the inclusion criteria were admitted to the experiment. Cardio-metabolic enzymes and a standard 12-lead ECG were utilized to evaluate the individuals who complained of chest pain (CK and CK-MB or Troponins). A thorough history of the chest pain, the presence of risk factors, as well as how long they had been present, were all acquired as appropriate. The results of coronary angiography were gathered. Based on the following ECG criteria, culprit vessel was identified:

- ST-segment elevation in Lead II, III, aVF
- ST-segment elevation in Lead III>Lead II (right coronary artery occlusion)
- ST-segment depression in V3/ ST-segment elevation in Lead III 0.5–1.2 mm (distal right coronary artery occlusion)
- ST-segment depression in V3/ ST-segment elevation in Lead III <0.5 mm (proximal right coronary artery occlusion)
- ST-segment depression in V1, V2, V3 • ST-segment depression in V3/ ST-segment elevation in Lead III >1.2mm (Left circumflex artery occlusion)
- ST-segment elevation in V2 and isoelectric or ST depression in V3, V4, V5, V6 (first diagonal branch of left anterior descending coronary artery)
- ST-segment depression in aVL (distal part of left anterior descending coronary artery).

Total blockage or significant stenosis (> 70%) of a coronary artery was used to identify the infarct-related artery (IRA).

1 Low-density lipoprotein (LDL) level was calculated from the Friedwald equation:

$$\text{LDL} = \text{Total cholesterol} - \left[\frac{\text{Triglyceride}}{5}\right]\text{HDL} \tag{23.1}$$

2 Very low-density lipoprotein (VLDL) level was calculated from the Friedwald equation:

$$VLDL = \frac{TG}{5} \tag{23.2}$$

and if TG > 400mg/dl, VLDL = 0.66TG.

23.4 STATISTICAL ANALYSIS

All of the information gathered was collected and presented in the form of a mean and standard deviation. Using SPSS version 23 software and OpenEpi version 2.3.1, the $\chi 2$ test was used to assess the ECG results between individuals with anterior and inferior wall, as appropriate. A p-value of less than 0.05 was used to indicate statistical significance. Calculations were made to determine each parameter's diagnostic accuracy like sensitivity, negative and predictive value, specificity, and diagnostic precision.

23.5 RESULTS

A total of 100 subjects with ST-segment elevation MI were included in the study out of which 80 subjects (80%) were males and 20 subjects (20%) were females. In the study, 8 subjects (8%) were in the age group of 18–40 years, 60 patients (60%) were in the age group of 40–60 years, and 32 patients (32%) were in the age group of >60 years. Mean age in years was 56.08, ranging from 34–75 years with SD ±10.74. Table 23.1 represents the distribution of study population on the basis of co-morbidities Around 24 patients (24%) had type 2 diabetes mellitus (T2DM), 36 patients (36%) were hypertensives, and 18 patients (18%) had both the co-morbidities, that is, T2DM and hypertension.

Table 23.1 Distribution of study population on the basis of co-morbidities

Co-morbidities	*n = 100*	*Percent*
Type 2 diabetes mellitus	24	24%
Hypertension	36	36%
T2DM and hypertension	18	1

Consequently, 26 patients (26%) had addiction of tobacco, 16 patients (16%) had addiction of alcohol, and 12 patients (12%) were addicted to both, that is, tobacco and alcohol.

Sixty-eight patients (68%) had anterior wall MI (AWMI) and 32 patients (32%) had inferior wall MI (IWMI).

Figure 23.1 represents the study population on the basis of type of MI.

23.5.1 Overall finding

Out of 68 patients with ECG findings suggestive of AWMI, 52 patients (76.5%) had an occlusion in the left anterior descending (LAD) artery upon confirmation on angiography. Out of 32 patients (32%) with ECG findings suggestive of IWMI, 20 patients (62.5%) had an occlusion in the right coronary artery (RCA) while 4 patients (12.5%) had an occlusion in the left circumflex (LCx) artery upon confirmation on angiography. It was observed that in the study population, a majority of patients had an occlusion in the culprit vessel on angiography which was previously predicted by ECG findings. ECG is a good modality for predicting the culprit vessel occlusion in patients with STEMI (see Tables 23.2 and 23.3).

Among 20 patients with Q-wave in aVL on ECG, 12 patients had an occlusion proximal to D1 and 8 patients had no occlusion proximal to D1 on angiography. It was observed that Q-wave in aVL on ECG showed a sensitivity of 60%, specificity of 100%, PPV of 100%, NPV of 85.7%, and accuracy of 88.2% in predicting an occlusion proximal to D1 in AWMI when compared with angiographic findings (see Figure 23.2).

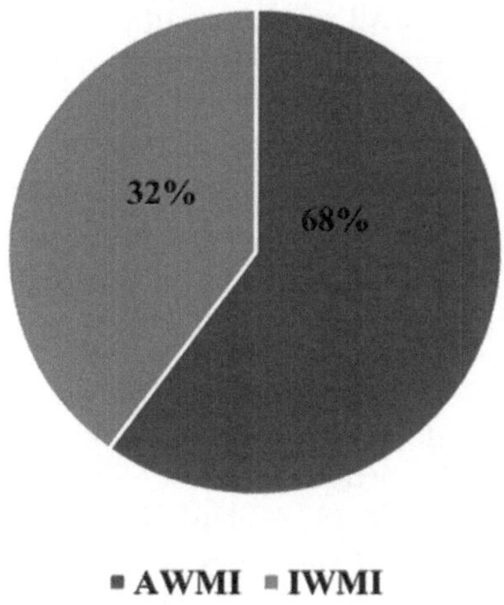

Figure 23.1 Study population on the basis of type of MI.

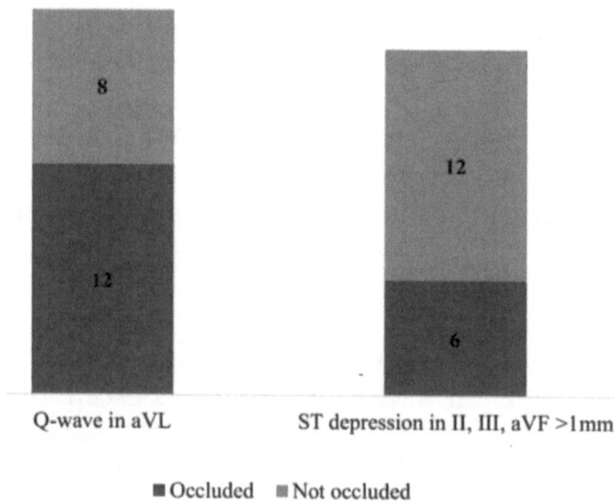

Figure 23.2 Distribution and correlation of ECG findings for localizing an occlusion proximal to first diagonal branch of LAD artery with angiographic findings in patients with AWMI.

Table 23.2 Distribution of study population on the basis of type of STEMI

Type of STEMI	*n = 100*	*Percent*
AWMI	68	68%
IWMI	32	32%

ECG findings included ST-segment elevation in lead V1-V4 with ST-segment depression in aVL. All of them had an occlusion distal to D1 on angiography. It was observed that ST-segment depression in aVL on ECG showed a sensitivity of 100%, specificity of 96.43%, PPV of 85.71%, NPV of 100%, and accuracy of 97.06% in predicting an occlusion distal to D1 in AWMI on ECG when compared with angiographic findings (see Table 23.3).

23.6 DISCUSSION

The predominance of STEMI in patient in India was determined to be 61%, according to a research done in 2014 by Chakraborty et al. [5]. Out of 100 STEMI patients in the current research, 68 patients (68%) had AWMI, while the remaining 32 patients (32%) had IWMI. According to research by Salunke et al., [9] there were 16 instances of IWMI and 34 cases of AWMI.

For ST-elevation in lead V1 > 2.5 mm, Manjunath et al.'s [11] study discovered a specificity of 66% and sensitivity of 71%. According to Kamal

Table 23.3 Distribution and correlation of ECG findings for localizing an occlusion distal to first diagonal branch of LAD artery with angiographic findings in patients with AWMI

Occlusion Distal to First Diagonal Branch (D1) of Lad Artery				*Sensitivity*	*Specificity*	*Ppv*	*Npv*	*Accuracy*
ECG findings	*Angiographic finding*		*No. of patients*					
	Occluded	Not-occluded						
ST-segment depression in lead aVL	12	0	12	100%	96.4%	85.7%	100%	97%

(LAD: Left anterior descending artery).

et al.'s, [12] study, lead aVR ST-segment elevation had a sensitivity of 43% and a specificity of 95%.

In a relative study by Manjunath et al., sensitivity and specificity were both determined to be 50% and 100%, respectively. In a study by Patil et al. [13], ST-segment elevation in lead aVR was identified in 100% of proximal LAD lesions, 85% of left main coronary artery (LMCA) lesions, and 40% of TVD lesions. For ST-segment depression in lead V5, sensitivity was found to be 17% and specificity to be 98% in a research by Shama et al. [14], but for ST depression in lead V5, sensitivity was found to be 8% and specificity to be 100% in the study by Manjunath et al.

When an occlusion in the proximal RCA was verified on CAG, it was shown that ST-segment elevation in lead V4R > 1mm on ECG had a sensitivity of 87.5%, specificity of 62.5%, PPV of 70%, NPV of 83.33%, and accuracy of 75% in predicting the occlusion. The results are in line with earlier research by Zimetbaum et al., who demonstrated that RCA occlusion was the sole circumstance in which lead III's ST-segment elevation was greater than lead II's.

According to a research by Pandey et al. [16], the RCA and LAD coronary arteries had 100% and 0%, respectively, sensitivity of ECG to identify the culprit vessel in AMI. The LCx coronary artery has the highest specificity (100%), followed by the RCA (91.67%) including LAD coronary artery (90.91%).

23.7 CONCLUSION

Electrocardiogram results of proximal coronary artery blockage show relatively significant myocardial infarction, which is best treated by comprehensive but rather early revascularization techniques like angioplasty. The ECG offers a cost-effective, dependable, and rapid means of discriminating the infarct-related artery in AMI, even if it is not a replacement for invasive treatments for identifying the culprit artery in AMI. In the current research, it was shown that patients suffering from acute STEMI, which was later validated by a coronary angiography, may benefit from using an electrocardiogram as a diagnostic instrument to forecast the location of coronary artery blockage.

REFERENCES

1. Estel C, Conti CR. Global burden of cardiovascular disease. *Cardiovascular Innovations and Applications*. 2016 Sep 1;1(4):369–377.
2. Kumar A, Thompson EW, Lefieux A, Molony DS, Davis EL, Chand N, Fournier S, Lee HS, Suh J, Sato K, Ko YA. High coronary shear stress in patients with coronary artery disease predicts myocardial infarction. *Journal of the American College of Cardiology* 2018;72(16):1926–1935.
3. Miranda DF, Lobo AS, Walsh B, Sandoval Y, Smith SW. New insights into the use of the 12-lead electrocardiogram for diagnosing acute myocardial infarction in the emergency department. *The Canadian Journal of Cardiology* 2018;34(2):132–145.

4. Lindow T, Pahlm O, Nikus K. A patient with non-ST-segment elevation acute coronary syndrome: Is it possible to predict the culprit coronary artery?. *Journal of Electrocardiology* 2016;49(4):614–619.
5. Chakraborty S, Majumder B, Sarkar D, Chatterjee S. A simple non-invasive ECG technique to localize culprit vessel occlusion site in ST-elevation myocardial infarction (STEMI) patients. *Journal of Clinical & Experimental Cardiology* 2017;8(556):2.
6. Wiśniewski P, Rostoff P, Gajos G, Nessler J, Kruszelnicka O. Predictive value of electrocardiographic ST-segment elevation myocardial infarction equivalents for detecting acute coronary artery occlusion in patients with nonST-segment elevation myocardial infarction. *Kardiologia Polska* 2019 Jun 25;77(6):624–631.
7. Sponder M, Ehrengruber S, Berghofer A, Schönbauer R, Toma A, Silbert BI, Hengstenberg C, Lang I, Richter B. New ECG algorithms with improved accuracy for prediction of culprit vessel in inferior ST-Segment elevation myocardial infarction. *Panminerva Medica* 2021, 65(3):303–311.
8. Liu Q, Zhang Y, Zhang P, Zhang J, Cao X, He S, Yang D. Both baseline Selvester QRS score and change in QRS score predict prognosis in patients with acute ST-segment elevation myocardial infarction after percutaneous coronary intervention. *Coronary Artery Disease* 2020;31(5):403.
9. Salunke KK, Khyalappa RJ. Role of electrocardiogram in identification of culprit vessel occlusion in acute ST elevation myocardial infarction in relation to coronary angiography. *Journal of Preventive Cardiology* 2017;6:128–132.
10. Sanaani A, Yandrapalli S, Jolly G, Paudel R, Cooper HA, Aronow WS. Correlation between electrocardiographic changes and coronary findings in patients with acute myocardial infarction and single-vessel disease. *Annals of translational medicine*. 2017;5(17), 10.21037/atm.2017.06.33
11. Abhisekh Mohanty RK Saran. Assessment of validity of the 'Culprit Score' for predicting the culprit lesion in patients with acute inferior wall myocardial infarction. *Indian Heart Journal* 2016; 68(6):776–779.
12. Kamal AM, Soltan GM, Ali MA. Electrocardiographic prediction of culprit artery in acute ST-segment elevation myocardial infarction. *Menoufia Medical Journal* 2018;31:1463–1469
13. Patil V, Pandere K, Damle S, Avhad A. Utility of aVR electrocardiogram lead for identifying the culprit lesion in patient with acute coronary syndrome. *ournal of Datta Meghe Institute of Medical Sciences University* 2019;14:383–390.
14. Shama MA, Hussaien MN, Elsaiedy MA, Elsheikh RG. Usefulness of the Electrocardiogram as a Tool to Localize Culprit Vessel Occlusion Site in Acute ST-Segment Elevation Myocardial Infarction. *International Journal of Current Microbiology and Applied Sciences* 2019;8(6):1988–1995.
15. Redfors B, Kosmidou I, Crowley A, Maehara A, Ben-Yehuda O, Arif A, Dizon JM, Mintz GS, Stone GW. Prognostic significance of QRS fragmentation and correlation with infarct size in patients with anterior ST-segment elevation myocardial infarction treated with percutaneous coronary intervention: Insights from the INFUSE-AMI trial. *International Journal of Cardiology* 2018;253:20–24.
16. Madan, P., Singh, V., Singh, D. P., Diwakar, M., & Kishor, A. (2022). Denoising of ECG signals using weighted stationary wavelet total variation. *Biomedical Signal Processing and Control*, *73*, 103478. http://dx.doi.org/10.1016/j.bspc.2021.103478

Chapter 24

Correlation of early post-cataract surgery-related OCT changes with its intra-operative surgical complications

Girish Gadre

24.1 INTRODUCTION

Cataract surgery is one of the most commonly performed surgeries all over the world as well as in India and cataract accounts for the most common cause of treatable blindness. As every surgery, cataract surgery also has various complications: one of the most common cause of suboptimal vision after cataract surgery is pseudophakic cystoid macular edema (PCME). Pseudophakic cystoid macular edema is also known as Irvine-Gass syndrome and is studied to occur in 1–4% of eyes undergoing cataract surgery in various studies across present literature. Surprisingly the appearance of angiographic macular edema is said to be around 20–30% and in some studies as high as 70% of the eyes undergoing cataract surgery. Various risk factors have been held accountable for macular edema after cataract surgery which includes pre-operative risk factors like preexisting uveitis, diabetes mellitus, hypertension, use of topical prostaglandin analogues, use of systemic thiazolidinedione, existing epiretinal membrane, and intra-operative factors includes type of surgery, surgical manipulations and excess iris handling, location of lens placement, posterior capsular rupture leading to intra-operative vitreous loss.

Fluorescein angiography used to be the gold standard method for diagnosing macular edema especially in cases of subclinical macular edema where central vision of the patient is unaffected but fluorescein angiography shows leakage in fovea. With time, addition of newer technology like spectral domain (SD) OCT, the scans obtained are of superior quality and high resolution which enrich us with accurate quantification helping to diagnose slightest change in anatomy of retina which is not detectable by indirect ophthalmoscopy. Due to this non-invasiveness and reliability, OCT can be a boon in early diagnosis of PCME especially in cases of subclinical macular edema which can be easily missed by indirect ophthalmoscopy [1].

In modern day setting of phacoemulsification cataract surgery, the incidence of PCME has been reduced significantly but the presence of subclinical macular edema has been observed to occur more frequently than expected and its early diagnosis is necessary to achieve a desirable visual

DOI: 10.1201/9781003536352-24

outcome following cataract surgery. For this, OCT will play a very important tool, and hence, it is mandatory to observe changes in macula following eventful and uneventful cataract surgery mainly SICS and phacoemulsification which are the most commonly performed surgeries in India [2].

Primary or first line of treatment for pseudophakic macular edema has emerged as topical NSAIDs which have been tried and tested by time and has been approved by FDA for the same. Intractable edema can be treated with other modalities and drugs via different routes mainly posterior subtenons and intravitreal.

Although subclinical macular edema is a self-limiting condition in most of the cases, an eye should be kept on progression of the edema and treat accordingly, so as to prevent permanent vision loss due to chronic macular edema.

24.2 REVIEW OF LITERATURE

24.2.1 Retina

Retina is derived from the Latin word 'rete' meaning net. It is a 10 layered network comprising supporting cells, photoreceptors, neural cell bodies, and their axons forming a transparent membrane lining the innermost layer of the eye. It covers a surface area of 266 m^2. The thickness of retina at the posterior pole in peripapillary region is approximately 0.56 mm, becomes thinner toward the periphery, and the thickness reduces to 0.18 mm at the equator and 0.1 mm at the ora serrata [3].

24.2.2 Gross anatomy

The major landmarks of retina include the optic disc, retinal blood vessels, area centralis, peripheral retina, and ora serrata.

24.2.3 Optic disc

It is pale pink, circular to slightly oval structure which is about 1.5 mm in diameter. Optic disc is made of the nerve fibers as they traverse through the lamina cribrosa. All other retinal layers terminate here.

24.2.4 Area centralis

Also called the central retina, this consists of perifovea, parafovea, fovea, and the foveola. Measuring approximately 5.5 mm, area centralis is located in the posterior fundus temporal to the optic disc. It is demarcated by the upper and lower arcuate fibers, and temporal retinal vessels. An oval yellowish area of 3 mm in diameter is referred to as macula lutea which contains the foveola at the center [3].

24.2.5 Fovea or fovea centralis

It is the central depressed part of the macula. It is located 0.8 mm below the horizontal meridian and 4 mm temporal from the center of the optic disc. It is about 1.85 mm in diameter which represents 50 of visual field and has an average thickness of 0.25 mm [3]. The term clivus refers to the sides of depression leading to foveola. It denotes the shift from vascular to avascular retina (FAZ). The exact location of which can be determined only by fluorescein angiography.

24.2.6 Foveola and UMBO

It is the central floor of the fovea, measuring 0.35 mm in diameter, 0.25 mm in depth, and 0.13 mm in thickness and represents the highest visual acuity in the retina corresponding to 10 of the visual field [3].

The foveola has no rods. There is a tiny depression in the center of foveola measuring 150 μ called the umbo. Due to the total internal reflection in this region, foveolar reflex is seen ophthalmoscopically.

24.2.7 Parafovea and perifovea

Surrounding the fovea is parafovea which is about 0.5 mm in diameter. It contains less retinal vessels, and compared to other parts of retina, the ganglion cell layer, inner nuclear layer, and inner plexiform layer are thicker [3].

The outer most region of the macula surrounding the parafovea is perifovea which is 1.5 mm in diameter with high rod-cone ratio and rich retinal blood vessels. Here the ganglion cell layer is more than a single cell layer thick and the cone density is more compared to peripheral retina.

24.2.8 The peripheral retina

This region is divided into four regions: the near periphery, the mid periphery, the far periphery, and extreme periphery.

Near periphery: It is about 1.5 mm wide, which surrounds the area centralis.

Mid periphery: It is a 3 mm wide zone around the near periphery.

Far periphery: It is a 6 mm wide zone around the mid periphery and from the optic disc, it is 9–10 mm on the temporal side and 16 mm on the nasal side, as the optic disc is located nasally. The sensory retina is attached firmly both to the vitreous and RPE in this region. It is 2.1 mm wide temporally, 0.8 mm wide nasally, and is at a distance of 7 mm and 6 mm, respectively, from the limbus. Ora serrata is 25 mm from the optic disc and 6–8 mm from the equator on the nasal side [3].

24.2.9 Retinal pigment epithelium

It consists of hexagonal cells arranged in a single layer which contains the pigment. It is the outermost layer of retina. The granular appearance of fundus is due to the unequal distribution of pigmentation of these cells and gives it a fine mottling appearance. It attaches loosely to the layer of rods and cones and firmly to the underlying Bruch's membrane [4–6]. The space between the RPE and sensory retina is a potential space known as the subretinal space where the subretinal fluid accumulates. The outer blood retinal barrier is constituted by the adjacent RPE cells which are connected to each other by zonula occludens and zonula adherence. Fovea consists of RPE cells which are taller and thinner, and contains larger pigment granules when compared to the rest of fundus, therefore responsible for giving a dark color to this area. On cross-section, RPE cells have two parts: the apical and the basal. The apical part is formed by the microvilli which project between the rods and cones and consists melanin granules. The basal part of the RPE cells has an increased surface area as a result of convoluted infolds which helps in absorption and secretion of materials [7, 8].

24.2.10 Neurosensory retina

It consists of rods and cones which are the photoreceptor cells of retina, and they are the primary neurons in the visual pathway. Visual purple or rhodopsin is a photosensitive substance present in the rods and is responsible for peripheral vision and scotopic vision, whereas cones are responsible for central vision and color vision. The rods outnumber cones in the total retina with a ratio of 125 million rods to 6.5 million cones. The density of the cones is highest at the fovea with an average of 150,000 per square millimeter. The number of cones decreases rapidly at the rate of 75,000 per square millimeter and at 130 μm from the foveal center and rods begin to appear. The rods are present at their highest density at 3 mm from the foveal center and the cone density is reduced to 6000 cones per square millimeter. The rods are absent at the fovea in an area of 0.35mm which corresponds to 1.25° of the visual field [9–13].

24.2.11 External limiting membrane

It is formed by the junctions between the cell membrane of photoreceptors and Muller's cell and the layer extends from ora serrata to the optic disc edge through which the processes of rods and cones pass. In low magnification, it appears as a fenestrated membrane [14, 15].

24.2.12 Outer nuclear layer

It is a single layer composed of the nuclei of rods and cones. The nuclei of cones are larger (6–7μm) when compared to rod nuclei (5.5 μm). The thickness of this layer as well as the number of nuclei varies from region to region. Eight to nine layers of nuclei with a thickness of 45μm are present nasal to the disc, whereas only four layers of nuclei with 22 μm thickness are present temporal to the disc. Foveal region consists of 10 layers of nuclei with a thickness of 50μm. Rest of the retina except ora serrata consists of one row of cone nuclei and four rows of rod nuclei with a thickness of 27μm.

24.2.13 Outer plexiform layer

It contains synapses between the dendrites of the bipolar cells and processes of horizontal cells with rod spherules and cone pedicles. It consists of first-order neurons in the retina. The layer is the thickest at the macula (51μm) and mainly consists of oblique fibers that have deviated from the fovea and is called Henle's layer [16, 17].

24.2.14 Inner nuclear layer

This layer is absent at the fovea. It consists of bipolar cells, horizontal cells, amacrine cells, the soma of Muller's cell, and capillaries of the central retinal vessels. The bipolar cells are the neurons of first order of vision. Their axons arborize with the ganglion cell dendrites and their dendrites arborize with the cone pedicles and rod spherules in the outer plexiform layer. The horizontal cells are flat neurons having many associative and neuronal interconnections between photoreceptors and bipolar cells in the outer plexiform layer. The amacrine cells are located in the innermost part of this layer and forms connections with the axons of bipolar cells and dendrites of the ganglion cells.

The Muller's cells play an important role in the metabolism of the sensory retina as well as provide structural support to it.

24.2.15 Inner plexiform layer

This layer is absent at the fovea and consists of synapses between the axon of bipolar cells, dendrites of ganglion cells, and processes of amacrine cells.

24.2.16 Ganglion cell layer

The ganglion cells form the second-order neurons of the visual pathway. It is multilayered (6–8 cell layers) at the macula, double layered temporal to the disc, and single layered throughout the rest of retina. Foveola lacks the ganglion cell layer.

24.2.17 Nerve fiber layer

It consists of the unmyelinated axons of the ganglion cells that converge at the level of optic nerve head, pass through lamina cribrosa, and become ensheathed by myelin posterior to lamina.

24.2.18 Internal limiting membrane

It forms an interface between retina and vitreous, and the internal lamellae of this layer merge with the vitreous fibrils. This layer has four elements namely collagen fibrils, basement membrane, proteoglycans, and plasma membrane of Muller's cells.

24.2.19 Available protocols

The Topcon 3D OCT-1 Maestro OCT offers various scan acquisition protocols designed for examination of the retina or glaucoma patients. The scan acquisition protocol can be selected from the scan tab in the main window.

The protocols can be grouped into four ways:

1. Glaucoma protocols
2. Retina protocols
3. All protocols
4. Custom protocols

24.3 METHODS

This prospective cohort study was conducted in the ophthalmology department, Krishna Hospital, Karad.

Type of study: Prospective cohort study
Period of collection of data: 18 months
Period of analysis and compilation: 6 months
Time of study: from Dec 2019 to May 2021
Rationale of sample size: p = 18 (reported prevalence)
q = 100-P = 82
L: Allowable error = 6% = 164.7

Sample size for my study is = 165

An informed written consent of the patient was taken and proforma of study was explained followed by a detailed history and examination.

Detailed history was taken followed by ocular examination which included:

- **Visual acuity:** tested by using Snellen's Distant Vision chart and Jaeger's Near Vision chart.
- **Intra-ocular pressure:** Taken on each visit on non-contact tonometer (Nidek NT-510).

- **Fundoscopy:** With the help of direct and indirect ophthalmoscope.
- **Optical coherence tomography (OCT)** – TOPCON 3D-OCT 1 Maestro machine was used to take radial 6-mm OCT scans pre-operatively,

Inclusion criteria:

- All patients undergoing cataract surgery (SICS and phacoemulsification).

Exclusion criteria:

- All patients where fundus examination and OCT are difficult.
- Patients who are already diagnosed and being treated for macular edema.
- Patients with diabetic retinopathy.
- Patients on prostaglandin analogue.
- Patients on thiazolidinedione drug for diabetes.
- Patient with history of uveitis.
- Patients who are on NSAID eye drops pre-operatively.
- Patients in which secondary surgical intervention was required.

24.4 OBSERVATIONS AND RESULTS

This prospective cohort study was conducted in Krishna Hospital, Karad. 165 eyes were included in this study that satisfied the inclusion criteria.

24.4.1 Distribution of patients according to age

Range of age distribution was 38–85years. The mean age was 62.51years and standard deviation was 8.74years. Majority of the patients were in the age range of 60–69 years (44%).

24.4.2 Distribution of patients according to gender

Study included 89 (53.93%), male patients, and 76 (46.06%) females with male to female ratio of 1.17:1.

24.4.3 Distribution of laterality

Study included 96 (58.18%) right eyes and 69 (41.81%).

24.4.4 Distribution of eyes according to type of surgery

132 (80%) of the eyes underwent SICS surgery and 33 (20%) of the eyes underwent phacoemulsification surgery.

24.4.5 Distribution of eyes with location of IOL implanted

162 (98.18%) eyes had IOL implanted in the bag and 3 (1.8%) eyes had IOL implanted in the sulcus.

24.4.6 Types of IOL implanted

131 (79.39%) eyes were implanted with a PMMA lens, 33 (20%) eyes with a foldable hydrophilic acrylic lens, and 1 (0.60%) eye with a foldable three-piece IOL.

24.4.7 Distribution of macular edema and types of IOLs

Of 131 eyes implanted with PMMA lenses, 38 (29%) had subclinical edema and 3 (2.29%) had clinical edema. Of 33 eyes implanted with foldable acrylic lenses, 6 (18.75%) had subclinical edema, and none had clinical edema. Of one eye implanted with a three-piece lens, none had subclinical or clinical edema.

24.4.8 Systemic Risk factors in patients

Patients with systemic risk factors include 18 (10.9%) had diabetes, 48 (29.09%) had hypertension, and 23 (13.93%) had diabetes and hypertension.

24.4.9 Incidence of macular edema in various systemic risk factors

Of all the patients with diabetes, 9 (50%) had subclinical macular edema and 2 (11.1%) had clinical edema. Ten (20.8%) patients with hypertension had subclinical edema. Twelve (52%) patients with diabetes and hypertension together had subclinical edema and 1 (4.3%) had clinical edema.

- Diabetes: $p = 0.000019$ was a statistically significant risk factor.
- Hypertension: $p = 0.81$ was statistically not a significant risk factor.

24.4.10 Incidence of edema in the presence of systemic risk factors

Of the total patients with systemic risk factors, 31 (34.8%) had subclinical macular edema and 3(3.3%) had clinical macular edema. And those without systemic risk factors include 13 (17.1%) had subclinical edema and no patient had clinical edema.

24.4.11 Incidence of macular edema in the presence of intra-operative complications

Of the total 45 (27%) eyes with intra-operative complications, 12 (26.6%) had subclinical macular edema and 2 (4.4%) had clinical macular edema.

24.4.12 Incidence of macular edema in various intra-operative risk factors

Eight (29.62%) eyes of total 27 which had prolonged surgery time had subclinical edema, of the total 13 eyes with iris prolapse, 2 (15.3%) had subclinical edema and 1 (7.6%) had clinical edema. Of the total five cases of posterior capsular rupture, 2 (40%) had subclinical edema and 1 (20%) had clinical macular edema.

24.4.13 Incidence and classification of macular edema according to type of surgery

Of the total 37 (22.42%) cases of Grade 1 subclinical edema, 32 (86%) eyes had undergone SICS and 5 (13.5%) had undergone phacoemulsification surgery. Of total seven (4.24%) of Grade 2 subclinical edema, six (85.7%) had undergone SICS and 1 (14.2%) had undergone phacoemulsification surgery. Of three clinical edema eyes, three (100%) had undergone SICS surgery.

24.4.14 Incidence of edema in different types of surgery

Of all 132 SICS cases, 38 (28.7%) had subclinical edema and three (2.2%) had clinical edema. Of all the 33 phacoemulsification cases, six (18%) had subclinical edema.

24.4.15 Distribution of type of edema and location of implanted IOL

Of all the 162 eyes with IOL implanted in bag, 42 (25.92%) had subclinical edema and 2 (1.23%) had clinical edema. Of all the three eyes with IOL implanted in sulcus, two (66.66%) had subclinical edema and one (33.33%) had clinical edema.

24.4.16 Distribution of type of edema and location of implanted IOL

Of all the 162 eyes with IOL implanted in bag, 42 (25.92%) had subclinical edema and 2 (1.23%) had clinical edema. Of all the three eyes with IOL implanted in sulcus, two (66.66%) had subclinical edema and one (33.33%) had clinical edema.

24.5 DISCUSSION

Cataract as we know is one of the most commonly performed surgeries all over the world, so it is very crucial to study the immediate post-operative complications, one being incidence of pseudophakic cystoid macular edema which was previously reported to be around 1% to 30% of which clinical significant edema seen in 1% to 3% in patients with no risk factors and more so in cases having risk factors up to 20%. Incidence of angiographic CME is yet higher up to 30% following uneventful cataract surgery. But fluorescein angiography is known to be a potentially invasive method, with complications ranging from rash to anaphylactic reaction and in rare cases death. OCT is a non-invasive and less time-consuming diagnosis technique which gives accurate histological scan results and quantification of macular thickness. OCT nowadays has practically replaced FA except in certain scenarios. So, it is necessary to monitor the changes in macula after cataract surgery and to establish some guidelines for diagnosis for pseudophakic macular edema on OCT.

A prospective cohort study with 165 study eyes was included, of which 21 study eyes lost follow up on last visit (4th month).

The mean age of patients in the present study was 62.51 years ± 8.74 years, with majority of patients in the 60–69 years age group. In the study done by Irfan et al., the mean age of the patients was 64.32± 13.84 years, whereas in the study by Meri Vukicevic et al. [8] the mean age of the patients was 78.18±8.58 years.

89 (53.93%) were male, 76 (46.06%) were female, and the male to female ratio was 1.17:1.

In the present study, 96 (58.18%) cases were right eye, and 69 (41.81%) were left eye.

132 (80%) of the eyes underwent small incision cataract surgery (SICS) and 33 (20%) underwent phacoemulsification.

In the present study, 44 (26.66%) out of 165 eyes had subclinical macular edema and three (1.81%) eyes had clinical macular edema as per the criteria defined earlier. In a retrospective study of 81984 eyes done by Chu et al. [2], the incidence of pseudophakic cystoid macular edema (clinical) was found out to be 1.17%–4.04%, whereas Henderson et al.'s [4]. study showed the incidence of clinical macular edema 0.1%–2.35% which was found out to be similar to our study. According to a study done by Hartnett et al., optical coherence tomography (OCT) for post-cataract macular edema evaluation was performed and CME was found in 22% of patients with diabetes at one month post-cataract extraction. In other studies done by Perente et al. [11]; Bélair et al.; Vukicevic et al. [8], the incidence of subclinical pseudophakic CME diagnosed by optical coherence tomography (OCT) varies between 4 and 10.9%. Whereas Wright PL et al. [6] reported the incidence of angiographic CME as 30%. The appearance of angiographic CME is much more frequent, with varying incidences up to 70%.

162 (98.18%) eyes had IOL implanted in the bag and 3 (1.8%) eyes had IOL implanted in the sulcus.

132 (80%) eyes were implanted with PMMA lens of which 38 (27.78%) had subclinical edema and 3 (2.27%) had clinical edema, 32 (19.39%) eyes with foldable hydrophilic acrylic lens of which 6 (18.75%) had subclinical edema and none had clinical edema and 1 (0.60%) eye with a three-piece IOL where no edema was observed.

Of the total 89 patients with systemic risk factors, 31(34.8%) had subclinical macular edema and 3 (3.3%) had clinical macular edema. And those 76 patients without systemic risk factors include 13 (17.1%) who had subclinical edema and no patient had clinical edema.

In the present study, systemic risk factors include 18 (10.9%) who had diabetes of which 9 (50%) had subclinical macular edema and 2 (11.1%) had clinical edema, 48(29.09%) had hypertension of which 10 (20.8%) had subclinical edema, 23 (13.93%) had diabetes and hypertension of which 12 (52%) had subclinical macular edema and 1 (4.3%) had clinical macular edema.

In the present study, diabetes has found out to be very significant risk factor for development of macular edema, and hypertension has found out to be a nonsignificant risk factor for development of macular edema, which was in accordance with the study done by Wright et al. [6], where in diabetes incidence of CME varied from 31% to 81%. In a retrospective study on 81,984 eyes by Chu et al. [2], it was found out that the incidence of edema was four times more in diabetic patients. On the contrary in Hartnett ME et al's. study, the incidence was 22%. In Flach et al.'s [7] study, hypertension apparently increases the risk of PCME.

In the present study, 45(27%) eyes had intra-operative complications of which 12 (26.6%) had subclinical macular edema and 2 (4.4%) had clinical macular edema. This did not turn out to be statistically significant but were significant in Chu et al.'s study [2].

Eight (29.62%) eyes of total 27 which had prolonged surgery time had subclinical edema, of the total 13 eyes with iris prolapse, 2 (15.3%) had subclinical edema and 1 (7.6%) had clinical edema. Of the total five cases of posterior capsular rupture, two (40%) had subclinical edema and one (20%) had clinical macular edema. There was no statistical significance to this, but it was observed that posterior capsular rupture could be a major risk factor for the development of macular edema which was also noted in Chu et al.'s [2] study.

Nowadays with the advent of OCT, fluorescein angiography has a very little role in diagnosis of subclinical edema. In the past, many studies demonstrated high incidence of subclinical macular edema after cataract surgery which was detected by fluorescein angiography; hence, it is important to set up criteria for diagnosis and classification of different subclinical macular edema on OCT. Due to lack of standardized definition and classification of subclinical macular edema, in the present study, some criteria were put forward so as to classify subclinical macular edema and to justify the high incidence of angiographic subclinical macular edema seen in the past.

- Cases in which baseline increase in thickness (CMT or Average macular thickness) was more than 1 standard deviation (14µm) and VA≥0.30 were labeled as Grade 1 subclinical macular edema.
- Cases in which baseline increases in thickness (CMT or Average macular thickness) was more than 2, standard deviation (25µm) or appearance in intra-retinal microcysts and VA≥0.30 were labeled as Grade 2 subclinical macular edema.
- Clinical cystoid macular edema was defined as clinically detectable using a slit lamp biomicroscope or an indirect ophthalmoscope and a typical cystoid pattern with CMT >350 µm on OCT and VA <6/12.

In the present study, cases were classified as per criteria described above and found that of the total 37 (22.42%) cases of Grade 1 subclinical edema, 32(86%) eyes had undergone SICS and 5 (13.5%) had undergone phacoemulsification surgery. Of total seven (4.24%) of Grade 2 subclinical edema 6 (85.7%) had undergone SICS and 1 (14.2%) had undergone phacoemulsification surgery. Of three clinical edema eyes, three (100%) had undergone SICS surgery.

Of all 132 SICS cases, 38 (28.7%) had subclinical edema and 3 (2.2%) had clinical edema. Of all the 33 phacoemulsification cases, six (18%) had subclinical edema. No statistical significance was seen in between different types of surgery and incidence of macular edema similar to Pragati et al.'s [12] study.

But the incidence of macular edema is seen more in cases of SICS which is probably due to excess handling of ocular tissues also proposed by Lobo et al. [13] and Andrez et al. [14].

Of all the 162 eyes with IOL implanted in the bag, 42 (25.92%) had subclinical edema and 2 (1.23%) had clinical edema. Of all the three eyes with IOL implanted in sulcus, two (66.66%) had subclinical edema and one (33.33%) had clinical edema. Statistical significance was seen between implanted IOL location and macular edema.

Median BCVA (LogMAR) during pre-op was 0.78±0.37, 0.18±0.15 at post-op day 7, 0±0.15 at post-op 1 month and 0±0.05 at post-op 4 month.

The present study shows significant improvement in VA after the surgery which was reduced in cases of clinical macular edema at post-operative 1 month which then returned to normal or near normal in majority cases by the end of 4th month. In cases of subclinical macular edema, there was hardly any difference as compared to VA in patients with no edema, suggesting that subclinical macular edema need not be vision threatening if diagnosed early.

Mean pre-operative BCVA in all the patients was 0.7 (LogMAR), post-op 1 month mean BCVA was 0.0±0.1, 0.1±.0.1 and 0.9±0.2 in cases of no macular edema, subclinical macular edema, and clinical macular edema, respectively. Statistically significant improvement in VA was seen post-operatively. Similar statistical results were seen in Pragati et al.'s [12] and Charu et al.'s [15] study.

The trend of VA in all cases of macular edema after post-op 1 month was toward baseline or near normal.

CMT was mapped on each visit and had a mean of 225.96±19.42 during pre-op, 230.49±24.24 during post-op day 7, 241.44±44.19 at post-op 1 month, and 232.17±22.57 at post-op 4 month. Whereas in Pragati et al.'s [12] study, CMT at pre-op was 234.1±17, 235.9±24.3 at 1st day, 246.7±25.3 at 1st month, and 239.4±26.3 at 3rd month, which were almost similar to this study.

AMT had a mean of 256.60±14 during pre-op, 261.08±14.75 during post-op day7, 270.10±18.13 at post-op 1 month, and 260.62±13.82 at post-op 4 month. Whereas in Pragati et al.'s study [12] 244.9±22.5 during pre-op, 248.5±21.1 at 1st day, 261.0±20.9 at 1st month, and 252.0±20.8 at 3rd month which were similar to our study.

Statistically significant difference was seen between the differences in mean CMT and mean AMT at per-op and post-op 1 month. Similar results were seen in other studies like Vukicevic et al. [8], Pragati et al. [12], and Charu et al. [15]. On the contrary, Despande et al.'s [16] study shows the difference of CMT was statistically not significant, but the difference of mean macular volume in diabetic patients at pre-op and post-op 1 month was statistically significant.

In the present study, it was seen that CMT and AMT were maximum at post-op 1 month which then returned to the baseline (pre-op) value at around post-op 4th month, validating the previous studies Vukicevic et al. [8], Pragati et al. [12] and Charu et al. [15].

The present study shows a positive correlation between VA and CMT throughout the follow-up. Pearson's correlation r = 0.120 for pre-op, 0.302 at post-op day 7, 0.564 at post-op 1month, and 0.114 at post-op 4 month. This signifies that VA is better when CMT is near baseline values, and post-op 4 months VA was normal in majority patients. In Pragati et al. [12], r = 0.085 at pre-op, 0.273 at postop day 1, 0.134 at post-op 1st month, and 0.112 at post of 3rd month.

Topical NSAID 0.1% nepafenac eye drop was used in patients having pseudophakic macular edema in our study which resolved the macular edema very effectively and similar results seen in Warren & Fox et al.'s [9] study and Singh et al.'s [10] study proved that there is significantly lower rate of PCME in diabetic patients using nepafenac eye drop.

24.6 CONCLUSIONS

In our study, incidence of pseudophakic cystoid macular edema (clinical) was 1.81% with peak incidence at post-op 1M. Incidence of subclinical macular edema was 26.66% of which nine cases showed a significant increase in baseline thickness and or intra-retinal microcysts which were diagnosed as early as post-op D7 and were treated accordingly. All the patients were successfully treated with topical NSAID 0.1% nepafenac eye drops thrice a day dosing. However, cases with clinical macular edema took 1–2 months for thickness to come back to baseline. Diabetes has occurred as statistically significant pre-op risk factors in our study most probably due to the inflammatory nature of the diseases. In spite of high incidence of intra-operative complications seen in this study, the incidence of clinical PCME is very less. Occurrence of subclinical macular edema is far more than expected but in a varied manner which needs to be explored and classified with the help of OCT. The average macular thickness is found to be more at post-op 1month which then returns to baseline at around 4 months. High incidence of subclinical macular edema following SICS and phacoemulsification surgery is not an alarming cause but as the progression suggests, at least postoperative 1 month, OCT can be done to look for reversible subclinical or clinical PCME which can be detected as early as post-op day 7 with the help of OCT. With the advent of OCT which is non-invasive and benefits quantification of macular thickness, early diagnosis of pseudophakic cystoid macular edema (PCME) can be beneficial to alter the progression of edema, hence preventing vision loss due to long-standing macular edema.

REFERENCES

1. Zur D, Loewenstein A. Postsurgical cystoid macular edema. *Developments in Ophthalmology* 2017;58:178–190. doi: 10.1159/000455280
2. Chu CJ, Johnston RL, Buscombe C, Sallam AB, Mohamed Q, Yang YC; United Kingdom Pseudophakic Macular Edema Study Group. Risk factors and incidence of macular edema after cataract surgery: A database study of 81984 eyes. *Ophthalmology* 2016 Feb;123(2):316–323. doi: 10.1016/j.ophtha.2015.10.001
3. Anthony J Bron, Ramesh C. Tripathi and Brenda J. Tripathi, editors. Wolff anatomy of the eye and orbit.8th ed. Chapman and Hall;1997.
4. Henderson BA, Kim JY, Ament CS, Ferrufino-Ponce ZK, Grabowska A, Cremers SL (2007) Clinical pseudophakic cystoids macular edema. Risk factors for development and duration after treatment. *Journal of Cataract and Refractive Surgery* 33:1550–1558
5. Perente I, Utine CA, Ozturker C, Cakir M, Kaya V, Eren H, Kapran Z, Yilmaz OF (2007) Evaluation of macular changes after uncomplicated phacoemulsification surgery by optical coherence tomography. *Current Eye Research* 32:241–247
6. Wright PL, Wilkinson CP, Balyeat HD, Popham J, Reinke M (1988) Angiographic cystoid macular edema after posterior chamber lens implantation. *Archives of Ophthalmology* 106:740–744.

7. Flach AJ: The incidence, pathogenesis and treatment of cystoid macular edema following cataract surgery. *Transactions of the American Ophthalmological Society* 1998; 96: 557–634
8. Vukicevic M, Gin T, Al-Qureshi S: Prevalence of optical coherence tomography diagnosed postoperative cystoid macular oedema in patients following uncomplicated phaco-emulsification cataract surgery. *Clinical & Experimental Ophthalmology* 2012; 40: 282–287.
9. Warren KA, Fox JE: Topical nepafenac as an alternative for cystoid macular edema in steroid responsive patients. *Retina* 2007; 28: 1427– 1434.
10. Singh R, Alpern L, Jaffe GJ, Lehmann RP, Lim J, Reiser HJ, Sall K, Walters T, Sager D. Evaluation of nepafenac in prevention of macular edema following cataract surgery in patients with diabetic retinopathy. *Clinical Ophthalmology* 2012; 6: 1259–1269. doi: 10.2147/OPTH.S31902
11. Perente I, Utine CA, Ozturker C, Cakir M, Kaya V, Eren H, Kapran Z, Yilmaz OF. Evaluation of macular changes after uncomplicated phacoemulsification surgery by optical coherence tomography. *Current Eye Research* 2007 Mar;32(3):241–247. doi: 10.1080/02713680601160610
12. Garg, Pragati. (2019). Foveal thickness alteration following uncomplicated cataract surgery- An OCT based study. *Journal of Medical Science And clinical Research* 7. doi: 10.18535/jmscr/v7i6.133
13. Lobo CL, Faria PM, Soares MA, Bernardes RC, Cunha-Vaz JG. Macular alterations after small-incision cataract surgery. *Journal of Cataract and Refractive Surgery* 2004 Apr;30(4):752–760. doi: 10.1016/S0886-3350(03)00582-0
14. Grzybowski, Andrzej et al. Pseudophakic cystoid macular edema: update 2016. *Clinical Interventions in Aging* vol. 11 1221–1229. 9 Sep. 2016,doi: 10.2147/CIA.S111761
15. Chaudhary, Charu & Bahadhur, Harsh & Gupta, Neeti. (2014). Study of cystoid macular edema by optical coherent tomography following uneventful cataract surgery. *International Ophthalmology* 35, 685–691.
16. Deshpande, Aditi. (2018). Incidence of clinical and subclinical cystoid macular edema in diabetic and non-diabetic patients after cataract surgery by means of optical coherence tomography. *Delhi Journal of Ophthalmology* 29. doi: 10.7869/djo.395
17. Sharma, R., Kim, M., & Gupta, A. (2022). Motor imagery classification in brain-machine interface with machine learning algorithms: Classical approach to multi-layer perceptron model. *Biomedical Signal Processing and Control*, *71*, 103101, doi: 10.1016/j.bspc.2021.103101

Index

Pages in *italics* refer to figures and pages in **bold** refer to tables.